Antibiotics Manual

A Guide to Commonly Used Antimicrobials

Antibiotics Manual

A Guide to Commonly Used Antimicrobials

Second Edition

David Schlossberg, MD, FACP, FIDSA, FCPP
The Lewis Katz School of Medicine at Temple University
Philadelphia, PA, USA

Rafik Samuel, MD, FACP, FIDSA, FCPP
The Lewis Katz School of Medicine at Temple University
Philadelphia, PA, USA

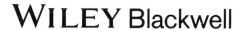

Edition History
PMPH-USA, Ltd (1e, 2011)

Registered Office(s)
John Wiley & Sons, Inc., 111 River Street, Hoboken, NJ 07030, USA
John Wiley & Sons Ltd, The Atrium, Southern Gate, Chichester, West Sussex, PO19 8SQ, UK

Editorial Office
9600 Garsington Road, Oxford, OX4 2DQ, UK

For details of our global editorial offices, customer services, and more information about Wiley products visit us at www.wiley.com.

Wiley also publishes its books in a variety of electronic formats and by print-on-demand. Some content that appears in standard print versions of this book may not be available in other formats.

Library of Congress Cataloging-in-Publication Data

Names: Schlossberg, David, author. | Samuel, Rafik, author.
Title: Antibiotics manual : a guide to commonly used antimicrobials / by David Schlossberg, Rafik Samuel.
Description: Second edition. | Hoboken, NJ : Wiley, 2017. | Includes bibliographical references and index.
Identifiers: LCCN 2017028213 (print) | LCCN 2017029407 (ebook) | ISBN 9781119220770 (pdf) | ISBN 9781119220763 (epub) |
    ISBN 9781119220756 (pbk.)
Subjects: | MESH: Anti-Bacterial Agents–administration & dosage | Anti-Bacterial Agents–therapeutic use | Handbooks
Classification: LCC RM267 (ebook) | LCC RM267 (print) | NLM QV 39 | DDC 615/.329–dc23
LC record available at https://lccn.loc.gov/2017028213

Cover Design: Wiley
Cover Image: © everything possible/Shutterstock

Set in 11/13pt Myriad Pro Condensed, SPi Global, Pondicherry, India

10 9 8 7 6 5 4 3 2 1

Once again, for Yuan:

Shall I compare thee to a summer's day?
Thou art more lovely and more temperate.
Rough winds do shake the darling buds of May,
And summer's lease hath all too short a date.
. . . .
But thy eternal summer shall not fade,
Nor lose possession of that fair thou ow'st

Shakespeare, Sonnet 18.

David Schlossberg

This book is dedicated to my family, Farid, Leila, Dalia, Ed, and Matt.
Thank you all; you are the reason I am the person I am today.

Rafik Samuel

We are pleased to present the Second Edition of our book. The development of new antimicrobials since the First Edition has been explosive, necessitating the addition of 36 new chapters, comprising new antiretroviral, anti-HCV, antimycobacterial, antifungal and antibacterial drugs and combinations. All the older chapters have been updated as necessary, and new tables have been added that highlight salient antimicrobial toxicities and indicate potential specific coverage of difficult pathogens. As with the First Edition, we intend this book to fill an important particular niche in the clinician's arsenal: it is a compilation of individual brief chapters, each dedicated to a specific antimicrobial. The final chapter of formulas, equations, and useful definitions now also includes the toxicity and coverage tables mentioned above. Each antimicrobial chapter lists the drug's class, mechanism of action, mechanism of resistance, metabolic route, indications and off-label uses, pertinent toxicities, significant drug interactions, and dosage for routine and special populations. The emphasis of this book is not on recommendations for specific organisms or clinical syndromes; rather, it is a compendium of clinically helpful information about available antimicrobials.

We have included the FDA-approved indications as they exist currently; additional off-label uses are also included. For many agents, the toxicities and drug interactions are numerous and complex; frequently, the clinician must research several sites or even multiple locations in the drug label itself to identify significant toxicities. We have tried to organize the most frequent and important toxicities and drug interactions in a convenient, user-friendly format.

Dosage information includes the special populations of renal failure, hepatic dysfunction, and pediatrics, and each chapter concludes with a list of clinical pearls, adding practical tips to the preceding discussion. When possible, we have used the official drug label as a primary source of information, supplemented by the various print and electronic sources in the References; further details may be sought in these resources.

In addition to FDA-approved indications, we have also listed off-label uses of selected agents; further, since many of the antiparasitic drugs are difficult to acquire in the United States, we have supplied relevant contact information for the CDC or compounding pharmacies, when appropriate.

The primary table of contents lists the antimicrobials alphabetically by brand name followed by the generic name; this is followed by a second table of contents, which lists the antimicrobials by generic name followed by the brand name. Thus, drug information is conveniently accessed via both brand and generic names. The chapter on formulas, definitions, and equations provides classifications for liver disease, formulas for computing creatinine clearance and body surface area, and a discussion of the varied terminology for continuous renal replacement therapy (CRRT). This is followed by tables of individual types of drug toxicity and specific antimicrobial–organism coverage for selected and challenging organisms.
We hope this book will help the clinician navigate – in a convenient and clinically useful format – the increasingly complex details of antimicrobial prescribing.

We gratefully acknowledge the vision and expertise of Claire Bonnett, Deirdre Barry, Teresa Netzler, M.R. Shobana, Patricia Bateson, and Sonali Melwani.

David Schlossberg, MD, FACP, FIDSA, FCPP
Rafik Samuel, MD, FACP, FIDSA, FCPP

BASIC CHARACTERISTICS

Class: Polyene.

Mechanism of Action: Amphotericin B inserts into the cytoplasmic membrane through ergosterol, leading to increased permeability of the fungal membrane and loss of intracellular ions.

Amphotericin B also affects oxidation and may cause fungal death in this manner.

Mechanism of Resistance: Resistance is rare, but is due to changes in the cell membrane that prevent amphotericin from inserting into the membrane.

Metabolic Route: Amphotericin B is excreted very slowly by the kidneys, with 2 to 5% of a given dose being excreted in the biologically active form. After discontinuation of treatment, amphotericin is detectable in urine for at least seven weeks. Details of possible metabolic pathways are not known.

 FDA-APPROVED INDICATIONS

Invasive fungal infections in patients who are refractory to or intolerant of conventional amphotericin B therapy.

 SIDE EFFECTS/TOXICITY

Side effects are similar to those seen with amphotericin B deoxycholate but tend to be less frequent or less severe.

Contraindicated in patients who have shown hypersensitivity to amphotericin B or any other component in the formulation.

Acute reactions including fever, shaking chills, hypotension, anorexia, nausea, vomiting, headache, and tachypnea are common 1 to 3 hours after starting an intravenous infusion. Rapid intravenous infusion has been associated with hypotension, hypokalemia, arrhythmias, and shock and should, therefore, be avoided.

Amphotericin B should be used with care in patients with reduced renal function; frequent monitoring of renal function is recommended.

Since acute pulmonary reactions have been reported in patients given amphotericin B during or shortly after leukocyte transfusions, it is advisable to temporarily separate these infusions as far as possible and to monitor pulmonary function.

Leukoencephalopathy has been reported following use of amphotericin B.

 DRUG INTERACTIONS

Antineoplastic agents may enhance the potential for renal toxicity, bronchospasm and hypotension and should be given concomitantly only with great caution.

Corticosteroids and **corticotropin** (**ACTH**): closely monitor serum electrolytes and cardiac function.

Digitalis glycosides: amphotericin B-induced hypokalemia may potentiate digitalis toxicity.

Flucytosine: concomitant use may increase the toxicity of flucytosine.

Antibiotics Manual: A Guide to Commonly Used Antimicrobials, Second Edition. David Schlossberg and Rafik Samuel.
© 2017 John Wiley & Sons Ltd. Published 2017 by John Wiley & Sons Ltd.

Imidazoles (e.g., **fluconazole**): imidazoles may induce fungal resistance to amphotericin B. Combination therapy should be administered with caution.

Other nephrotoxic medications: may enhance the potential for drug-induced renal toxicity and should be used concomitantly only with great caution.

Skeletal muscle relaxants: amphotericin B-induced hypokalemia may enhance the curariform effect of skeletal muscle relaxants.

Leukocyte transfusions: acute pulmonary toxicity has been reported in patients receiving intravenous amphotericin B and leukocyte transfusions.

 ## DOSING

5 mg/kg/day given as a single infusion.

 ## SPECIAL POPULATIONS

RENAL IMPAIRMENT: Monitor renal function closely. No dosage adjustment recommended for renal impairment or for dialysis.

HEPATIC IMPAIRMENT: Liver tests should be monitored routinely.

PEDIATRICS: As for adults.

 ## THE ART OF ANTIMICROBIAL THERAPY

Clinical Pearls

1. There are various forms of amphotericin with many important differences: amphotericin B deoxycholate, amphotericin B lipid dispersion, amphotericin B lipid complex or liposomal amphotericin B. This section pertains only to amphotericin B lipid complex. **Side effects of amphotericin B lipid complex are similar to those seen with amphotericin B deoxycholate but tend to be less frequent or less severe.**

2. Premedication with acetaminophen, diphenhydramine, meperidine, and even hydrocortisone can decrease infusion-related toxicity.

3. Hydration and sodium repletion prior to amphotericin B administration may reduce the risk of developing nephrotoxicity.

4. *Candida lusitaniae*, *Pseudallescheria boydii*, and *Fusarium* spp. are often resistant to amphotericin B. Voriconazole is frequently used for these infections.

5. It is advisable to monitor on a regular basis liver function, serum electrolytes (particularly magnesium and potassium), blood counts, and hemoglobin concentrations.

BASIC CHARACTERISTICS

Class: Broad-spectrum antihelminthic.

Mechanism of Action: Inhibits tubulin polymerization, resulting in loss of cytoplasmic microtubules.

Metabolic Route: Converted in the liver to Albendazole sulfoxide and is excreted in the feces.

 FDA-APPROVED INDICATIONS

Treatment of neurocysticersosis and hydatid disease (the larval forms of *Taenia solium*). Also *Echinococcus granulosus*.

Also Used for: Ancylostoma, Ascariasis, cutaneous larva migrans, *Enterobius vermicularis*, *Clonorchis sinensis*, gnathostomiasis, hookworm, microsporidiosis, strongyloidiasis, trichinellosis, trichuriasis, and visceral larval migrans.

 SIDE EFFECTS/TOXICITY

Granulocytopenia, agranulocytosis, and pancytopenia; increased hepatic enzymes in over 15% of patients.

 DRUG INTERACTIONS/FOOD INTERACTIONS

Albendazole should be administered with food.

Albendazole induces the cytochrome P450-1A enzymes and should be given with caution when used with theophylline, cimetidine, dexamethasone, and praziquantel.

 DOSING

Albendazole is administered in 200 mg tablets.

Hydatid disease: 400 mg twice daily with meals, for 28 days, followed by 14 days without meds. This cycle is repeated twice to complete 3 cycles.

Neurocysticercosis: 400 mg twice daily with meals given for 8–30 days. For those under 60 kg, the dose is 15 mg/kg/day in divided doses with a maximum of 800 mg daily dose.

Ancylostoma: 400 mg × 1 dose.

Ascariasis: 400 mg × 1 dose.

Clonorchis: 10 mg/kg once daily for 7 days.

Cutaneous larva migrans: 400 mg once daily for 3 days.

Emterobiasis: 400 mg × 1 dose.

Gnathostomiasis: 400 mg twice daily for 21 days.

Hookworm: 400 mg × 1 dose.

Microsporidiosis: 400 mg twice in one day.

Strongyloidiasis: 400 mg × 1 dose.

Trichinosis: 400 mg twice daily for 14 days.

Antibiotics Manual: A Guide to Commonly Used Antimicrobials, Second Edition. David Schlossberg and Rafik Samuel.
© 2017 John Wiley & Sons Ltd. Published 2017 by John Wiley & Sons Ltd.

Trichuriasis: 400 mg × 1 dose.

Visceral larva migrans: 400 mg twice daily for 5 days.

 SPECIAL POPULATIONS

RENAL IMPAIRMENT: There is no dose adjustment for renal insufficiency.

HEPATIC DYSFUNCTION: There are increases in levels of albendazole in those with extrahepatic obstruction, though no dose adjustment is necessary.

PEDIATRICS: 15 mg/kg/day, divided into 2 doses.

 THE ART OF ANTIMICROBIAL THERAPY

Clinical Pearls

1. In the treatment of neurocysticercosis, steroids should be given before the albendazole is administered.
2. Albendazole should be given with food.
3. For children, the pill should be crushed because children often have trouble swallowing the tablet.
4. CBC and liver function tests should be checked every 2 weeks while on therapy.

BASIC CHARACTERISTICS

Class: Antiprotozoal agent.

Mechanism of Action: Inhibition of pyruvate ferredoxin oxidoreductase in protozoa.

Metabolic Route: One third of the administered dose excreted in the urine and two thirds in the feces.

 ## FDA-APPROVED INDICATIONS

Nitazoxanide for oral suspension (patients 1 year of age and older) and tablets (patients 12 years and older) are indicated for the treatment of diarrhea caused by *Giardia lamblia* or *Cryptosporidium parvum*.

Also Used for: *Entamoeba histolytica, Cyclospora cayetanensis, Trichomonas vaginalis, Encephalitozoon intestinalis, Isospora belli, Blastocystis hominis, Balantidium coli, Enterocytozoon bieneusi, Ascaris lumbricoides, Trichuris trichura, Taenia saginata, Hymenolepis nana*, and *Fasciola hepatica*.

 ## SIDE EFFECTS/TOXICITY

Nausea, vomiting, diarrhea, and abdominal pain.

 ## DRUG INTERACTIONS/FOOD INTERACTIONS

Food will increase the absorption of nitazoxanide.

 ## DOSING

Treatment of diarrhea caused by *Giardia lamblia* or *Cryptosporidium parvum*	1–3 years	5 mL (100 mg nitazoxanide) every 12 hours with food	3 days
	4–11 years	10 mL (200 mg nitazoxanide) every 12 hours with food	
	≥12 years	1 tablet (500 mg nitazoxanide) every 12 hours with food or 25 mL (500 mg nitazoxanide) every 12 hours with food	

SPECIAL POPULATIONS

RENAL IMPAIRMENT: No dose adjustment is necessary.

HEPATIC DYSFUNCTION: No dose adjustment is necessary.

PEDIATRICS: See dosing table above.

Antibiotics Manual: A Guide to Commonly Used Antimicrobials, Second Edition. David Schlossberg and Rafik Samuel.
© 2017 John Wiley & Sons Ltd. Published 2017 by John Wiley & Sons Ltd.

THE ART OF ANTIMICROBIAL THERAPY

Clinical Pearls

1. Nitazoxanide has not been shown to be superior to placebo for the treatment of diarrhea caused by *Cryptosporidium parvum* in HIV-infected or immunodeficient patients.

BASIC CHARACTERISTICS

Class: Lyophilized polyene.

Mechanism of Action: Amphotericin B inserts into the cytoplasmic membrane through ergosterol, leading to increased permeability of the fungal membrane and loss of intracellular ions.

Amphotericin B also affects oxidation and may cause fungal death in this manner.

Mechanism of Resistance: Resistance is rare, but is due to changes in the cell membrane that prevent amphotericin from inserting into the membrane.

Metabolic Route: Details of possible metabolic pathways are not known.

 FDA-APPROVED INDICATIONS

Empirical therapy for presumed fungal infection in febrile, neutropenic patients.

Cryptococcal meningitis in HIV infected patients.

Aspergillus, Candida, or *Cryptococcus* species infections refractory to amphotericin B deoxycholate, or in patients where renal impairment or unacceptable toxicity precludes the use of amphotericin B deoxycholate.

Treatment of visceral leishmaniasis.

 SIDE EFFECTS/TOXICITY

Side effects are similar to those seen with amphotericin B deoxycholate but tend to be less frequent or less severe.

Contraindicated in patients who have shown hypersensitivity to amphotericin B or any other component in the formulation.

Acute reactions including fever, shaking chills, hypotension, anorexia, nausea, vomiting, headache, and tachypnea are common 1 to 3 hours after starting an intravenous infusion. Rapid intravenous infusion has been associated with hypotension, hypokalemia, arrhythmias, and shock and should therefore be avoided.

Amphotericin B should be used with care in patients with reduced renal function; frequent monitoring of renal function is recommended.

Since acute pulmonary reactions have been reported in patients given amphotericin B during or shortly after leukocyte transfusions, it is advisable to temporarily separate these infusions as far as possible and to monitor pulmonary function.

Leukoencephalopathy has been reported following use of amphotericin B.

 DRUG INTERACTIONS

Antineoplastic agents may enhance the potential for renal toxicity, bronchospasm, and hypotension and should be given concomitantly only with great caution.

Corticosteroids and **corticotropin** (**ACTH**): closely monitor serum electrolytes and cardiac function.

Digitalis glycosides: amphotericin B-induced hypokalemia may potentiate digitalis toxicity.

Flucytosine: concomitant use may increase the toxicity of flucytosine.

Antibiotics Manual: A Guide to Commonly Used Antimicrobials, Second Edition. David Schlossberg and Rafik Samuel.
© 2017 John Wiley & Sons Ltd. Published 2017 by John Wiley & Sons Ltd.

Imidazoles (e.g., **fluconazole**): imidazoles may induce fungal resistance to amphotericin B. Combination therapy should be administered with caution.

Other nephrotoxic medications may enhance the potential for drug-induced renal toxicity and should be used concomitantly only with great caution.

Skeletal muscle relaxants: amphotericin B-induced hypokalemia may enhance the curariform effect of skeletal muscle relaxants.

Leukocyte transfusions: acute pulmonary toxicity has been reported in patients receiving intravenous amphotericin B and leukocyte transfusions

 DOSING

Indication	Dose
Empirical therapy	3 mg/kg/day
Systemic fungal infection	3–5 mg/kg/day
Cryptococcal meningitis	6 mg/kg/day
Visceral leishmaniasis (immunocompetent)	3 mg/kg/day for 5 days; then again on days 14 and 21
(immunocompromised)	4 mg/kg/day for 5 days; then again on days 10, 17, 24, 31, and 38

 SPECIAL POPULATIONS

RENAL IMPAIRMENT: Monitor renal function closely. No dosage adjustment recommended for renal impairment or for dialysis.

HEPATIC IMPAIRMENT: Liver tests should be monitored routinely.

PEDIATRICS: Use similar dose as adults.

 THE ART OF ANTIMICROBIAL THERAPY

Clinical Pearls

1. There are various forms of amphotericin with many important differences: amphotericin B deoxycholate, amphotericin B lipid dispersion, amphotericin B lipid complex, or liposomal amphotericin B. This section pertains only to liposomal amphotericin B. **Side effects with liposomal amphotericin B are similar to those seen with amphotericin B deoxycholate but tend to be less frequent or less severe.**

2. Premedication with acetaminophen, diphenhydramine, meperidine, and even hydrocortisone can decrease infusion related toxicity.

3. Hydration and sodium repletion prior to amphotericin B administration may reduce the risk of developing nephrotoxicity.

4. *Candida lusitaniae*, *Pseudallescheria boydii*, and *Fusarium* sp. are often resistant to amphotericin B. Voriconazole is frequently used for these infections.

5. It is advisable to monitor on a regular basis liver function, serum electrolytes (particularly magnesium and potassium), blood counts, and hemoglobin concentrations.

BASIC CHARACTERISTICS

Class: Aminoglycoside.

Mechanisms of Action:

1. Rearranges lipopolysaccharide in the outer membrane of the bacterial cell wall, resulting in disruption of the cell wall.
2. Binds the 30S subunit of the bacterial ribosome, which terminates protein synthesis.

Mechanism of Resistance:

1. Gram-negative bacteria inactivate aminoglycosides by acetylation.
2. Some bacteria alter the 30S ribosomal subunit, which prevents amikacin's interference with protein synthesis.
3. Low-level resistance may result from inhibition of amikacin uptake by the bacteria.

Metabolic Route: The drug is excreted unchanged in the urine.

 FDA-APPROVED INDICATIONS

Treatment of susceptible gram-negative bacteria causing bacteremia, pneumonia, osteomyelitis, arthritis, meningitis, skin and soft tissue infection, intra-abdominal infections, in burns and postoperative infections, urinary tract infections.

Also Used for: *Mycobacterium tuberculosis*, *Mycobacterium avium*-intracellulare lung disease, and *Nocardia*; combination therapy with beta-lactams for the treatment of gram-positive endovascular infections.

 SIDE EFFECTS/TOXICITY

WARNING: Ototoxicity: vestibular toxicity and auditory ototoxicity, especially in patients with renal damage, those treated with higher doses, and those with prolonged treatment. Avoid use with potent diuretics such as ethacrynic acid because of additive ototoxicity.

Nephrotoxicity: especially in patients with impaired renal function and those treated with higher doses or prolonged treatment. Avoid concurrent use with other nephrotoxic agents and potent diuretics, which can cause dehydration.

Neuromuscular blockade: especially in those receiving anesthetics, neuromuscular blocking agents or massive transfusions. Other neurotoxicity may include numbness, skin tingling, muscle twitching, and convulsions.

Other adverse effects include rash, fever, headache, paresthesia, tremor, seizures, nausea and vomiting, eosinophilia, arthralgia, anemia, hypotension and hypomagnesemia. Macular infarction sometimes leading to permanent loss of vision has been reported following intravitreous administration (injection into the eye) of amikacin.

 DRUG INTERACTIONS

Amikacin should not be administered with other medications that are nephrotoxic or ototoxic.

Antibiotics Manual: A Guide to Commonly Used Antimicrobials, Second Edition. David Schlossberg and Rafik Samuel.
© 2017 John Wiley & Sons Ltd. Published 2017 by John Wiley & Sons Ltd.

DOSING

Total dose: 15 mg/kg/day IM or IV, either once daily or in divided doses every 8–12 hours.
Intrathecal dose: 10–40 mg/24 hours.

 SPECIAL POPULATIONS

RENAL IMPAIRMENT: Adjust dose either by increased interval (serum creatinine multiplied by 9, based on q 12 hour dosing) or by lowering the dose by multiplying the dose by the ratio of observed creatinine clearance/normal creatinine clearance.

Hemodialysis: 10 mg/kg loading dose followed by 2.5–3.75 mg/kg after hemodialysis.
Peritoneal dialysis: 2.5 mg/kg/day IV or 3–4 mg/2 L dialysate removed.
CRRT: 10 mg/kg loading dose followed by 7.5 mg/kg q 24–48 hours.

HEPATIC DYSFUNCTION: No dose adjustment necessary.

PEDIATRICS: Amikacin should be used with caution in children.

 THE ART OF ANTIMICROBIAL THERAPY

Clinical Pearls

1. Amikacin is more likely to be active against gram-negative rods when compared to the other aminoglycosides.
2. Aminoglycosides require oxygen to be active and thus are less effective in anaerobic environments such as an abscess or infected bone.
3. Aminoglycosides have decreased activity in low pH environments such as respiratory secretions or abscesses.
4. When dosing aminoglycosides, use the ideal body weight not true body weight.
5. Amikacin has a postantibiotic effect, which allows it to be used once daily.
6. Aminoglycosides are concentration-dependent and therefore are more effective if given at longer intervals and with higher doses. For example, giving amikacin at 15 mg/kg/day may be more effective than 5 mg/kg/8 hours.
7. The IV dose should be infused over 60 minutes to avoid neuromuscular blockade.
8. Renal and eighth-nerve function should be closely monitored.
9. Targeted serum levels: multiple daily dosing – peak 15–30 mcg/mL, trough 5–10 mcg/mL. With once-daily dosing – peak 56–64 mcg/mL, trough <1 mcg/mL.

BASIC CHARACTERISTICS

Class: Aminopenicillin.

Mechanism of Action: Binds penicillin-binding protein, disrupting cell wall synthesis.

Mechanisms of Resistance:

1. The PBP can be altered, with reduced affinity.
2. Production of a beta-lactamase, resulting in hydrolysis of the beta-lactam ring.
3. Decreased ability of the antibiotic to reach the PBP when bacteria decrease porin production, resulting in a decrease of the drug concentration within the cell.

Metabolic Route: Amoxicillin is excreted unchanged in the urine.

 FDA-APPROVED INDICATIONS

Amoxicillin is indicated in the treatment of infections due to susceptible (only beta-lactamase negative) strains of microorganisms in the conditions listed below:

Infections of the ear, nose, and throat

Infections of the genitourinary tract

Infections of the skin and skin structure

Infections of the lower respiratory tract

Gonorrhea, acute uncomplicated (ano-genital and urethral infections)

***H. pylori* eradication:**

   Triple therapy: Amoxicillin/clarithromycin/lansoprazole

   Dual therapy: Amoxicillin/lansoprazole

 SIDE EFFECTS/TOXICITY

A history of allergic reaction to any of the penicillins is a **contraindication**.

Side effects include *Clostridium difficile*-associated diarrhea (CDAD), mucocutaneous candidiasis, nausea, vomiting, diarrhea, black hairy tongue, hypersensitivity reactions including rashes, erythema multiforme, and Stevens–Johnson syndrome, rise in AST (SGOT) and/or ALT (SGPT), crystalluria, anemia, thrombocytopenia, eosinophilia, leukopenia, hyperactivity, and convulsions.

 DRUG INTERACTIONS/FOOD INTERACTIONS

Amoxicillin capsules, chewable tablets, and oral suspensions may be given without regard to meals.

Concurrent use of amoxicillin and probenecid may result in increased and prolonged blood levels of amoxicillin.

Chloramphenicol, macrolides, sulfonamides, and tetracyclines may interfere with the bactericidal effects of penicillins.

High urine concentrations of amoxicillin may result in false-positive reactions when testing for the presence of glucose in urine using *Clinitest®*; it is recommended that glucose tests based on enzymatic glucose oxidase reactions (such as *Clinistix®*) be used.

Antibiotics Manual: A Guide to Commonly Used Antimicrobials, Second Edition. David Schlossberg and Rafik Samuel.
© 2017 John Wiley & Sons Ltd. Published 2017 by John Wiley & Sons Ltd.

DOSING

Each capsule contains 250 mg or 500 mg; each tablet contains 500 mg or 875 mg; each chewable tablet contains 125 mg, 200 mg, 250 mg, or 400 mg; the oral suspension contains 200 mg per 5 mL or 400 mg per 5 mL.

Infection	Dose
Ear/nose/throat (mild/moderate)	500 mg q 12 hours or 250 mg q 8 hours
Ear/nose/throat (severe)	875 mg q 12 hours or 500 mg q 8 hours
Lower respiratory tract	875 mg q 12 hours or 500 mg q 8 hours
Skin/skin structure (mild/moderate)	500 mg q 12 hours or 250 mg q 8 hours
Skin/skin structure (severe)	875 mg q 12 hours or 500 mg q 8 hours
Genitourinary (mild/moderate)	500 mg q 12 hours or 250 mg q 8 hours
Genitourinary (severe)	875 mg q 12 hours or 500 mg q 8 hours
H. pylori eradication	1 gram amoxicillin, 500 mg clarithromycin, and 30 mg lansoprazole, all given twice daily (q 12 h) for 14 days **or**
	1 gram amoxicillin and 30 mg lansoprazole, each given three times daily (q 8 h) for 14 days

 SPECIAL POPULATIONS

RENAL IMPAIRMENT: Patients with a glomerular filtration rate of < 30 mL/minute should not receive the 875 mg tablet.

Creatinine clearance, mL/min	Dose
10–30	250–500 mg every 12 hours
<10	250 mg–500 mg daily
Hemodialysis	250–500 mg every 24 hours and an additional dose after dialysis
CAPD	250 mg every 12 hours
CRRT	N/A

HEPATIC DYSFUNCTION: No dose adjustment is necessary.

PEDIATRICS: **Neonates and infants aged ≤ 12 weeks (≤ 3 months):** The recommended upper dose of amoxicillin is 30 mg/kg/day divided q 12 h.

Pediatric patients > 3 months:

25–45 mg/kg/day in divided doses every 12 hours **or**

20–40 mg/kg/day in divided doses every 8 hours, depending on severity of the infection.

 THE ART OF ANTIMICROBIAL THERAPY

Clinical Pearls

1. Amoxicillin needs to be dose adjusted for renal dysfunction.

2. Patients with mononucleosis who receive amoxicillin may develop an erythematous skin rash.

BASIC CHARACTERISTICS

Class: Polyene.

Mechanism of Action: Amphotericin B inserts into the cytoplasmic membrane through ergosterol, leading to increased permeability of the fungal membrane and loss of intracellular ions. Amphotericin B also affects oxidation and may cause fungal death in this manner.

Mechanism of Resistance: Resistance is rare, but is due to changes in the cell membrane that prevent amphotericin from inserting into the membrane.

Metabolic Route: Details of possible metabolic pathways are not known.

 ## FDA-APPROVED INDICATIONS

Treatment of invasive aspergillosis in patients where renal impairment or unacceptable toxicity precludes the use of amphotericin B deoxycholate in effective doses and in patients with invasive aspergillosis where prior amphotericin B deoxycholate therapy has failed.

 ## SIDE EFFECTS/TOXICITY

Contraindicated in patients who have shown hypersensitivity to amphotericin B or any other component in the formulation.

Acute reactions including fever, shaking chills, hypotension, anorexia, nausea, vomiting, headache, and tachypnea are common 1 to 3 hours after starting an intravenous infusion. Rapid intravenous infusion has been associated with hypotension, hypokalemia, arrhythmias, and shock and should therefore be avoided.

Amphotericin B should be used with care in patients with reduced renal function; frequent monitoring of renal function is recommended.

Since acute pulmonary reactions have been reported in patients given amphotericin B during or shortly after leukocyte transfusions, it is advisable to temporarily separate these infusions as far as possible and to monitor pulmonary function.

Leukoencephalopathy has been reported following use of amphotericin B.

 ## DRUG INTERACTIONS

Antineoplastic agents may enhance the potential for renal toxicity, bronchospasm, and hypotension and should be given concomitantly only with great caution.

Corticosteroids and **corticotropin (ACTH)**: closely monitor serum electrolytes and cardiac function.

Digitalis glycosides: amphotericin B-induced hypokalemia may potentiate digitalis toxicity.

Flucytosine: concomitant use may increase the toxicity of flucytosine.

Imidazoles (e.g., **fluconazole**): imidazoles may induce fungal resistance to amphotericin B. Combination therapy should be administered with caution.

Other nephrotoxic medications may enhance the potential for drug-induced renal toxicity and should be used concomitantly only with great caution.

Antibiotics Manual: A Guide to Commonly Used Antimicrobials, Second Edition. David Schlossberg and Rafik Samuel.
© 2017 John Wiley & Sons Ltd. Published 2017 by John Wiley & Sons Ltd.

Skeletal muscle relaxants: amphotericin B-induced hypokalemia may enhance the curariform effect of skeletal muscle relaxants.

Leukocyte transfusions: acute pulmonary toxicity has been reported in patients receiving intravenous amphotericin B and leukocyte transfusions

 DOSING

3–4 mg/kg once a day.

 SPECIAL POPULATIONS

RENAL IMPAIRMENT: Monitor renal function closely. No dosage adjustment recommended for renal impairment or for dialysis

HEPATIC IMPAIRMENT: Liver tests should be monitored routinely.

PEDIATRICS: Doses (mg/kg) similar to those given to adults.

 THE ART OF ANTIMICROBIAL THERAPY

Clinical Pearls

1. There are various forms of amphotericin with many important differences: Amphotericin B deoxycholate, amphotericin B lipid dispersion, amphotericin B lipid complex, or liposomal amphotericin B. This section pertains only to amphotericin B lipid dispersion.

2. Premedication with acetaminophen, diphenhydramine, meperidine, and even hydrocortisone can decrease infusion-related toxicity.

3. Hydration and sodium repletion prior to amphotericin B administration may reduce the risk of developing nephrotoxicity.

4. *Candida lusitaniae*, *Pseudallescheria boydii*, and *Fusarium* spp. are often resistant to amphotericin B. Voriconazole is frequently used for these infections.

5. It is advisable to monitor on a regular basis liver function, serum electrolytes (particularly magnesium and potassium), blood counts, and hemoglobin concentrations.

BASIC CHARACTERISTICS

Class: Aminopenicillin.

Mechanism of Action: Binds penicillin-binding protein, disrupting cell wall synthesis.

Mechanisms of Resistance:

1. The PBP can be altered, with reduced affinity.
2. Production of a beta-lactamase resulting in hydrolysis of the beta lactam ring.
3. Decreased ability of the antibiotic to reach the PBP when bacteria decrease porin production, resulting in a decrease of the drug concentration within the cell.

Metabolic Route: Ampicillin is excreted unchanged in the urine.

 FDA-APPROVED INDICATIONS

1. Ampicillin for **injection** is indicated in the treatment of infections due to susceptible (only beta-lactamase negative) strains of microorganisms in the conditions listed below:

   Respiratory tract infections

   Bacterial meningitis

   Septicemia and endocarditis

   Urinary tract infections

   Gastrointestinal infections

2. Ampicillin **capsules** are indicated in the treatment of infections due to susceptible (only beta-lactamase negative) strains of microorganisms in the conditions listed below:

   Infections of the genitourinary tract

   Infections of the respiratory tract

   Infections of the gastrointestinal tract

 SIDE EFFECTS/TOXICITY

A history of allergic reaction to any of the penicillins is a **contraindication**.

Side effects include *Clostridium difficile*-associated diarrhea (CDAD), hypersensitivity reactions, including rashes, erythema multiforme, toxic epidermal necrolysis and Stevens–Johnson syndrome, nausea, vomiting, diarrhea, hepatic and renal dysfunction, crystalluria, anemia, thrombocytopenia, eosinophilia, leucopenia.

 DRUG INTERACTIONS/FOOD INTERACTIONS

Ampicillin capsules are stable in the presence of gastric acid.

The concurrent administration of allopurinol and ampicillin increases the incidence of rash; concurrent use of ampicillin and probenecid may result in increased and prolonged blood levels of ampicillin.

Antibiotics Manual: A Guide to Commonly Used Antimicrobials, Second Edition. David Schlossberg and Rafik Samuel.
© 2017 John Wiley & Sons Ltd. Published 2017 by John Wiley & Sons Ltd.

Chloramphenicol, macrolides, sulfonamides, and tetracyclines may interfere with the bactericidal effects of penicillins.

High urine concentrations of ampicillin may result in false-positive reactions when testing for the presence of glucose in urine using *Clinitest®*. It is recommended that glucose tests based on enzymatic glucose oxidase reactions (such as *Clinistix®*) be used.

 ## DOSING

IV ampicillin

Infection	Dose for patients weighing 40 kg or more
Infections of the respiratory tract	250 to 500 mg every 6 hours IV or IM
Infection of soft tissues	250 to 500 mg every 6 hours IV or IM
Infections of the gastrointestinal tract	500 mg every 6 hours IV or IM
Infections of the genitourinary tract	500 mg every 6 hours IV or IM
Bacterial meningitis	150 to 200 mg/kg/day IV divided q 3 to 4 h
Septicemia	150 to 200 mg/kg/day IV divided q 3 to 4 h

Oral ampicillin

Ampicillin is supplied as 250 mg and 500 mg capsules. It is also supplied as an oral suspension with two concentrations: 125 mg/5 mL and 250 mg/5 mL.

Infection	Dose
Genitourinary or gastrointestinal tract	500 mg qid
Respiratory tract infections	250 mg qid

 ## SPECIAL POPULATIONS

RENAL IMPAIRMENT

Creatinine clearance, mL/min	Dose
10 to 30	500 mg or 250 mg every 12 hours
< 10	500 mg or 250 mg every 24 hours
Hemodialysis	500 mg or 250 mg every 24 hours
	An additional dose during and at the end of dialysis should be administered.
CAPD	250 mg every 12 hours
CRRT	1 gram every 8 hours

HEPATIC DYSFUNCTION: No dose adjustment is necessary.

PEDIATRICS

IV ampicillin

Infection	Dose for patients weighing 40 kg or less
Infections of the respiratory tract	20 to 50 mg/kg/day divided every 6–8 hours IV or IM
Infection of soft tissues	20 to 50 mg/kg/day divided every 6–8 hours IV or IM
Infections of the gastrointestinal tract	50 mg/kg/day divided every 6–8 hours IV or IM
Infections of the genitourinary tract	50 mg/kg/day divided every 6–8 hours IV or IM
Bacterial meningitis	150 to 200 mg/kg/day IV divided q 3 to 4 hours
Septicemia	150 to 200 mg/kg/day IV divided q 3 to 4 hours

Oral ampicillin
Children weighing 20 kg or less

Infection	Dose
Genitourinary infections	25 mg/kg qid
Gastrointestinal infections	25 mg/kg qid
Respiratory infections	50 mg/kg/day divided 3–4 times daily

 THE ART OF ANTIMICROBIAL THERAPY

Clinical Pearls

1. Ampicillin needs to be dose adjusted for renal dysfunction.
2. A high percentage (43 to 100%) of patients with infectious mononucleosis who receive ampicillin develop a skin rash.

■ ANCEF (Cefazolin)

 BASIC CHARACTERISTICS

Class: First generation cephalosporin.

Mechanism of Action: Binds penicillin-binding protein, disrupting cell wall synthesis.

Mechanisms of Resistance:

1. The PBP can be altered, with reduced affinity.

2. Production of a beta-lactamase, resulting in hydrolysis of the beta-lactam ring.

3. Decreased ability of the antibiotic to reach the PBP when bacteria decrease porin production, resulting in a decrease of the drug concentration within the cell.

Metabolic Route: Excreted unchanged in the urine.

 FDA-APPROVED INDICATIONS:

Treatment of the following infections due to *susceptible organisms*:

Respiratory tract infections

Urinary tract infections

Skin and skin structure infections

Biliary tract infections

Bone and joint infections

Genital infections

Septicemia

Endocarditis

Perioperative prophylaxis

 SIDE EFFECTS/TOXICITY

Cefazolin is **contraindicated** in patients with known allergy to cephalosporins and should be used with caution if hypersensitivity exists to penicillin.

Toxicity includes fever, anaphylaxis, rash including Stevens–Johnson syndrome, erythema multiforme and toxic epidermal necrolysis, angioedema, flushing, serum-sickness like reactions, encephalopathy, seizures, diarrhea, *Clostridium difficile*-associated diarrhea and pseudomembranous colitis, oral candidiasis, anorexia, nausea, vomiting, stomach cramps, flatulence, hepatitis, renal impairment, genital moniliasis, vaginitis, hemorrhage, prolonged prothrombin time, pancytopenia, thrombocytosis, hemolytic anemia, positive Coombs test; cephalosporins may cause false-positive urine glucose determinations when using cupric sulfate solution (Benedict's solution, *Clinitest®*). Tests utilizing glucose oxidase (*Tes-Tape®*, *Clinistix®*) are not affected by cephalosporins.

 DRUG INTERACTIONS/FOOD INTERACTIONS

Probenecid may decrease renal tubular secretion of cephalosporins when used concurrently, resulting in increased and more prolonged cephalosporin blood levels.

Antibiotics Manual: A Guide to Commonly Used Antimicrobials, Second Edition. David Schlossberg and Rafik Samuel.
© 2017 John Wiley & Sons Ltd. Published 2017 by John Wiley & Sons Ltd.

DOSING

Usual adult dosage

Type of infection	Dose*	Frequency
Moderate to severe infections	500 mg–1 gram	Every 6–8 hours
Mild infections – gram positive	250–500 mg	Every 8 hours
Acute urinary tract infections	1 gram	Every 12 hours
Pneumococcal pneumonia	500 mg	Every 12 hours
Severe life-threatening infections (such as endocarditis or sepsis)	1–1.5 grams	Every 6 hours
Perioperative prophylactic use	1 gram	1/2 hour to 1 hour prior to the start of surgery

*For lengthy operations (e.g., 2 hours or more), 500 mg to 1 gram during surgery; *then* 500 mg to 1 gram every 6 to 8 hours for 24 hours postoperatively.

 SPECIAL POPULATIONS

RENAL IMPAIRMENT:

Creatinine clearance	Dose adjustment
>55 mL/min	Full dose
35 to 54 mL/min	Full dose, but at least 8 hours between doses
11 to 34 mL/min	1/2 the usual dose every 12 hours
10 mL/min or less	1/2 the usual dose every 18 to 24 hours
Hemodialysis	500 mg–1 gram after dialysis
CAPD	500 mg every 12 hours
CRRT	1 gram every 12 hours

HEPATIC DYSFUNCTION: No dose adjustment is necessary.

PEDIATRICS: Safety and effectiveness for use in premature infants and neonates have not been established.

A total daily dosage of 25 to 50 mg per kg divided into 3 or 4 equal doses is effective for most mild to moderately severe infections. Total daily dosage may be increased to 100 mg per kg (45 mg per pound) of body weight for severe infections.

Renal adjustment in children

Creatinine clearance	Dose adjustment*
40–70 mL/min	60% of the normal daily dose every 12 hours
20–39 mL/min	25% of the normal daily dose every 12 hours
<20 mL/min	10% of the normal daily dose every 24 hours

*All dosage recommendations apply after an initial loading dose.

THE ART OF ANTIMICROBIAL THERAPY

Clinical Pearls

1. Cefazolin must be renally adjusted.
2. Cross allergy with penicillins is <10% and can be used in life-threatening infections with caution if the allergy is not severe.
3. When using cefazolin for surgical prophylaxis, it should be started 30 min prior to incision and continued no longer than 24 hours after surgery.

BASIC CHARACTERISTICS

Class: Fluorinated pyrimidine analog.

Mechanism of Action: Flucytosine is taken up by fungal organisms and is rapidly converted to fluorouracil. Fluorouracil is converted into several active metabolites, which inhibit protein synthesis by being falsely incorporated into fungal RNA or interfere with the biosynthesis of fungal DNA through the inhibition of the enzyme thymidylate synthetase.

Flucytosine exhibits *in vitro* activity against *Candida* species and *Cryptococcus neoformans*.

Mechanism of Resistance: Flucytosine resistance may arise from a mutation of an enzyme necessary for the cellular uptake or metabolism of flucytosine or from increased synthesis of pyrimidines, which compete with the active metabolites of flucytosine. Resistance to flucytosine has been shown to develop during monotherapy after prolonged exposure to the drug.

Metabolic Route: Flucytosine is excreted via the kidneys.

 FDA-APPROVED INDICATIONS

Serious infections caused by susceptible strains of *Candida* (septicemia, endocarditis, urinary tract infection and pneumonia) or *Cryptococcus* (meningitis, pneumonia). Flucytosine should be used in combination with amphotericin B because of the emergence of resistance to flucytosine when it is used alone.

 SIDE EFFECTS/TOXICITY

> **WARNING:** Use with extreme caution in patients with impaired renal function and monitor renal, hematologic, and hepatic status of all patients.
>
> Flucytosine should not be used in patients with a known hypersensitivity to the drug.
>
> Flucytosine must be given with extreme caution to patients with bone marrow depression. Bone marrow toxicity with anemia, leucopenia or granulocytopenia can be irreversible and may lead to death in immunosuppressed patients.

Other adverse reactions: These include nausea, vomiting, diarrhea, hepatitis, renal failure, cardiac arrest, respiratory arrest, chest pain, rash, photosensitivity, ataxia, peripheral neuropathy, seizure, psychosis, hypoglycemia, hypokalemia.

 DRUG INTERACTIONS

Cytosine arabinoside can inactivate the antifungal activity of flucytosine by competitive inhibition.Drugs that impair glomerular filtration may prolong the biological half-life of flucytosine.

 DOSING

Flucytosine is administered in 250 mg and 500 mg capsules.

50 to 150 mg/kg/day administered in divided doses at 6-hour intervals.

Antibiotics Manual: A Guide to Commonly Used Antimicrobials, Second Edition. David Schlossberg and Rafik Samuel.
© 2017 John Wiley & Sons Ltd. Published 2017 by John Wiley & Sons Ltd.

SPECIAL POPULATIONS

HEPATIC IMPAIRMENT: Monitor liver function tests routinely.

RENAL IMPAIRMENT: Use with extreme caution in patients with impaired renal function.

Creatinine clearance, mL/min	Dose
50–80	500 mg q 12 h
10–50	500 mg q 18 h
< 10	500 mg/day
CAPD	0.5-1.0 gm q 24 h
Hemodialysis	Give additional dose after dialysis

PEDIATRICS: Safety and dosing has not been systematically studied in children.

 THE ART OF ANTIMICROBIAL THERAPY

Clinical Pearls

1. Flucytosine should be used in combination with amphotericin compounds to minimize resistance.
2. Flucytosine is active only against *Candida* and *Cryptococcus* strains.
3. Nausea or vomiting may be reduced or avoided if the capsules are given a few at a time over a 15-minute period.
4. Frequent monitoring of hepatic, renal, and hematopoietic function is indicated during therapy.
5. Serum levels should be between 25 mcg/mL and 100 mcg/mL.

BASIC CHARACTERISTICS

Class: Tetrahydropyrimidine.

Mechanism of Action: Depolarizing the neuromuscular junction of the nematode causing muscular contraction followed by paralysis.

Metabolic Route: Poorly absorbed from the gastrointestinal tract. Predominantly eliminated unchanged in the feces.

Used for: *Enterobius vermicularis, Trichostrongylus orientalis, Ancylostoma duodenale* and *Necator americanus, Moniliformis,* and *Oesophagostomum bifurcum*.

 SIDE EFFECTS/TOXICITY

Abdominal cramps, nausea, vomiting, diarrhea, anorexia, headache, dizziness, pruritus, and insomnia.

 DRUG INTERACTIONS/FOOD INTERACTIONS

Pyrantel is antagonistic with piperazine and should not be co-administered.

 DOSING

Enterobius, Trichostrongylus: 11 mg/kg base PO once (maximum 1 g); repeat in 2 weeks.

Ancylostoma, Necator, Oesophagostomum: 11 mg/kg base (maximum 1 g) PO daily × 3 days.

Moniliformis: 11 mg/kg base (maximum 1 g); repeat twice, 2 weeks apart.

 SPECIAL POPULATIONS

RENAL IMPAIRMENT: There is no dose adjustment.

HEPATIC DYSFUNCTION: There is no dose adjustment.

PEDIATRICS: Safety in children less than 2 years of age has not been established.

 THE ART OF ANTIMICROBIAL THERAPY

Clinical Pearls

1. Pyrantel is not available commercially in the US. It may be obtained through compounding pharmacies via the National Association of Compounding Pharmacies (800-687-7850) or the Professional Compounding Centers of America (800-331-2498, www.pccarx.com).
2. Pyrantel is not effective against *Trichuris trichiura*.
3. Available without a prescription.
4. Pyrantel pamoate suspension can be mixed with milk or fruit juice.

Antibiotics Manual: A Guide to Commonly Used Antimicrobials, Second Edition. David Schlossberg and Rafik Samuel.
© 2017 John Wiley & Sons Ltd. Published 2017 by John Wiley & Sons Ltd.

■ ARALEN (Chloroquine Phosphate and Hydroxychloroquine)

 BASIC CHARACTERISTICS

Class: 4-Aminoquinolone.

Mechanism of Action: Forms toxic complexes with heme molecules, depriving the parasite of hemoglobin.

Mechanism of Resistance: Mutation in transport molecule of digestive vacuole membrane (PfCRT), reducing the amount of drug that accumulates in the digestive vacuoles.

Metabolic Route: Half is excreted in the urine and the rest is degraded to multiple metabolic products.

 FDA-APPROVED INDICATIONS

Chloroquine: Suppressive treatment and acute attacks of malaria due to *P. vivax*, *P. malariae*, *P. ovale*, and susceptible strains of *P. falciparum*.

Treatment of extraintestinal amebiasis.

Hydroxychloroquine: Suppressive treatment and treatment of acute attacks of malaria due to *Plasmodium vivax*, *P. malariae*, *P. ovale*, and susceptible strains of *P. falciparum*

 SIDE EFFECTS/TOXICITY

> **WARNING:** For malaria and extraintestinal amebiasis.

Other **toxicities**: Psoriasis, porphyria, hypotension, tachycardia, bradycardia, A-V block or other transient conduction altera-tions, rash including Stevens–Johnson syndrome and toxic epidermal necrolysis, psychiatric symptoms including anxiety, paranoia, depression, hallucinations and psychosis, nausea, vomiting, diarrhea, hepatitis, seizures, nerve deafness, tinnitus, visual disturbances, myopathy, retinopathy, anemia, leucopenia, and thrombocytopenia.

 DRUG INTERACTIONS/FOOD INTERACTIONS

Antacids and kaolin can reduce the absorption of chloroquine; separate by 4 hours.

Concomitant use of cimetidine should be avoided.

An interval of at least two hours between intake of ampicillin and chloroquine should be observed.

May increase cyclosporine levels; close monitoring of the serum cyclosporine level is recommended.

 DOSING

Chloroquine phosphate is calculated as the base. Each 250 mg tablet of chloroquine phosphate is equivalent to the 150 mg base and each 500 mg tablet of chloroquine phosphate is equivalent to the 300 mg base.

Malaria prophylaxis: 500 mg (= 300 mg base) on exactly the same day of each week. Prophylactic therapy should begin two weeks prior to exposure and continued for eight weeks after leaving the endemic area.

Antibiotics Manual: A Guide to Commonly Used Antimicrobials, Second Edition. David Schlossberg and Rafik Samuel.
© 2017 John Wiley & Sons Ltd. Published 2017 by John Wiley & Sons Ltd.

Malaria treatment: An initial dose of 1 g (= 600 mg base) followed by an additional 500 mg (= 300 mg base) after six to eight hours and a single dose of 500 mg (= 300 mg base) on each of two consecutive days. This represents a total dose of 2.5 g chloroquine phosphate or 1.5 g base in three days.

Extraintestinal amebiasis: 1 g (600 mg base) daily for two days, followed by 500 mg (300 mg base) daily for at least two to three weeks.

Hydroxychloroquine: One tablet of 200 mg of hydroxychloroquine is equivalent to 155 mg base.

Malaria prophylaxis: *In adults*, 400 mg (= 310 mg base) on exactly the same day of each week. If circumstances permit, suppressive therapy should begin two weeks prior to exposure. The suppressive therapy should be continued for eight weeks after leaving the endemic area.

Treatment: An initial dose of 800 mg (= 620 mg base) followed by 400 mg (= 310 mg base) in six to eight hours and 400 mg (= 310 mg base) on each of two consecutive days (total 2 g hydroxychloroquine sulfate or 1.55 g base). An alternative method, employing a single dose of 800 mg (= 620 mg base), has also proved effective.

SPECIAL POPULATIONS

RENAL IMPAIRMENT: There is no adjustment needed.

HEPATIC DYSFUNCTION: Use with caution.

PEDIATRICS:

Chloroquine phosphate

The weekly **prophylactic** dosage is 5 mg calculated as base, per kg of body weight, but should not exceed the adult dose regardless of weight.

For treatment:

First dose: 10 mg base per kg (but not exceeding a single dose of 600 mg base).

Second dose: (6 hours after first dose) 5 mg base per kg (but not exceeding a single dose of 300 mg base).

Third dose: (24 hours after first dose) 5 mg base per kg.

Fourth dose: (36 hours after first dose) 5 mg base per kg.

Hydroxychloroquine

The weekly **prophylactic dosage** is 5 mg, calculated as base, per kg of body weight, but should not exceed the adult dose regardless of weight.

Treatment:

First dose: 10 mg base per kg (but not exceeding a single dose of 620 mg base).

Second dose: 5 mg base per kg (but not exceeding a single dose of 310 mg base) 6 hours after first dose.

Third dose: 5 mg base per kg 18 hours after second dose.

Fourth dose: 5 mg base per kg 24 hours after third dose.

THE ART OF ANTIMICROBIAL THERAPY

Clinical Pearls

1. *P. falcipirum* is usually resistant to chloroquine in all regions of the world except the Caribbean and the Middle East.

2. Chloroquine does not eliminate hepatic phase parasites and patients with acute *P. vivax* malaria are at high risk of relapse; to avoid relapse, after initial treatment of the acute infection, patients should subsequently be treated with an 8-aminoquinoline derivative (e.g., primaquine).

3. Chloroquine can induce hemolysis in patients with G6PD deficiency

4. Caution is urged when using chloroquine in patients with a history of epilepsy, auditory damage, liver disease, and alcoholism.

5. Since irreversible retinal damage may occur with prolonged or high dose therapy, ophthalmologic monitoring is advisable.

6. Concomitant use with mefloquine may increase the risk of seizures.

7. Complete blood cell counts should be made periodically if patients are given prolonged therapy.

BASIC CHARACTERISTICS

Class: Antimalarial agent.

Mechanism of Action: Inhibits nucleic acid and protein synthesis.

Metabolic Route: Metabolites eliminated in bile/feces and urine.

 FDA-APPROVED INDICATIONS

Not approved by FDA, but available through IND protocol on an emergency basis by the CDC Drug Service for patients with the following:

- Severe malaria disease
- High levels of malaria parasites in the blood
- Inability to take oral medications
- Lack of timely access to intravenous quinidine
- Quinidine intolerance or contraindications
- Quinidine failure

How to obtain Artesunate: To enroll a patient with severe malaria in this treatment protocol, contact the CDC Malaria Hotline: 770-488-7788 (M-F, 8 am–4:30 pm, Eastern time), or after hours call 770-488-7100 and request to speak with a CDC Malaria Branch clinician.

 SIDE EFFECTS/TOXICITY

Nausea, vomiting, diarrhea, seizures, tinnitus, rash, sinus bradycardia and first-degree heart block, prolongation of QTc, **potential cerebellar toxicity,** ataxia, and slurred speech.

 THE ART OF ANTIMICROBIAL THERAPY

Clinical Pearls

1. To avoid development of resistance, artesunate should be given with atovaquone/proguanil, doxycycline (not in children), clindamycin, or mefloquine.
2. Data on safety in pregnancy incomplete. Some recommend avoidance during first trimester.
3. Artesunate is also available in oral and rectal formulations, but only the IV form is provided by CDC.

Antibiotics Manual: A Guide to Commonly Used Antimicrobials, Second Edition. David Schlossberg and Rafik Samuel.
© 2017 John Wiley & Sons Ltd. Published 2017 by John Wiley & Sons Ltd.

■ ATABRINE (Quinacrine HCl)

 ## BASIC CHARACTERISTICS

Class: Acridine derivative.
Mechanism of Action: Unknown.
Metabolic Route: Excreted in the urine.
Used for: *Giardia lamblia* infections.

 ## SIDE EFFECTS/TOXICITY

Quinacrine should not be given to patients with a history of psychosis or to patients with psoriasis because of possible exacerbations.

Dizziness, abdominal pain, nausea, vomiting, diarrhea, and headache.

Yellow discoloration of the skin and urine.

 ## DRUG INTERACTIONS/FOOD INTERACTIONS

Quinacrine should not be administered with primaquine because it increases the plasma concentration of primaquine.

 ## DOSING

100 mg tid for 5–7 days.

 ## SPECIAL POPULATIONS

RENAL IMPAIRMENT: Unknown.

HEPATIC DYSFUNCTION: Unknown.

PEDIATRICS: 2 mg/kg tid for 5–7 days (maximum 300 mg/d).

 ## THE ART OF ANTIMICROBIAL THERAPY

Clinical Pearls

1. Quinacrine should not be used for malaria or tapeworm infections.
2. Quinacrine should not be given to patients with a history of psychosis or psoriasis.
3. Not available commercially in the US. It may be available through a compounding pharmacy: Call the National Association of Compounding Pharmacies (800-687-7850) or Professional Compounding Centers of America (800-331-2498, www.pccarx.com).

Antibiotics Manual: A Guide to Commonly Used Antimicrobials, Second Edition. David Schlossberg and Rafik Samuel.
© 2017 John Wiley & Sons Ltd. Published 2017 by John Wiley & Sons Ltd.

BASIC CHARACTERISTICS

Class: Combination of a nonnucleoside reverse transcriptase inhibitor (efavirenz), a nucleotide reverse transcriptase inhibitor (tenofovir), and a nucleoside reverse transcriptase inhibitor (emtricitabine)

Mechanism of Action: Tenofovir and emtricitabine are converted by cellular enzymes to their active drugs tenofovir biphosphate (an analog of adenosine triphosphate) and emtricitabine triphosphate (an analog of cytosine triphosphate). These drugs compete with the naturally occurring nucleotides for incorporation in newly forming HIV DNA. Since they do not have a terminal hydroxyl group, they halt transcription and replication of the virus. Efavirenz inhibits reverse transcriptase activity by binding the enzyme.

Mechanism of Resistance: Changes in the structure of reverse transcriptase leads to the inability of efavirenz to bind the enzyme and allow transcription to continue. The most frequent resistance mutations include K103N and Y181C.

Changes in the structure of HIV reverse transcriptase leads to preferred incorporation of adenosine triphosphate and cytosine triphosphate and decreased incorporation of tenofovir biphosphate and emtricitabine triphosphate, which allows transcription of DNA to continue. Resistance mutations include K65R, M184V, and TAMS.

Metabolic Route: Efavirenz is metabolized by the cytochrome P450 system to hydroxylated metabolites with subsequent glucuronidation.

Tenofovir and emtricitabine are excreted in the urine unchanged.

 ## FDA-APPROVED INDICATIONS

Treatment of HIV-1 as a single regimen tablet.

 ## SIDE EFFECTS/TOXICITY

> **WARNING: Lactic acidosis and severe hepatomegaly with steatosis**, including fatal cases, have been reported with the use of nucleoside analogs, including tenofovir disoproxil fumarate, a component of atripla, in combination with other antiretrovirals.

Atripla is not approved for the treatment of chronic hepatitis B virus (HBV) infection and the safety and efficacy of atripla have not been established in patients coinfected with HBV and HIV-1. Severe acute exacerbations of hepatitis B have been reported in patients who have discontinued emtricitabine or tenofovir, which are components of atripla. Hepatic function should be monitored closely with both clinical and laboratory follow-up for at least several months in patients who are coinfected with HIV-1 and HBV and discontinue atripla. If appropriate, initiation of antihepatitis B therapy may be warranted.

Other toxic effects include serious psychiatric toxicity, including severe depression, suicidal ideation, nonfatal suicide attempts, aggressive behavior, paranoid reactions, manic reactions, insomnia, impaired concentration, somnolence, abnormal dreams, and hallucinations; headache, rash, diarrhea, nausea, abdominal pain, elevated liver enzymes, cough, and rhinitis; convulsions, elevated cholesterol, immune reconstitution inflammatory syndrome, fat redistribution including central obesity and dorsocervical fat enlargement, peripheral wasting, facial wasting, and breast enlargement; renal impairment, including acute renal failure and Fanconi syndrome; decreased bone mineral density has been seen with tenofovir.

Antibiotics Manual: A Guide to Commonly Used Antimicrobials, Second Edition. David Schlossberg and Rafik Samuel.
© 2017 John Wiley & Sons Ltd. Published 2017 by John Wiley & Sons Ltd.

DRUG INTERACTIONS/FOOD INTERACTIONS

Atripla should be administered on an empty stomach.

Atripla should not be administered concurrently with astemizole, bepridil, cisapride, midazolam, pimozide, triazolam, ergot derivatives, St John's wort, voriconazole or etravirine, adefovir, simepravir, tenofovir, emtricitabine, lamivudine, efavirenz, or truvada.

Atripla should not be administered with any medication containing lamivudine because lamivudine and emtricitabine are both cytosine analogs and may be antagonistic.

Atripla causes hepatic enzyme induction of CYP3A4; coadministration of efavirenz with drugs primarily metabolized by 2C9, 2C19, and 3A4 isozymes may result in altered plasma concentrations of the coadministered drug; drugs that induce CYP3A4 activity would be expected to increase the clearance of efavirenz, resulting in lowered plasma concentrations. Because of these metabolic activities, the following drug interactions warrant consideration of dosage adjustment and monitoring of clinical effects and serum levels of affected drugs:

Medication	Adjustment or action
Clarithromycin	Consider alternative agent
Rifabutin	Increase rifabutin to 450–600/q d or 600 3 × week
Rifampin	Add efavirenz 200/day to the atripla in those who weigh more than 50 kg
Contraceptives	Use alternative or additional method
Phenobarbitol, phenytoin, or carbamazepine	Monitor anticonvulsant level and consider alternative
Methadone	Opiate withdrawal common, titrate methadone
Warfarin	Monitor INR closely
Fosamprenavir	fAPV 1400 + RTV 300 daily or usual BID dose
Darunavir	Monitor levels with normal dosing
Indinavir	IDV 800 bid + RTV 100 bid
Maraviroc	Maraviroc dose should be 600 mg bid
Didanosine	Decrease didanosine to 250 mg daily
Atazanavir	ATV 300 mg + RTV 100 mg (naïve only)

 DOSING

Each tablet contains 600 mg of efavirenz, 200 mg of emtricitabine, and 300 mg of tenofovir disoproxil fumarate. The recommended dose is one tablet at bedtime.

 SPECIAL POPULATIONS

RENAL IMPAIRMENT: It is not recommended to be administered in patients with creatinine clearance less than 50 mL/min.

HEPATIC DYSFUNCTION: In patients with a known or suspected history of hepatitis B or C infection and in patients treated with other medications associated with liver toxicity, monitoring of liver enzymes is recommended.

PEDIATRICS: **For treatment**: Atripla should not be given to those under 12 years of age or under 40 kg.

THE ART OF ANTIMICROBIAL THERAPY

Clinical Pearls

1. Atripla is a standalone antiretroviral regimen.
2. Atripla should be dosed at bedtime to decrease the CNS adverse events.
3. If atripla is given without food, less is absorbed and side effects can be decreased.
4. Women receiving atripla should use two methods of birth control.
5. Atripla contains tenofovir, emtricitabine, and efavirenz. It should not be administered with Viread, Emtriva, Truvada, Sustiva, Odefsey, Descovy, Complera, Genvoya, Stribild, or Vemlidy.
6. Patients with HIV-1 should be tested for hepatitis B virus before initiating antiretroviral therapy with atripla.
7. Atripla and didanosine combinations should be administered with caution.

■ AUGMENTIN, AUGMENTIN 600ES, AUGMENTIN XR (Amoxicillin-Clavulanate Potassium)

 BASIC CHARACTERISTICS

Class: Aminopenicillin + beta-lactamase inhibitor.

Mechanism of Action: Binds penicillin-binding protein, disrupting cell wall synthesis.

Mechanisms of Resistance:

1. The PBP can be altered, with reduced affinity.
2. Decreased ability of the antibiotic to reach the PBP when bacteria decrease porin production, resulting in a decrease of the drug concentration within the cell.

Metabolic Route: Amoxicillin and clavulanate are excreted unchanged in the urine.

 FDA-APPROVED INDICATIONS

1. **Augmentin** Indicated in the treatment of infections due to susceptible strains of microorganisms in the conditions listed below:

   Lower respiratory tract infections

   Otitis media

   Sinusitis

   Skin and skin structure infections

   Urinary tract infections

2. **Augmentin ES 600** Indicated for the treatment of **pediatric patients** with recurrent or persistent acute otitis media, with the following risk factors: antibiotic exposure for acute otitis media within the preceding 3 months, plus either age of 2 years or less or daycare attendance.

3. **Augmentin XR** Indicated for the treatment of adults with community acquired pneumonia or acute bacterial sinusitis.

 SIDE EFFECTS/TOXICITY

A history of allergic reaction to any of the penicillins is a **contraindication**.

Side effects include *Clostridium difficile*-associated diarrhea (CDAD), hypersensitivity reactions, including rashes, erythema multiforme, toxic epidermal necrolysis and Stevens–Johnson syndrome, nausea, vomiting, diarrhea, hepatic and renal dysfunction, crystalluria, anemia, thrombocytopenia, eosinophilia, leukopenia, hyperactivity, and seizures.

 DRUG INTERACTIONS/FOOD INTERACTIONS

Augmentin capsules may be given without regard to meals.

Augmentin XR should be taken at the start of the meal.

Concurrent use of amoxicillin-clavulanate and probenecid may result in increased and prolonged blood levels of amoxicillin.

Chloramphenicol, macrolides, sulfonamides, and tetracyclines may interfere with the bactericidal effects of penicillins.

Amoxicillin-clavulanate may reduce the efficacy of oral contraceptives.

Antibiotics Manual: A Guide to Commonly Used Antimicrobials, Second Edition. David Schlossberg and Rafik Samuel.
© 2017 John Wiley & Sons Ltd. Published 2017 by John Wiley & Sons Ltd.

High urine concentrations of amoxicillin may result in false-positive reactions when testing for the presence of glucose in urine using *Clinitest®*; it is recommended that glucose tests based on enzymatic glucose oxidase reactions (such as *Clinistix®*) be used.

 DOSING

1. Augmentin

Augmentin is supplied in multiple formulations as follows:

Dose and formulation	Amoxicillin	Clavulanate
875 mg tablet	875 mg	125 mg
500 mg tablet	500 mg	125 mg
250 mg tablet	250 mg	125 mg
125 mg chewable tablet	125 mg	31.25 mg
200 mg chewable tablet	200 mg	28.5 mg
250 mg chewable tablet	250 mg	62.5 mg
400 mg chewable tablet	400 mg	57.0 mg
125 mg/5 cc	125 mg	31.25 mg
250 mg/5 cc	250 mg	62.5 mg
200 mg/5 cc	200 mg	28.5 mg
400 mg/5 cc	400 mg	57.0 mg

The usual adult dose is one 500-mg tablet every 12 hours or one 250-mg tablet every 8 hours.

For severe infections and infections of the respiratory tract, the dose should be one 875-mg tablet every 12 hours or one 500-mg tablet every 8 hours.

2. Augmentin XR

Augmentin XR is supplied as a 1 g/67.5 mg tablet and the recommended dose is 2 tablets every 12 hours.

 SPECIAL POPULATIONS

RENAL IMPAIRMENT

Augmentin

Creatine clearance, mL/min	Dose and formulation
10–30	250–500 mg every 12 hours
<10	250–500 mg every 24 hours
Hemodialysis	250–500 mg every 24 hours and an additional dose during and at the end of dialysis
CAPD	No recommendation

Augmentin XR and Augmentin 875 mg are **contraindicated** in patients with a creatinine clearance of <30 mL/min and in hemodialysis patients.

HEPATIC DYSFUNCTION: No dose adjustment but use with caution.

PEDIATRICS:

Augmentin

Neonates and infants aged <12 weeks: 30 mg/kg/day divided q 12 h, based on the amoxicillin component. The 200 mg/5 mL formulation in this age group is not recommended.

Patients aged 12 weeks (3 months) and older

Infection	Dose*,**,***,****
Otitis media, sinusitis	45 mg/kg/12 hours* or 40 mg/kg/8 hours**
Lower respiratory infections	45 mg/kg/12 hours* or 40 mg/kg/8 hours**
Less severe infections	25 mg/kg/12 hours* or 20 mg/kg/8 hours**

*Use the 200 mg/5 mL or 400 mg/5 mL formulations for this dose.
**Use the 125 mg/5 mL or 250 mg/5 mL formulations for this dose.
***The q 12 h regimen is associated with less diarrhea.
****Pediatric patients weighing 40 kg and more should be dosed following adult doses.

Augmentin ES-600

Supplied as a suspension with 600 mg amoxicillin and 42.9 mg of clavulanate per 5 mL.

Pediatric patients 3 months and older

The recommended dose is 45 mg/kg/12 hours, administered for 10 days.

For pediatric patients weighing 40 kg and more follow the Augmentin adult dosing recommendation.

Augmentin XR

Safety and effectiveness in pediatric patients younger than 16 years have not been established.

 THE ART OF ANTIMICROBIAL THERAPY

Clinical Pearls

1. Amoxicillin/clavulanate needs to be dose adjusted for renal dysfunction.
2. Augmentin XR and Augmentin 875 mg are contraindicated in patients with a creatinine clearance of <30 mL/min and in hemodialysis patients.
3. Augmentin XR is not recommended for patients under 16 years.
4. Augmentin ES is recommended only for children.
5. The 400 and 200 mg suspension formulations contain aspartame.
6. A high percentage of patients with mononucleosis who receive ampicillin develop an erythematous skin rash. Thus, ampicillin class antibiotics should not be administered to patients with mononucleosis.
7. Amoxicillin-clavulanate should be used with caution in patients with evidence of hepatic dysfunction.

BASIC CHARACTERISTICS

Class: Fluoroquinolone.

Mechanism of Action: Inhibition of bacterial topoisomerase IV and DNA gyrase.

Mechanisms of Resistance: Mutations in DNA gyrase and/or topoisomerase IV, or through altered efflux.

Metabolic Route: Moxifloxacin is metabolized via glucuronide and sulfate conjugation by the liver and the metabolites are excreted in the feces and urine.

 FDA-APPROVED INDICATIONS

Moxifloxacin is indicated for the treatment of serious infections caused by susceptible strains of microorganisms in the diseases listed below:

Acute bacterial sinusitis

Acute bacterial exacerbation of chronic bronchitis

Community acquired pneumonia

Uncomplicated skin and skin structure infections

Complicated intra-abdominal infections

Complicated skin and skin structure infections

Also Used for: Treatment of tuberculosis.

 SIDE EFFECTS/TOXICITY

WARNING: Serious adverse reactions including tendinitis, tendon rupture, peripheral neuropathy, central nervous system effects, and exacerbation of myasthenia gravis. Fluoroquinolones, including moxifloxacin, have been associated with disabling and potentially irreversible serious adverse reactions that have occurred together, including tendinitis and tendon rupture, peripheral neuropathy and central nervous system effects.

Discontinue moxifloxacin immediately and avoid the use of fluoroquinolones, including moxifloxacin, in patients who experience any of these serious adverse reactions. Fluoroquinolones, including moxifloxacin, may exacerbate muscle weakness in patients with myasthenia gravis. Avoid moxifloxacin in patients with a known history of myasthenia gravis.

Because fluoroquinolones, including moxifloxacin, have been associated with serious adverse reactions, reserve moxifloxacin for use in patients who have no alternative treatment options for the following indications: acute bacterial exacerbation of chronic bronchitis and acute bacterial sinusitis.

Moxifloxacin is **contraindicated** in persons with a history of hypersensitivity associated with the use of moxifloxacin or any quinolone.

Other adverse effects include anaphylactic reactions and allergic skin reactions including toxic epidermal necrolysis and Stevens–Johnson syndrome, photosensitivity, tendinitis and tendon rupture, renal toxicity, hepatotoxicity (sometimes fatal), central nervous system effects including headache, dizziness, seizures, anxiety, confusion, depression, and insomnia (use with

Antibiotics Manual: A Guide to Commonly Used Antimicrobials, Second Edition. David Schlossberg and Rafik Samuel.
© 2017 John Wiley & Sons Ltd. Published 2017 by John Wiley & Sons Ltd.

caution in patients at risk of seizures), peripheral neuropathy, nausea, diarrhea, constipation, *Clostridium difficile*-associated colitis, prolongation of the QT interval and torsade de pointes (avoid use in patients with known prolongation of QT, hypokalemia, and with other drugs that prolong the QT interval), and pancytopenia.

 DRUG INTERACTIONS/FOOD INTERACTIONS

1. Moxifloxacin should be taken 4 hours before or 8 hours after antacids containing calcium, magnesium, or aluminum; sucralfate; divalent or trivalent cations such as iron; or multivitamins containing zinc.
2. The concomitant administration of a nonsteroidal anti-inflammatory drug with a quinolone may increase the risk of CNS stimulation and seizures.
3. Disturbances of blood glucose, including hyperglycemia and hypoglycemia, may be seen in patients treated concurrently with antidiabetic agents

 DOSING

Moxifloxacin can be administered as 400 mg tablets or via intravenous injection.

Infection	Dose	Duration
Acute bacterial sinusitis	400 mg q 24 h	10 days
Acute exacerbation of chronic bronchitis	400 mg q 24 h	5 days
Community acquired pneumonia	400 mg q 24 h	7–14 days
Uncomplicated skin infections	400 mg q 24 h	7 days
Complicated skin infections	400 mg q 24 h	7–21 days
Complicated intra-abdominal Infections	400 mg q 24 h	5–14 days

For complicated intra-abdominal infections, therapy should usually be initiated with the intravenous formulation.

 SPECIAL POPULATIONS

RENAL IMPAIRMENT: No dose adjustment is necessary.

HEPATIC DYSFUNCTION: No dose adjustment is necessary.

PEDIATRICS: Safety and efficacy in pediatric patients less than 18 years of age have not been established.

 THE ART OF ANTIMICROBIAL THERAPY

Clinical Pearls
1. Moxifloxacin should be given at least 4 hours before or 8 hours after ingestion of cations.
2. All fluoroquinolones can cause tendon rupture, especially in patients over 60 years of age.
3. Caution should be used when given with medications that affect QT intervals.
4. All fluoroquinolones can cause phototoxicity.
5. All fluoroquinolones can cause seizures.

6. Moxifloxacin should be avoided if possible in children, pregnant women, and nursing mothers because of concerns for cartilage developmental problems.

7. Moxifloxacin has activity against Mycobacteria; therefore moxifloxacin monotherapy should be avoided if mycobacterial infection is possible.

8. Treatment of gonorrhea with fluoroquinolones should be undertaken with caution because of rising resistance.

9. Moxifloxacin is not indicated for urinary tract infections.

10. Unlike the other fluoroquinolones, moxifloxacin has significant activity against gram-negative anaerobes.

11. In 2016, an FDA Safety Communication advised that the serious side effects associated with fluoroquinolones generally outweigh the benefits for patients with sinusitis, bronchitis, and uncomplicated urinary tract infections who have other treatment options.

AVYCAZ (Ceftazidime and Avibactam Sodium Powder)

 BASIC CHARACTERISTICS

Class: Cephalosporin plus beta-lactamase inhibitor.

Mechanism of Action: Binds penicillin-binding protein, disrupting cell wall synthesis.

Mechanisms of Resistance:

1. The PBP can be altered, with reduced affinity.
2. Production of a beta-lactamase, resulting in hydrolysis of the beta-lactam ring.
3. Decreased ability of the antibiotic to reach the PBP when bacteria decrease porin production, resulting in a decrease of the drug concentration within the cell.

Metabolic Route: Excreted, unchanged in the urine.

 FDA-APPROVED INDICATIONS

Treatment of the following infections when caused by susceptible organisms:

Complicated intra-abdominal infections (in combination with metronidazole)

Complicated urinary tract infections, including pyelonephritis

 SIDE EFFECTS/TOXICITY

Contraindicated in patients who have shown immediate hypersensitivity reactions to other beta-lactam antibiotics or avibactam. If other forms of hypersensitivity to beta-lactams exist, use with caution.

Toxicity includes inflammation at the site of injection, fever, anaphylaxis, rash including Stevens–Johnson syndrome, erythema multiforme and toxic epidermal necrolysis, angioedema, flushing, serum-sickness like reactions, encephalopathy, seizures, myoclonus, diarrhea, *Clostridium difficile*-associated diarrhea and pseudomembranous colitis, oral candidiasis, anorexia, nausea, vomiting, stomach cramps, flatulence, hepatitis, renal impairment, genital moniliasis, vaginitis, hemorrhage, prolonged prothrombin time, pancytopenia, hemolytic anemia, eosinophilia, thrombocytopenia, hypokalemia, positive Coombs test, increased gamma-glutamyltransferase, and renal impairment.

 DRUG INTERACTIONS/FOOD INTERACTIONS

Nephrotoxicity has been reported following concomitant administration of cephalosporins with aminoglycoside antibiotics or potent diuretics such as furosemide. Cephalosporins may cause false-positive urine glucose determinations when using cupric sulfate solution (Benedict's solution, *Clinitest*®). Tests utilizing glucose oxidase (*Tes-Tape*®, *Clinistix*®) are not affected by cephalosporins.

Coadministration with probenecid may decrease elimination of avibactam and is not recommended.

DOSING

Type of infection	Dose	Duration
Intra-abdominal infection	2.5 grams q 8 hours	5–14 days
UTI	2.5 grams q 8 hours	7–14 days

Antibiotics Manual: A Guide to Commonly Used Antimicrobials, Second Edition. David Schlossberg and Rafik Samuel.
© 2017 John Wiley & Sons Ltd. Published 2017 by John Wiley & Sons Ltd.

SPECIAL POPULATIONS

RENAL IMPAIRMENT:

Creatinine clearance	Doses (administered over 2 hours)
31–50 mL/min	1.25 grams q 8 hours
16–30 mL/min	0.94 grams q 12 hours
6–15 mL/min	0.94 grams q 24 hours
5 mL/min or less	0.94 grams q 48 hours
HD	Hemodialyzable; therefore give after hemodialysis on dialysis days
CAPD	Data incomplete
CRRT	Data incomplete

HEPATIC DYSFUNCTION: No dose adjustment is necessary.

PEDIATRICS: Safety and effectiveness in pediatric patients below the age of 18 years have not been established.

GERIATRICS: Because of limited data, differences in outcomes or specific risks with ceftazidime/avibactam cannot be ruled out for patients 65 years of age and older.

 ## THE ART OF ANTIMICROBIAL THERAPY

Clinical Pearls:

1. There may be a decreased clinical response in patients with a baseline creatinine clearance of 30 to ≤ 50 mL/min.
2. Ceftazidime/avibactam is dose adjusted for renal dysfunction.
3. Cross allergy with penicillins is <10% and can be used in life-threatening infections with caution if the allergy is not severe.
4. Avibactam is a beta-lactamase inhibitor resistant to ESBL and KPC beta-lactamases.

BASIC CHARACTERISTICS

Class: Monobactam.

Mechanism of Action: Binds penicillin-binding protein (PBP), disrupting cell wall synthesis.

Mechanisms of Resistance:

1. The PBP can be altered, with reduced affinity
2. Production of a beta-lactamase, resulting in hydrolysis of the beta-lactam ring.
3. Decreased ability of the antibiotic to reach the PBP when bacteria increase porins, resulting in a decrease of the drug concentration within the cell.

Metabolic Route: Excreted unchanged in the urine.

 FDA-APPROVED INDICATIONS

Treatment of the following infections caused by susceptible gram-negative organisms:

Urinary tract infections

Lower respiratory tract Infections

Septicemia

Skin and skin-structure infections

Intra-abdominal infections

Gynecologic infections

Adjunctive therapy to surgery in the management of infections caused by susceptible organisms, including abscesses, infections complicating hollow viscus perforations, cutaneous infections and infections of serous surfaces.

 SIDE EFFECTS/TOXICITY

Clostridium difficile-associated diarrhea, phlebitis/thrombophlebitis, hypersensitivity, anaphylaxis, fever, rash including toxic epidermal necrolysis and erythema multiforme, seizure, confusion, tinnitus, altered taste, diarrhea, nausea, hepatitis, vomiting, bronchospasm, arrhythmias, hypotension, myalgia, vaginitis, breast tenderness, increased serum creatinine, pancytopenia, neutropenia, eosinophilia, thrombocytopenia, anemia, leukocytosis, thrombocytosis, prolonged prothrombin time.

 DRUG INTERACTIONS/FOOD INTERACTIONS

If an aminoglycoside is used concurrently with aztreonam the renal function should be monitored.

 DOSING

Aztreonam may be administered intravenously or by intramuscular injection.

Antibiotics Manual: A Guide to Commonly Used Antimicrobials, Second Edition. David Schlossberg and Rafik Samuel.
© 2017 John Wiley & Sons Ltd. Published 2017 by John Wiley & Sons Ltd.

Type of infection	Dose
Urinary tract infections	500 mg or 1 g q 8–12 hours
Moderately severe systemic infections	1–2 g q 8–12 hours
Severe systemic infections	2 g q 6–8 hours
Pseudomonas infections	2 g q 6–8 hours

 SPECIAL POPULATIONS

RENAL IMPAIRMENT: The dosage of aztreonam should be halved in patients with estimated creatinine clearances between 10 mL/min/1.73 m^2 and 30 mL/min/1.73 m^2 after an initial loading dose of 1 g or 2 g.

In patients with creatinine clearance less than 10 mL/min/1.73 m^2, such as those supported by **hemodialysis**, the usual dose of 500 mg, 1 g, or 2 g should be given **initially**.

The **maintenance** dose should be one-fourth of the usual initial dose given at the usual fixed interval of 6, 8, or 12 hours.

For serious or life-threatening infections, in addition to the maintenance doses, one-eighth of the initial dose should be given after each hemodialysis session.

CRRT: Administer 50–75% of the dose every 8–12 hours.

HEPATIC DYNFUNCTION: No dose adjustment is necessary.

PEDIATRICS: The safety and effectiveness of aztreonam has been established in the age groups 9 months to 16 years.

Type of infection	Dose
Mild to moderate infections	30 mg/ kg q 8 hours
Moderate to severe systemic infections	30 mg/kg q 6–8 hours

 THE ART OF ANTIMICROBIAL THERAPY

Clinical Pearls

1. While cross-reactivity of aztreonam with other beta-lactam antibiotics is rare, this drug should be administered with caution to any patient with a history of hypersensitivity to beta-lactams.

2. Aztreonam is similar in structure to ceftazidime and cross-allergies may occur.

3. Aztreonam has no activity against gram-positive organisms.

■ BACTRIM, BACTRIM DS, SEPTRA, SEPTRA DS (Trimethoprim/Sulfamethoxazole)

 BASIC CHARACTERISTICS

Class: Antimetabolite/sulfonamide.

Mechanism of Action: Sulfamethoxazole inhibits bacterial synthesis of dihydrofolic acid by competing with *para*-aminobenzoic acid. Trimethoprim blocks the production of tetrahydrofolic acid from dihydrofolic acid by binding to and reversibly inhibiting the required enzyme, dihydrofolate reductase.

Mechanisms of Resistance:

1. Plasmid mediated alterations in dihydrofolate reductase and changes in cell permeability.
2. Overproduction of *para*-aminobenzoic acid.
3. Structural change in dihydropteroate synthesis.

Metabolic Route: Both trimethoprim and sulfamethoxazole are excreted in the urine.

 FDA-APPROVED INDICATIONS

Urinary tract infections

Acute otitis media

Acute exacerbations of chronic bronchitis in adults

Shigellosis

Pneumocystis jirovecii pneumonia: treatment and prophylaxis

Traveler's diarrhea in adults

Also Used for: Infections due to *Listeria*, *Nocardia*, *Salmonella*, *Brucella*, *Paracoccidioides*, melioidosis, *Burkholderia*, *Stenotrophomonas*, cyclospora, isospora, Whipple's disease, and alternative therapy for toxoplasmosis and community-acquired MRSA skin infections.

 SIDE EFFECTS/TOXICITY

Contraindicated

Patients with a known hypersensitivity to trimethoprim or sulfonamides.

Patients with a history of drug-induced immune thrombocytopenia with use of trimethoprim and/or sulfonamides.

Patients with documented megaloblastic anemia due to folate deficiency.

Pregnant patients.

Nursing mothers.

Pediatric patients less than 2 months of age.

Patients with marked hepatic damage or with severe renal insufficiency when renal function status cannot be monitored.

Adverse reactions include Stevens–Johnson syndrome, toxic epidermal necrolysis, fulminant hepatic necrosis, stomatitis, glossitis, nausea, emesis, abdominal pain, pancreatitis, diarrhea, *Clostridium difficile*-associated diarrhea anorexia, hepatitis, renal failure, interstitial nephritis, aseptic meningitis, convulsions, peripheral neuritis, ataxia, vertigo, tinnitus, headache, hallucinations, depression, apathy, nervousness, weakness, fatigue, insomnia, rhabdomyolysis, lung hypersensitivity reactions,

Antibiotics Manual: A Guide to Commonly Used Antimicrobials, Second Edition. David Schlossberg and Rafik Samuel.
© 2017 John Wiley & Sons Ltd. Published 2017 by John Wiley & Sons Ltd.

diuresis, periarteritis, lupus, arthralgia, myalgias, hypoglycemia, hypoprothrombinemia, methemoglobinemia, eosinophilia, hypoglycemia, hyperkalemia, crystalluria, megaloblastic anemia, thrombocytopenia, agranulocytosis, aplastic anemia and other blood dyscrasias.

DRUG INTERACTIONS/FOOD INTERACTIONS

Trimethoprim/sulfamethoxazole can be given with or without food.

Reported interactions include thrombocytopenia with thiazides.

Increased effect of phenytoin, methotrexate, digoxin, oral hypoglycemics and warfarin.

Increased sulfamethoxazole levels with indomethacin; decreased efficacy of tricyclic antidepressants and hyperkalemia with ACE inhibitors.

DOSING

Trimethoprim/sulfamethoxazole is in a fixed dose ratio of 1:5.

Bactrim and Septra contain 400 mg sulfamethoxazole and 80 mg trimethoprim.

Bactrim DS and Septra DS contain 800 mg sulfamethoxazole and 160 mg trimethoprim.

Oral suspension contains 200 mg sulfamethoxazole and 40 mg trimethoprim per teaspoon.

Intravenous formulation contains 400 mg sulfamethoxazole and 80 mg trimethoprim/5 mL.

Urinary tract infections, shigellosis, acute exacerbations of chronic bronchitis: The usual adult dosage in the treatment of urinary tract infections is 1 DS tablet, 2 tablets, four teaspoonfuls (20 mL) or 10 ml IV every 12 hours × 10–14 days.

Pneumocystis jirovecii pneumonia

Treatment: 75 to 100 mg/kg sulfamethoxazole and 15 to 20 mg/kg trimethoprim per 24 hours given in equally divided doses every 6 hours × 14–21 days. Thus, a patient weighing 64 kg would take 4 tablets, 2 DS tablets, or 20 ml IV every 6 h.

Prophylaxis: The recommended dosage for prophylaxis in adults is 1 DS or single strength tablet daily. Alternatively, 1 DS tablet every Monday, Wednesday, and Friday.

Traveler's diarrhea: The usual adult dosage is 1 DS tablet, 2 tablets or four teaspoonfuls (20 mL) every 12 hours for 5 days.

SPECIAL POPULATIONS

RENAL IMPAIRMENT:

Creatinine clearance, mL/min	Dose
15–30	Use half the usual dose
<15, hemodialysis, CAPD, CRRT	Use not recommended

HEPATIC DYSFUNCTION: No dose adjustment is necessary.

PEDIATRICS: TMP/SMX is not recommended for infants younger than 2 months of age.

The recommended dose for children with urinary tract infections or acute otitis media is 40 mg/kg sulfamethoxazole and 8 mg/kg trimethoprim per 24 hours, given in two divided doses every 12 hours for 10 days. An identical daily dosage is used for 5 days in the treatment of shigellosis.

Pneumocystis jirovecii pneumonia

Treatment: 75 to 100 mg/kg sulfamethoxazole and 15 to 20 mg/kg trimethoprim per 24 hours given in equally divided doses every 6 hours × 14–21 days.

Prophylaxis: The recommended dose is 750 mg/m²/day sulfamethoxazole with 150 mg/m²/day trimethoprim given orally in equally divided doses twice a day, on 3 consecutive days per week. The total daily dose should not exceed 1600 mg sulfamethoxazole and 320 mg trimethoprim.

 ## THE ART OF ANTIMICROBIAL THERAPY

Clinical Pearls

1. Because sulfamethoxazole and trimethoprim may interfere with folic acid metabolism, it should be used during pregnancy only if the potential benefit justifies the potential risk to the fetus.

2. The sulfonamides should not be used for treatment of group A β-hemolytic streptococcal infections.

3. Although not FDA approved, the usual dose of TMP/SMX for systemic infections due to typical bacteria is 10 mg/kg/day of trimethoprim and 50 mg/day of sulfamethoxazole.

4. Clinical signs such as rash, sore throat, fever, arthralgia, pallor, purpura, or jaundice may be early indications of serious reactions.

5. Patients taking trimethoprim/sulfamethoxazole should drink adequate amounts of water to decrease the likelihood of crystalluria and stone formation.

BASIC CHARACTERISTICS

Class: Nucleoside reverse transcriptase inhibitor for hepatitis B.

Mechanism of Action: Entecavir is a guanosine nucleoside analog that is phosphorylated to the active triphosphate form. It competes with guanosine triphosphate to inhibit all three activities of the HBV polymerase (reverse transcriptase): (1) base priming, (2) reverse transcription of the negative strand from the pregenomic messenger RNA, and (3) synthesis of the positive strand of HBV DNA.

Mechanism of Resistance: Lamivudine-resistant HBV caries 8- to 30-fold reduction in entecavir susceptibility. The mutations rtM204I/V with or without rtL180M in HBV polymerase lead to decreased incorporation of entecavir.

Metabolic Route: Entecavir is excreted unchanged in the urine.

 FDA-APPROVED INDICATIONS

Treatment of chronic hepatitis B virus infection with evidence of active viral replication and either evidence of persistent elevations in serum aminotransferases (ALT or AST) or histologically active disease.

 SIDE EFFECTS/TOXICITY

> **WARNING:** Severe acute exacerbations of hepatitis B have been reported in patients who have discontinued antihepatitis B therapy, including entecavir. Hepatic function should be monitored closely with both clinical and laboratory follow-up for at least several months in patients who discontinue antihepatitis B therapy. If appropriate, initiation of antihepatitis B therapy may be warranted.
>
> Limited clinical experience suggests there is a potential for the development of resistance to HIV (human immunodeficiency virus) nucleoside reverse transcriptase inhibitors if entecavir is used to treat chronic hepatitis B virus (HBV) infection in patients with HIV infection that is not being treated. Therapy with entecavir is not recommended for HIV/HBV coinfected patients who are not also receiving highly active antiretroviral therapy (HAART).
>
> **Lactic acidosis and severe hepatomegaly with steatosis**, including fatal cases, have been reported with the use of nucleoside analog inhibitors alone or in combination with antiretrovirals.

Other adverse effects include headache, fatigue, rash, dizziness, and nausea.

 DRUG INTERACTIONS/FOOD INTERACTIONS

Entecavir should be administered at least 2 hours after a meal and 2 hours before the next meal.

There are no significant drug interactions.

 DOSING

Entecavir is supplied in 0.5-mg, 1-mg tablets and an orange-flavored, clear, colorless to pale yellow aqueous solution containing 0.05 mg/mL.

Antibiotics Manual: A Guide to Commonly Used Antimicrobials, Second Edition. David Schlossberg and Rafik Samuel.
© 2017 John Wiley & Sons Ltd. Published 2017 by John Wiley & Sons Ltd.

The recommended dose in nucleoside-treatment-naive adults and adolescents 16 years of age and older is 0.5 mg once daily. The recommended dose in those who are receiving lamiviudine or have virus resistant to either lamivudine or telbivudine is 1 mg once daily.

 SPECIAL POPULATIONS

RENAL IMPAIRMENT:

Creatinine clearance, mL/min	Naïve dose	Lamivudine-resistant dose
≥50	0.5 mg once daily	1 mg once daily
30 to <50	0.25 mg once daily or 0.5 mg every 48 hours	0.5 mg once daily or 1 mg every 48 hours
10 to <30	0.15 mg once daily or 0.5 mg every 72 hours	0.3 mg once daily or 1 mg every 72 hours
<10, hemodialysis or PD	0.05 mg once daily or 0.5 mg every 7 days	0.1 mg once daily or 1 mg every 7 days

HEPATIC DYSFUNCTION: Recommended dose with hepatic decompensation is 1 mg once daily.

PEDIATRICS: Children 2 years and older who weigh at least 10 kg can be treated with entecavir liquid as follows:

Weight, kg	Daily dose, mL, naïve	Daily dose, mL, lamvudine-resistant
10 to 11	3	6
>11 to 14	4	8
>14 to 17	5	10
>17 to 20	6	12
>20 to 23	7	14
>23 to 26	8	16
>26 to 30	9	18
>30	10	20

 THE ART OF ANTIMICROBIAL THERAPY

Clinical Pearls

1. Lamivudine resistance leads to decreased susceptibility to entecavir.
2. Resistance mutations are similar for entecavir and telbivudine.
3. Before initiating entecavir therapy, HIV testing should be offered to all patients.
4. Do not initiate entecavir in HIV coinfected patients unless they are on HAART; M184V mutations on HIV reverse transcriptase have been reported.

■ BENZATHINE PENICILLIN, PENICILLIN G, PENICILLIN V, PROCAINE PENICILLIN (Penicillin)

 ## BASIC CHARACTERISTICS

Class: Penicillin.

Mechanism of Action: Binds penicillin-binding protein, disrupting cell wall synthesis.

Mechanisms of Resistance:

1. The PBP can be altered, with reduced affinity.
2. Production of a beta-lactamase, resulting in hydrolysis of the beta-lactam ring.
3. Decreased ability of the antibiotic to reach the PBP when bacteria decrease porin production, resulting in a decrease of the drug concentration within the cell.

Metabolic Route: Penicillin is excreted unchanged in the urine.

 ## FDA-APPROVED INDICATIONS

Penicillin G potassium injection is indicated in the treatment of susceptible strains of microorganisms causing **septicemia**, **empyema**, **pneumonia**, **pericarditis**, **endocarditis**, and **meningitis. It is indicated for** pneumococcal infection, fusospiro-chetosis, anthrax, actinomycosis, clostridial infections, erysipelothrix, spirochetal infections, listeriosis, *Pasteurella multocida*, rat-bite fever, syphilis, susceptible gonococcal and meningococcal infection, and prevention of rheumatic fever.

Penicillin V is indicated for **mild-to-moderate** infections due to susceptible organisms, including streptococcal infections (without bacteremia) of the upper respiratory tract, scarlet fever, and mild erysipelas, pneumococcal infections, fusospiroche-tosis, and prevention of rheumatic fever. Severe pneumonia, empyema, bacteremia, pericarditis, meningitis, and arthritis should not be treated with penicillin V during the acute stage.

Penicillin G procaine is indicated in the treatment of **moderately severe** infections susceptible to low serum levels of penicillin G, including upper respiratory tract infections, skin and soft-tissue infections, scarlet fever, erysipelas, fusospi-rochetosis, pneumococcal infection, syphilis, yaws, bejel, pinta, an adjunct to antitoxin for prevention of the carrier stage of diphtheria, anthrax, rat-bite fever, *Erysipelothrix rhusiopathiae*, and subacute bacterial endocarditis due to Group A Streptococci.

Penicillin G benzathine is indicated in the treatment of infections that are susceptible to low and prolonged serum levels: upper respiratory tract streptococcal infection, syphilis, yaws, bejel, pinta, and prevention of rheumatic fever.

 ## SIDE EFFECTS/TOXICITY

A history of allergic reaction to any of the penicillins is a **contraindication**.

Side effects include hypersensitivity, including rashes, ranging from maculopapular eruptions to exfoliative dermatitis, urticaria, serum-sicknesslike reactions, including chills, fever, edema, arthralgia, prostration, anaphylaxis, *Clostridium difficile*-associated diarrhea (CDAD), mucocutaneous candidiasis, nausea, vomiting, diarrhea, black hairy tongue, rise in AST (SGOT) and/or ALT (SGPT), crystalluria, interstitial nephritis, anemia, thrombocytopenia, eosinophilia, leukopenia, hyperac-tivity, and convulsions.

Procaine side effects: Anxiety, confusion, agitation, depression, weakness, seizures, hallucinations, combativeness, and expressed "fear of impending death".

Antibiotics Manual: A Guide to Commonly Used Antimicrobials, Second Edition. David Schlossberg and Rafik Samuel.
© 2017 John Wiley & Sons Ltd. Published 2017 by John Wiley & Sons Ltd.

Procaine and benzathine penicillin injection side effects: Inadvertent intravascular administration has resulted in severe neurovascular damage, transverse myelitis, gangrene, and necrosis. Others include pallor, mottling, or cyanosis of the extremity, severe edema, quadriceps femoris fibrosis, and atrophy.

 DRUG INTERACTIONS/FOOD INTERACTIONS

Penicillin tablets and oral suspensions may be given without regard to meals.

Concurrent use of penicillin and probenecid may result in increased and prolonged blood levels of penicillin.

Chloramphenicol, macrolides, sulfonamides, and tetracyclines may interfere with the bactericidal effects of penicillin.

 DOSING

Penicillin G potassium injection

Clinical indication	Dosage
Septicemia, empyema, pneumonia, pericarditis, endocarditis and meningitis	12 to 24 million units/day in equally divided doses every 4–6 hours
Anthrax	8 million units/day in divided doses every 6 hours
Actinomycosis	
Cervicofacial disease	1 to 6 million units/day
Thoracic and abdominal disease	10 to 20 million units/day
Clostridial infections	20 million units/day
Diphtheria	2 to 3 million units/day in divided doses
Erysipelothrix endocarditis	12 to 20 million units/day
Fusospirochetosis	5 to 10 million units/day
Listeria infections	
Meningitis	15 to 20 million units/day
Endocarditis	15 to 20 million units/day
Pasteurella infections	4 to 6 million units/day
Rat-bite fever	12 to 20 million units/day
Disseminated gonococcal infections	10 million units/day
Syphilis (neurosyphilis)	12 to 24 million units/day, as 2-4 MU every 4 hours
Meningococcal meningitis and/or septicemia	24 million units/day as 2 million units every 2 hours

Penicillin V

Penicillin V potassium is administered as 250 mg (400 000 units) or 500 mg (800 000 units) tablets and an oral solution containing 125 mg (200 000 units) per 5 mL and 250 mg (400 000 units) per 5 mL.

Streptococcal infections: 125 to 250 mg every 6 to 8 hours for 10 days.

Pneumococcal infections, fusospirochetosis or staphylococcal infections: 250 to 500 mg every 6 hours.

For the **prevention** of recurrence following rheumatic fever and/or chorea: 125 to 250 mg twice daily on a continuing basis.

Penicillin G procaine

Should be administered by intramuscular injection in the upper, outer quadrant of the buttock. It is supplied in 600 000 and 1 200 000 unit injections.

Pneumonia, streptococcal, staphylococcal infections, bacterial endocarditis, cutaneous anthrax, fusospirochetosis, erysipeloid, and rat-bite fever: 600 000 to 1 000 000 units daily.

Primary, secondary, and latent syphilis: 600,000 units daily for total of 4 800 000 units.

Late (**tertiary, neurosyphilis**, and **latent syphilis** with positive spinal-fluid examination or no spinal-fluid examination): 600 000 units daily for 10 to 15 days with a total of 6 to 9 million units.

Diphtheria-adjunctive therapy with antitoxin: 300 000 to 600 000 units daily.

Diphtheria carrier state: 300 000 units daily for 10 days.

Anthrax-inhalational (postexposure): 1 200 000 units every 12 hours.

Benzathine penicillin

Should be administered in the upper, outer quadrant of the buttock. It comes in 600 000 units, 1 200 000 units and 2 400 000 units per syringe.

Upper respiratory infections: a single injection of 1 200 000 units.

Primary, secondary, and early latent syphilis: 2 400 000 units for 1 dose.

Late syphilis: 2 400 000 units at 7-day intervals for three doses.

Yaws, bejel, and pinta: 1 200 000 units.

Prophylaxis of rheumatic fever: 1 200 000 units once a month or 600 000 units every 2 weeks.

 SPECIAL POPULATIONS

RENAL IMPAIRMENT:

Penicillin G

Creatinine clearance, mL/min	Dose
10–50	1–2 million units q 4 hours
<10	1 million units q 6 hours
Hemodialysis	2 million units after dialysis
CAPD	1 million units q 6 hours
CRRT	1-2 million units q 4 hours

Penicillin V

Creatinine clearance, mL/min	Dose
10–50	No change
<10	250–500 mg q 8 hours
Hemodialysis	250 mg after dialysis
CAPD	250–500 mg
CRRT	N/A

HEPATIC DYSFUNCTION: No dose adjustment is necessary.

PEDIATRICS

Penicillin G

Clinical indication	Dosage
Serious infections	150 000–300 000 units/kg/day divided every 4–6 hours
Meningitis	250 000 units/kg/day divided in equal doses every 4 hours
Disseminated gonococcal infections	Weight less than 45 kg
Arthritis	100 000 units/kg/day in 4 equally divided doses
Meningitis	250 000 units/kg/day in equal doses every 4 hours
Endocarditis	250 000 units/kg/day in equal doses every 4 hours
Arthritis, meningitis, endocarditis	Weight 45 kg or greater: 10 million units/day in 4 doses
Syphilis (congenital and neurosyphilis) after the newborn period	200 000–300 000 units/kg/day (administered as 50 000 units/kg every 4–6 hours)
Diphtheria	150 000–250 000 units/kg/day in equal doses every 6 hours
Rat-bite fever	150,000–250 000 units/kg/day in equal doses every 4 hours

Penicillin G procaine

In neonates, infants, and small children, the midlateral aspect of the thigh may be preferable. When doses are repeated, vary the injection site.

In pneumonia, streptococcal, and staphylococcal infections in pediatric patients under 60 pounds: 300 000 units daily.

Congenital syphilis under 70 lb body weight: 50 000 units/kg/day for 10 days.

Anthrax-inhalational (postexposure): 25 000 units per kilogram of body weight (maximum 1 200 000 unit) every 12 hours in children.

Benzathine penicillin

Upper respiratory infections in older pediatric patients – a single injection of 900 000 units; infants and pediatric patients under 60 lb – 300 000 to 600 000 units.

Congenital syphilis: under 2 years of age: 50 000 units/kg/body weight; ages 2 to 12 years: adjust dosage based on adult dosage schedule.

 THE ART OF ANTIMICROBIAL THERAPY

Clinical Pearls

1. Penicillin needs to be dose adjusted for renal dysfunction.
2. The Jarisch–Herxheimer reaction can occur following treatment of syphilis as well as other spirochetal infections.
3. Penicillin G potassium, USP (1 million units contains 1.68 meq of potassium ion) may cause serious and even fatal electrolyte disturbances, i.e., hyperkalemia, when given intravenously in large doses, especially in patients with renal failure.
4. Chloramphenicol, macrolides, sulfonamides, and tetracyclines may interfere with the bactericidal effects of penicillins.

BASIC CHARACTERISTICS

Class: Nitroimidazole.

Mechanism of Action: Data incomplete.

Mechanism of resistance: Data incomplete.

Used for: Treatment of *Trypanosoma cruzii*.

 ## SIDE EFFECTS/TOXICITY

Peripheral neuropathy, rash, granulocytopenia.

Increased incidence of malignant tumors in patients given benznidazole after cardiac transplantation.

 ## DRUG INTERACTIONS/FOOD INTERACTIONS

Data incomplete.

 ## DOSING

The treatment dose is 5 mg/kg/day for a total of 60 days. This is the recommended dose and duration for all forms of *Trypanosoma cruzii*.

 ## SPECIAL POPULATIONS

RENAL IMPAIRMENT: Do not administer.

HEPATIC DYSFUNCTION: Do not administer.

PEDIATRICS: Same dose as adults.

 ## THE ART OF ANTIMICROBIAL THERAPY

Clinical Pearls

1. Benznidazole is available from the CDC Drug Service, 404-639-3670; evenings, weekends, and holidays: 770-488-7100; FAX 404-639-3717.
2. Benznidazole is considered the drug of choice for *Trypanosoma cruzii*.
3. Patients with severe cardiac or gastrointestinal Chagas disease should not be treated with benznidazole.

Antibiotics Manual: A Guide to Commonly Used Antimicrobials, Second Edition. David Schlossberg and Rafik Samuel.
© 2017 John Wiley & Sons Ltd. Published 2017 by John Wiley & Sons Ltd.

■ BIAXIN (Clarithromycin)

 BASIC CHARACTERISTICS

Class: Macrolide.

Mechanism of Action: Clarithromycin acts by binding to the 50S ribosomal subunit of susceptible microorganisms and, thus, interfering with microbial protein synthesis.

Mechanisms of Resistance:

1. Decreased permeability.
2. Active efflux.
3. Alteration of the 50S ribosomal unit.
4. Alteration of the 23S subunit of the 50S ribosomal unit.
5. Enzymatic inactivation of the macrolide.

Metabolic Route: About 30 % is excreted in the urine with the remainder excreted in the bile.

 FDA-APPROVED INDICATIONS

I. **Biaxin (tablets and oral suspension):** susceptible organisms causing

Pharyngitis/tonsillitis (adults and children)

Acute maxillary sinusitis (adults and children)

Acute bacterial exacerbation of chronic bronchitis (adults)

Community-acquired pneumonia (adults and children)

Uncomplicated skin and skin structure infections (adults and children)

Acute otitis media (children)

Disseminated infection due to *Mycobacterium avium* or *Mycobacterium intracellulare* (adults and children)

In combination with amoxicillin and lansoprazole or omeprazole delayed-release capsules, as triple therapy, are indicated for the treatment of patients with *H. pylori* infection and duodenal ulcer disease

In combination with omeprazole or ranitidine bismuth citrate tablets for the treatment of patients with an active duodenal ulcer associated with *H. pylori* infection.

Prevention of disseminated *Mycobacterium avium* complex (MAC) disease in patients with advanced HIV infection.

II. **Biaxin XL**

Acute maxillary sinusitis (adults)

Acute bacterial exacerbation of chronic bronchitis (adults)

Community-acquired pneumonia (adults)

 SIDE EFFECTS/TOXICITY

Contraindicated in patients with known hypersensitivity to clarithromycin, erythromycin, any macrolide or ketolide antibiotic.

Side effects include serious allergic reactions, including rash, photosensitivity, anaphylaxis, angioedema, Stevens–Johnson syndrome and toxic epidermal necrolysis, *Clostridium difficile*-associated diarrhea, tooth discoloration, nausea, vomiting,

Antibiotics Manual: A Guide to Commonly Used Antimicrobials, Second Edition. David Schlossberg and Rafik Samuel.
© 2017 John Wiley & Sons Ltd. Published 2017 by John Wiley & Sons Ltd.

diarrhea, abdominal pain, pancreatitis, hepatitis, cholestatic jaundice, dyspepsia, flatulence, melena, prolonged cardiac repolarization and QT interval, palpitations, chest pain, exacerbation of symptoms of myasthenia gravis and new onset of myasthenic syndrome, monilia, vaginitis, nephritis, dizziness, headache, vertigo, somnolence, fatigue, seizure, deafness, thrombocytopenia, and leucopenia.

 DRUG INTERACTIONS/FOOD INTERACTIONS

Clarithromycin can be administered with or without food.

Clarithromycin extended release tablets should be taken with food.

Clarithromycin and other macrolides are known to inhibit enzymes, particularly CYP3A; therefore, coadministration of clarithromycin and a drug primarily metabolized by CYP3A may be associated with elevations in concentrations of the latter. As a result:

1. It is **contraindicated** to use clarithromycin with terfenadine, oral midazolam, triazolam, alprazolam, ergotamine, dihydroergotamine, cisapride, pimozide, or astemizole.

2. Clarithromycin should be **used with caution** with theophylline, oral anticoagulants, digoxin, verapamil, zidovudine, colchicine, sildenafil, tadalafil and vardenafil, tolterodine, intravenous midazolam, itraconazole, HMG-CoA reductase inhibitors (e.g., lovastatin and simvastatin), cyclosporine, carbamazepine, tacrolimus, alfentanil, disopyramide, rifabutin, quinidine, methylprednisolone, cilostazol, bromocriptine, vinblastine, hexobarbital, phenytoin, and valproate.

3. If giving clarithromycin with **ritonavir** for patients with renal impairment, the following dosage adjustments should be considered. For patients with CLCR 30 to 60 mL/min, the dose of clarithromycin should be reduced by 50 %. For patients with CLCR < 30 mL/min, the dose of clarithromycin should be decreased by 75 %.

4. When using **atazanavir** in patients with moderate renal function (creatinine clearance 30 to 60 mL/min), the dose of clarithromycin should be decreased by 50 %. For patients with creatinine clearance <30 mL/min, the dose of clarithromycin should be decreased by 75 % using an appropriate clarithromycin formulation.

5. Doses of clarithromycin greater than 1000 mg per day should not be coadministered with protease inhibitors.

6. There have been reports of torsades de pointes occurring with concurrent use of clarithromycin and **quinidine or disopyramide**; if given, ECG and serum levels of these drugs should be monitored.

7. Clarithromycin in combination with **ranitidine bismuth citrate** therapy is not recommended in patients with creatinine clearance less than 25 mL/min. Clarithromycin in combination with ranitidine bismuth citrate should not be used in patients with a history of acute porphyria.

 DOSING

Biaxin is administered in 250 mg and 500 mg tablets; and as granules in 2 concentrations: 125 mg/5 mL and 250 mg/5 mL.

Biaxin XL is administered in 500 mg tablets.

Infection	Tablets		Extended-release	
	dosage (q 12 h)	Duration (days)	dosage (q 24 h)	Duration (days)
Pharyngitis/tonsillitis	250 mg	10	–	–
Acute maxillary sinusitis	500 mg	14	2 × 500 mg	14
Acute exacerbation of chronic bronchitis	500 mg	7–14	2 × 500 mg	7
Community-acquired pneumonia	250 mg	7	2 × 500 mg	7
Uncomplicated skin and skin structure	250 mg	7–14	–	–

For *H. pylori* eradication to reduce the risk of duodenal ulcer recurrence

I.   Triple therapy: clarithromycin/lansoprazole/amoxicillin: The recommended adult dose is 500 mg clarithromycin, 30 mg lansoprazole, and 1 gram amoxicillin, all given twice daily (q 12 h) for 10 or 14 days.

II. Triple therapy: clarithromycin/omeprazole/amoxicillin: The recommended adult dose is 500 mg clarithromycin, 20 mg omeprazole, and 1 gram amoxicillin, all given twice daily (q 12 h) for 10 days. In patients with an ulcer present at the time of initiation of therapy, an additional 18 days of omeprazole 20 mg once daily is recommended for ulcer healing and symptom relief.

III. Dual therapy: clarithromycin/omeprazole: The recommended adult dose is 500 mg clarithromycin given three times daily (q 8 h) and 40 mg omeprazole given once daily (q am) for 14 days. An additional 14 days of omeprazole 20 mg once daily is recommended for ulcer healing and symptom relief.

IV. Dual therapy: clarithromycin/ranitidine bismuth citrate: The recommended adult dose is 500 mg clarithromycin given twice daily (q 12 h) or three times daily (q 8 h) and 400 mg ranitidine bismuth citrate given twice daily (q 12 h) for 14 days. An additional 14 days of 400 mg twice daily is recommended for ulcer healing and symptom relief.

The recommended dose of clarithromycin for the prevention of disseminated *Mycobacterium avium* disease is 500 mg bid.

The recommended dose of clarithromycin for the treatment of disseminated *Mycobacterium avium* disease is 500 mg bid in combination with other medications.

 ## SPECIAL POPULATIONS

RENAL IMPAIRMENT:

Creatinine clearance, mL/min	Dose
<30	500 mg once daily
Hemodialysis	Give dose after dialysis
CAPD and CRRT	N/A

HEPATIC DYSFUNCTION: No adjustment is necessary.

PEDIATRICS: Safety and effectiveness of clarithromycin in pediatric patients under 6 months of age have not been established.

The usual recommended daily dosage is 15 mg/kg/day divided q 12 h for 10 days.

The recommended dose of clarithromycin for the prevention of disseminated *Mycobacterium avium* disease is 7.5 mg/kg bid up to 500 mg bid.

For treatment of MAC, the recommended dose is 7.5 mg/kg bid up to 500 mg bid. The safety of clarithromycin has not been studied in MAC patients under the age of 20 months.

 ## THE ART OF ANTIMICROBIAL THERAPY

Clinical Pearls

1. When treating MAC, clarithromycin must be combined with other agents to minimize resistance.

2. Macrolides prolong QT intervals and must be used with caution.

3. Clarithromycin should not be used in pregnant women unless there is no alternative.

BASIC CHARACTERISTICS

Class: Heterocyclic prazino-isoquinoline derivative.

Mechanism of Action: Praziquantel induces a rapid contraction of schistosomes and causes vacuolization and disintegration of the schistosome tegument.

Metabolic Route: Metabolized by the liver and excreted in the urine.

 ## FDA-APPROVED INDICATIONS

Indicated for the treatment of **Schistosoma** (e.g. *Schistosoma mekongi*, *Schistosoma japonicum*, *Schistosoma mansoni*, and *Schistosoma hematobium*), and infections due to the **liver flukes**, *Clonorchis sinensis* and *Opisthorchis viverrini*.

Also Used for: **Intestinal flukes**: *Fasciolopsis buski*, *Heterophyes heterophyes*, *Metagonimus yokogawai*.

Intestinal tapeworms, *Taenia saginata*, *Taenia solium*, *Diphyllobothrium latum*, *Dipylidium caninum*, *hymenolepsis nana*, *Cysticercus cellulosae*, and for hydatid cyst disease preoperatively or in case of spillage of cyst contents during surgery.

Lung flukes: Paragonimus.

 ## SIDE EFFECTS/TOXICITY

Praziquantel must not be given to patients who previously have shown hypersensitivity to the drug. Since parasite destruction within the eye may cause irreparable lesions, ocular cysticercosis should not be treated with this compound.

Common side effects include abdominal pain, nausea, diarrhea, malaise, headache and dizziness; also reported are hypersensitivity, polyserositis, arrhythmia (including bradycardia, ectopic rhythms, ventricular fibrillation, AV blocks), seizures, myalgia, somnolence, and vertigo.

 ## DRUG INTERACTIONS/FOOD INTERACTIONS

Praziquantel should be taken with food.

Since praziquantel is metabolized by the liver cytochrome P450 system, concomitant administration of drugs that increase the activity of these enzymes may reduce plasma levels of praziquantel, such as antiepileptic drugs (e.g., phenytoin, phenobarbital and carbamazepine), dexamethasone and rifampin. In addition, chloroquine may lower concentrations of praziquantel in blood (mechanism is unclear).

Concomitant administration of drugs that decrease the activity of drug metabolizing liver enzymes (cytochrome P 450), may increase plasma levels of praziquantel, e.g., cimetidine, ketoconazole, itraconazole, erythromycin; grapefruit juice may also increase plasma levels of praziquantel.

 ## DOSING

Praziquantel is supplied as 600 mg tablets. The tablets should be washed down unchewed with water during meals.

Antibiotics Manual: A Guide to Commonly Used Antimicrobials, Second Edition. David Schlossberg and Rafik Samuel.
© 2017 John Wiley & Sons Ltd. Published 2017 by John Wiley & Sons Ltd.

Treatment of schistosomiasis:

S. haematobium	40 mg/kg/d PO in 1 or 2 doses × 1 d
S. intercalatum	40 mg/kg/d PO in 1 or 2 doses × 1 d
S. japonicum	60 mg/kg/d PO in 2 or 3 doses × 1 d
S. mansoni	40 mg/kg/d PO in 1 or 2 doses × 1 d
S. mekongi	60 mg/kg/d PO in 2 or 3 doses × 1 d

Treatment of clonorchiasis and opisthorchiasis and intestinal flukes: 25 mg/kg bodyweight three times a day as a one day treatment, at intervals of not less than 4 hours and not more than 6 hours.

Other disease states:

Disease	Dose and duration
Intestinal tapeworms	5–10 mg/kg once (for *Hymenolepis nana*: 25 mg/kg once)
Cysticercus cellulosae	50 mg/kg/d PO × 15 d
Paragonimus westermani	75 mg/kg/day in 3 doses for 2 days

 SPECIAL POPULATIONS

RENAL IMPAIRMENT: There is no dose adjustment for renal insufficiency.

HEPATIC DYSFUNCTION: Caution should be exercised in the administration of patients with moderate to severe liver impairment (Child Pugh class B and C).

PEDIATRICS

S. haematobium	40 mg/kg/d PO in 2 doses × 1 d
S. intercalatum	40 mg/kg/d PO in 2 doses × 1 d
S. japonicum	60 mg/kg/d PO in 3 doses × 1 d
S. mansoni	40 mg/kg/d PO in 2 doses × 1 d
S. mekongi	60 mg/kg/d PO in 3 doses × 1 d

For other indications: same as adult dose.

 THE ART OF ANTIMICROBIAL THERAPY

Clinical Pearls

1. Although praziquantel is indicated only for the treatment of schistosomiasis and liver flukes, it is the treatment of choice for intestinal tapeworms and lung flukes.
2. Unlike the situation with other liver flukes, praziquantel is **not recommended** for the treatment of *Fasciola hepatica*.
3. Praziquantel tablets should be washed down unchewed with water during meals to avoid choking.
4. Strong inducers of cytochrome P450 enzymes, such as rifampin, may result in subtherapeutic levels of praziquantel and should be avoided if possible.

BASIC CHARACTERISTICS

Class: Chlorinated bis-phenol.

Mechanism of Action: Unclear; possibly an uncoupler of oxidative phosphorylation.

Metabolic Route: Excreted in the urine.

Used for: The treatment of acute and chronic *Fasciola hepatica* and *Paragonimus westermani*.

SIDE EFFECTS/TOXICITY

Nausea, diarrhea, abdominal pain, anorexia, and urticaria.

DRUG INTERACTIONS/FOOD INTERACTIONS

Unknown.

DOSING

30 to 50 mg/kg of body weight on alternate days for 10–15 doses for the treatment of fascioliasis and paragonimiasis.

SPECIAL POPULATIONS

RENAL IMPAIRMENT: Data incomplete.

HEPATIC DYSFUNCTION: Data incomplete.

PEDIATRICS: 30–50 mg/kg on alternate days for 10–15 doses.

THE ART OF ANTIMICROBIAL THERAPY

Clinical Pearls

1. Bithionol is not available in the US. It may be available through a compounding pharmacy: call the National Association of Compounding Pharmacies (800-687-7850) or Professional Compounding Centers of America (800-331-2498, www.pccarx.com).
2. Treatment with antispasmodics and antihistamines helps reduce side effects.
3. Giving bithionol in 2–3 divided doses and after meals decreases the incidence of toxicity.

Antibiotics Manual: A Guide to Commonly Used Antimicrobials, Second Edition. David Schlossberg and Rafik Samuel.
© 2017 John Wiley & Sons Ltd. Published 2017 by John Wiley & Sons Ltd.

BROACT, CEFROM KEITEN, CEFIR (Cefpirome)

 ## BASIC CHARACTERISTICS

Class: Fourth generation cephalosporin.

Mechanism of Action: Binds penicillin binding protein, disrupting cell wall synthesis.

Mechanisms of Resistance:

1. The PBP can be altered, with reduced affinity.

2. Production of a beta-lactamase, resulting in hydrolysis of the beta-lactam ring.

3. Decreased ability of the antibiotic to reach the PBP when bacteria decrease porin production, resulting in a decrease of the drug concentration within the cell.

Metabolic Route: Excreted unchanged in the urine.

Indications (not available in the US):

Lower respiratory tract infections

Complicated upper (pyelonephritis) and lower urinary tract infections

Skin and soft tissue infections

Bacteremia/septicemia

Infections in neutropenic and immunocompromised patients

 ## SIDE EFFECTS/TOXICITY

Cefpirome is **contraindicated** in patients who have shown immediate hypersensitivity reactions to cefpirome or cephalosporins, and in patients with porphyria. Caution in patients with penicillin allergy.

Toxicity includes fever, anaphylaxis, rash including Stevens–Johnson syndrome, erythema multiforme and toxic epidermal necrolysis, angioedema, flushing, serum-sickness-like reactions, encephalopathy, seizures, myoclonus, diarrhea, *Clostridium difficile*-associated diarrhea and pseudomembranous colitis, oral candidiasis, anorexia, nausea, vomiting, stomach cramps, flatulence, hepatitis, renal impairment, genital moniliasis, vaginitis, hemorrhage, prolonged prothrombin time, hypercalcemia, hypocalcemia, pancytopenia, hemolytic anemia, positive Coombs test.

 ## DRUG INTERACTIONS/FOOD INTERACTIONS

Renal function should be monitored carefully if high doses of aminoglycosides or diuretics are to be administered with cefpirome because of the increased potential of nephrotoxicity and ototoxicity of aminoglycoside antibiotics. Cephalosporins may cause false-positive urine glucose determinations when using cupric sulfate solution (Benedict's solution, *Clinitest*®). Tests utilizing glucose oxidase (*Tes-Tape*®, *Clinistix*®) are not affected by cephalosporins.

DOSING

Usual adult dose: 1–2 gm IV q 12 hours.

Antibiotics Manual: A Guide to Commonly Used Antimicrobials, Second Edition. David Schlossberg and Rafik Samuel.
© 2017 John Wiley & Sons Ltd. Published 2017 by John Wiley & Sons Ltd.

SPECIAL POPULATIONS

RENAL IMPAIRMENT:

Creatinine clearance, mL/min	Dose
<50	1–2 gram loading dose
Then	
20–50	500 mg–1 gram q 12 hours
5–20	500 mg–1 gram q 24 hours
<5, hemodialysis	500 mg–1 gram q 24 hours then half-dose postdialysis

HEPATIC DYSFUNCTION: No dose adjustment is necessary.

PEDIATRICS: Should not be used in children.

 THE ART OF ANTIMICROBIAL THERAPY

Clinical Pearls

1. Cefpirome is dose adjusted for renal dysfunction.

2. Cross allergy with penicillins is <10%.

3. Patients with creatinine clearance less than or equal to 50 mL/min must have dosage adjustment to avoid adverse reactions such as encephalopathy, myoclonus, and seizures.

4. Concomitant aminoglycosides increase the potential of nephrotoxicity and ototoxicity.

5. Nephrotoxicity has been reported with concomitant administration of other cephalosporins with potent diuretics such as furosemide.

■ CANCIDAS (Caspofungin)

 BASIC CHARACTERISTICS

Class: Echinocandin.

Mechanism of Action: Inhibition of synthesis of 1,3-beta-D-glucan, an essential component of fungal cell walls.

Mechanism of Resistance: Data incomplete.

Metabolic Route: Caspofungin is slowly metabolized by hydrolysis and *N*-acetylation and is eliminated in the feces and urine. It is not metabolized by the cytochrome P450 enzymes.

 FDA-APPROVED INDICATIONS

Empirical therapy for presumed fungal infections in febrile, neutropenic patients.

Treatment of candidemia and the following *Candida* infections: intra-abdominal abscesses, peritonitis, and pleural space infections.

Treatment of esophageal candidiasis.

Treatment of invasive aspergillosis in patients who are refractory to or intolerant of other therapies.

 SIDE EFFECTS/TOXICITY

Fever, chills, anaphylaxis, possible histamine-mediated symptoms, rash, facial swelling, pruritus, sensation of warmth, bronchospasm, pancreatitis, hepatic necrosis, diarrhea, renal failure, seizures, swelling and peripheral edema, hypotension, arrhythmias, thrombocytopenia, hypomagnesemia, hypercalcemia, hyperglycemia, and hypokalemia.

 DRUG INTERACTIONS

Tacrolimus: Standard monitoring of tacrolimus blood concentrations and appropriate tacrolimus dosage adjustments are recommended.

Cyclosporine: Transient increases in liver ALT and AST were noted when caspofungin and cyclosporine were coadministered. Monitoring of LFTs are recommended.

Rifampin: Adult patients on rifampin should receive 70 mg of caspofungin daily.

Nevirapine, efavirenz, carbamazepine, dexamethasone, or phenytoin: increase caspofungin dose to 70 mg daily.

 DOSING

Empiric therapy, *Candida* infections or *Aspergillus* infections: 70 mg IV loading dose and then 50 mg IV daily.

Esophageal candidiasis: 50 mg IV daily.

 SPECIAL POPULATIONS

RENAL IMPAIRMENT: No dose adjustment is necessary.

HEPATIC DYSFUNCTION: Adult patients with mild hepatic insufficiency (Child Pugh* score 5 to 6) do not need a dosage adjustment.

Antibiotics Manual: A Guide to Commonly Used Antimicrobials, Second Edition. David Schlossberg and Rafik Samuel.
© 2017 John Wiley & Sons Ltd. Published 2017 by John Wiley & Sons Ltd.

Adult patients with moderate hepatic insufficiency (Child Pugh* score 7 to 9), caspofungin 35 mg daily is recommended. However, a 70-mg loading dose should still be administered on day 1.

There is no clinical experience in adult patients with severe hepatic insufficiency (Child Pugh* score >9) and in pediatric patients with any degree of hepatic insufficiency.

*Child Pugh determination: see chapter on Helpful Formulas, Equations, and Definitions.

PEDIATRICS: Indicated for children over 3 months of age.

For all indications, a single 70-mg/m²** loading dose should be administered on day 1, followed by 50 mg/m² daily thereafter. The maximum loading dose and the daily maintenance dose should not exceed 70 mg, regardless of the patient's calculated dose.

When caspofungin is coadministered to pediatric patients with inducers of drug clearance, such as rifampin, efavirenz, nevirapine, phenytoin, dexamethasone, or carbamazepine, a caspofungin dose of 70 mg/m² daily (not to exceed 70 mg) should be considered.

**Mosteller formula for computing body surface area: see Helpful Formulas, Equations, and Definitions.

 THE ART OF ANTIMICROBIAL THERAPY

Clinical Pearls

1. Echinocandins have activity only against *Candida* species, *Pneumocystis jirovecii*, and *Aspergillus* species. They should not be used for any other fungal infections.

2. Caspofungin is active against all pathogenic *Candida* species, including those resistant to fluconazole.

3. Increasing resistance to echinocandins has been noted in *Candida glabrata* and *Candida parapsilosis*.

■ CAPASTAT (Capreomycin)

 BASIC CHARACTERISTICS

Class: Cyclic polypeptide.

Mechanisms of Action: Inhibits protein synthesis by binding to the 70S ribosomal unit.

Mechanisms of Resistance: Incompletely understood.

Metabolic Route: Excreted unchanged in the urine.

 FDA-APPROVED INDICATIONS

Treatment of pulmonary *M. tuberculosis* when the primary agents (isoniazid, rifampin, ethambutol, aminosalicylic acid, and streptomycin) have been ineffective or cannot be used because of toxicity or the presence of resistant tubercle bacilli

 SIDE EFFECTS/TOXICITY

> **WARNING:** Use in patients with renal insufficiency or preexisting auditory impairment must be undertaken with great caution, and the risk of additional cranial nerve VIII impairment or renal injury should be weighed against the benefits to be derived from therapy.
>
> Since other parenteral antituberculosis agents (e.g., streptomycin) also have similar and sometimes irreversible toxic effects, particularly on cranial nerve VIII and renal function, simultaneous administration of these agents with capreomycin is not recommended. Use with nonantituberculosis drugs (polymyxin A sulfate, colistin sulfate, amikacin, gentamicin, tobramycin, vancomycin, kanamycin, and neomycin) having ototoxic or nephrotoxic potential should be undertaken only with great caution.

Contraindicated in patients who are hypersensitive to capreomycin.

Nephrotoxicity and ototoxicity similar to aminoglycosides.

Hypokalemia, hypomagnesemia, hypocalcemia

 DRUG INTERACTIONS/FOOD INTERACTIONS

Use with caution when administering neuromuscular blocking agents, other nephrotoxic agents or ototoxic agents (polymyxin A sulfate, colistin sulfate, amikacin, gentamicin, tobramycin, vancomycin, kanamycin, and neomycin) because of possible additive effects. Use with great caution in patients with preexisting renal disease or auditory impairment.

 DOSING

15 m/kg/day (maximum 1 gm) IV or IM.

Over age 59: 10 mg/kg/day (maximum 750 mg).

After a period of daily administration, can be given 2–3 times/week.

Antibiotics Manual: A Guide to Commonly Used Antimicrobials, Second Edition. David Schlossberg and Rafik Samuel.
© 2017 John Wiley & Sons Ltd. Published 2017 by John Wiley & Sons Ltd.

SPECIAL POPULATIONS

RENAL IMPAIRMENT: Creatinine clearance <30 mL/min or in dialysis patients: 12–15 mg/kg/2–3 times weekly.

HEPATIC DYSFUNCTION: No adjustment necessary.

PEDIATRICS: 15–30 mg/kg/day with a maximum of 1 gram daily.

 THE ART OF ANTIMICROBIAL THERAPY

Clinical Pearls

1. Capreomycin should never be used alone in the treatment of active tuberculosis.
2. Capreomycin should only be used if resistance to first line antimycobacterial agents is noted.
3. Serum levels of capreomycin should be monitored, with a goal of peak levels (2 hours after a 15 mg/kg dose) of 35–45 mcg/mL. Trough concentrations should be <5 mcg/mL in patients with normal renal function.
4. Dose should be based on ideal body weight.
5. May demonstrate cross-resistance with amikacin and kanamycin.
6. Treatment of TB with capreomycin plus kanamycin or amikacin (double injectable therapy) is not recommended unless the situation is dire and there are no reasonable alternatives.

■ CEDAX (Ceftibuten)

 BASIC CHARACTERISTICS

Class: Third generation cephalosporin.

Mechanism of Action: Binds penicillin-binding protein, disrupting cell wall synthesis.

Mechanisms of Resistance:

1. The PBP can be altered, with reduced affinity.

2. Production of a beta-lactamase, resulting in hydrolysis of the beta-lactam ring.

3. Decreased ability of the antibiotic to reach the PBP when bacteria decrease porin production, resulting in a decrease of the drug concentration within the cell.

Metabolic Route: Ceftibuten is excreted predominantly in the urine, with a small amount in the feces.

 FDA-APPROVED INDICATIONS

Treatment of the following mild-to-moderate infections when caused by susceptible organisms:

Acute bacterial exacerbations of chronic bronchitis

Acute bacterial otitis media

Pharyngitis and tonsillitis

 SIDE EFFECTS/TOXICITY

Ceftibuten is **contraindicated** in patients with allergy to cephalosporins. Ceftibuten should be used with caution if hypersensitivity exists to penicillins.

Toxicity includes fever, anaphylaxis, rash including Stevens–Johnson syndrome, erythema multiforme and toxic epidermal necrolysis, angioedema, flushing, serum-sickness-like reactions, encephalopathy, seizures, aphasia, psychosis, stridor, diarrhea, *Clostridium difficile*-associated diarrhea and pseudomembranous colitis, oral candidiasis, anorexia, nausea, vomiting, stomach cramps, flatulence, hepatitis, renal impairment, genital moniliasis, vaginitis, hemorrhage, prolonged prothrombin time, pancytopenia, hemolytic anemia, and positive Coombs' test.

 DRUG INTERACTIONS/FOOD INTERACTIONS

Ceftibuten oral suspension must be administered at least 2 hours before or 1 hour after a meal. Probenecid inhibits the renal excretion of ceftibuten. Cephalosporins may cause false-positive urine glucose determinations when using cupric sulfate solution (Benedict's solution, *Clinitest®*). Tests utilizing glucose oxidase (*Tes-Tape®*, *Clinistix®*) are not affected by cephalosporins.

 DOSING

Ceftibuten is supplied as a 400 mg capsule and an off-white colored powder that, when reconstituted, contains 90 mg/5 mL of ceftibuten.

The usual adult dose of ceftibuten is 400 mg daily for 10 days.

Antibiotics Manual: A Guide to Commonly Used Antimicrobials, Second Edition. David Schlossberg and Rafik Samuel.
© 2017 John Wiley & Sons Ltd. Published 2017 by John Wiley & Sons Ltd.

SPECIAL POPULATIONS

RENAL IMPAIRMENT:

Creatinine clearance	Dose
30–49 mL/min	4.5 mg/kg or 200 mg daily
5–29 mL/min	2.25 mg/kg or 100 mg daily
Hemodialysis	9 mg/kg or 400 mg after HD
CAPD	N/A
CRRT	N/A

HEPATIC DYSFUNCTION: No dose adjustment is necessary.

PEDIATRICS: 9 mg/kg daily up to 400 mg a day. Safety and efficacy not established in infants less than 6 months of age.

 ## THE ART OF ANTIMICROBIAL THERAPY

Clinical Pearls

1. Ceftibuten must be adjusted for renal insufficiency.
2. Cross allergy with penicillins is <10%.
3. Diabetic patients should be informed that ceftibutin oral suspension contains 1 gram sucrose per teaspoon of suspension.

BASIC CHARACTERISTICS

Class: Second generation cephalosporin.

Mechanism of Action: Binds penicillin-binding protein, disrupting cell wall synthesis.

Mechanisms of Resistance:

1. The PBP can be altered, with reduced affinity.

2. Production of a beta-lactamase, resulting in hydrolysis of the beta-lactam ring.

3. Decreased ability of the antibiotic to reach the PBP when bacteria decrease porin production, resulting in a decrease of the drug concentration within the cell.

Metabolic Route: the majority of cefaclor is excreted unchanged in the urine.

 FDA-APPROVED INDICATIONS

Cefaclor is indicated in the treatment of the following infections when caused by susceptible organisms:

Otitis media

Lower respiratory tract infections

Pharyngitis and tonsillitis

Urinary tract infections

Skin and skin structure infections

 SIDE EFFECTS/TOXICITY

Cefaclor is **contraindicated** in patients with known allergy to cephalosporins and should be used with caution if hypersensitivity exists to penicillin.

Toxicity includes fever, anaphylaxis, rash including Stevens–Johnson syndrome, erythema multiforme and toxic epidermal necrolysis, angioedema, flushing, serum-sickness-like reactions, encephalopathy, seizures, diarrhea, *Clostridium difficile*-associated diarrhea and pseudomembranous colitis, oral candidiasis, anorexia, nausea, vomiting, stomach cramps, flatulence, hepatitis, renal impairment, genital moniliasis, vaginitis, hemorrhage, prolonged prothrombin time, pancytopenia, hemolytic anemia, positive Coombs' test; cephalosporins may cause false-positive urine glucose determinations when using cupric sulfate solution (Benedict's solution, *Clinitest®*). Tests utilizing glucose oxidase (*Tes-Tape®*, *Clinistix®*) are not affected by cephalosporins.

 DRUG INTERACTIONS/FOOD INTERACTIONS

Cefaclor can be taken with or without food.

Probenecid may decrease renal tubular secretion of cephalosporins when used concurrently, resulting in increased and more prolonged cephalosporin blood levels.

Antibiotics Manual: A Guide to Commonly Used Antimicrobials, Second Edition. David Schlossberg and Rafik Samuel.
© 2017 John Wiley & Sons Ltd. Published 2017 by John Wiley & Sons Ltd.

DOSING

Cefaclor is administered as 250 mg and 500 mg capsules. It can be administered as an oral suspension in the following concentrations: 125 mg/5 mL, 187 mg/5 mL, 250 mg/5 mL, and 375 mg/5 mL.

The usual adult dosage is 250 mg every 8 hours.

For more severe infections (such as pneumonia) or those caused by less susceptible organisms, doses may be doubled.

 SPECIAL POPULATIONS

RENAL IMPAIRMENT: Use with caution, but no dose adjustment is necessary.

HEPATIC DYSFUNCTION: No dose adjustment is necessary.

PEDIATRICS: Safety and effectiveness of this product for use in pediatric patients less than 1 month of age have not been established.

The usual recommended daily dosage for children is 20 mg/kg/day in divided doses every 8 hours.

In more serious infections, otitis media, and infections caused by less susceptible organisms, 40 mg/kg/day are recommended, with a maximum dosage of 1 g/day.

 THE ART OF ANTIMICROBIAL THERAPY

Clinical Pearls

1. Cefaclor is not dose adjusted for renal dysfunction.
2. Cross-hypersensitivity among β-lactam antibiotics may occur in up to 10 % of patients with a history of penicillin allergy
3. β-Lactamase-negative, ampicillin-resistant (BLNAR) strains of *Haemophilus influenzae* should be considered resistant to cefaclor despite apparent *in vitro* susceptibility of some BLNAR strains.

■ CEFIZOX (Ceftizoxime)

 BASIC CHARACTERISTICS

Class: Third generation cephalosporin.

Mechanism of Action: Binds penicillin-binding protein, disrupting cell wall synthesis.

Mechanisms of Resistance:

1. The PBP can be altered, with reduced affinity.
2. Production of a beta-lactamase, resulting in hydrolysis of the beta-lactam ring.
3. Decreased ability of the antibiotic to reach the PBP when bacteria decrease porin production, resulting in a decrease of the drug concentration within the cell.

Metabolic Route: Excreted unchanged in the urine.

 FDA-APPROVED INDICATIONS

Treatment of patients with infections caused by susceptible strains of organisms in the following diseases:

Lower respiratory tract infections

Urinary tract infections

Gonorrhea including uncomplicated cervical and urethral gonorrhea

Pelvic inflammatory disease

Intra-abdominal infections

Septicemia

Skin and skin structure infections

Bone and joint infections

Meningitis

 SIDE EFFECTS/TOXICITY

Ceftizoxime is **contraindicated** in patients who have shown hypersensitivity to ceftizoxime.

Ceftizoxime should be used with caution if hypersensitivity exists to other cephalosporins or penicillin.

Toxicity includes inflammation at the site of injection, fever, anaphylaxis, rash including Stevens–Johnson syndrome, erythema multiforme and toxic epidermal necrolysis, angioedema, flushing, serum-sickness-like reactions, encephalopathy, seizures, diarrhea, *Clostridium difficile*-associated diarrhea and pseudomembranous colitis, oral candidiasis, anorexia, nausea, vomiting, stomach cramps, flatulence, hepatitis, renal impairment, genital moniliasis, vaginitis, hemorrhage, prolonged prothrombin time, pancytopenia, hemolytic anemia, positive Coombs' test.

 DRUG INTERACTIONS/FOOD INTERACTIONS

Nephrotoxicity has been reported following concomitant administration of cephalosporins with aminoglycoside antibiotics or potent diuretics such as furosemide. Cephalosporins may cause false-positive urine glucose determinations when using cupric sulfate solution (Benedict's solution, *Clinitest®*). Tests utilizing glucose oxidase (*Tes-Tape®*, *Clinistix®*) are not affected by cephalosporins.

Antibiotics Manual: A Guide to Commonly Used Antimicrobials, Second Edition. David Schlossberg and Rafik Samuel.
© 2017 John Wiley & Sons Ltd. Published 2017 by John Wiley & Sons Ltd.

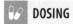 **DOSING**

Infection	Dose
Uncomplicated urinary tract	500 mg IM or IV q 12 hours
Other infections	1 gram IM or IV q 8–12 hours
Severe infections	1–2 grams IM or IV q 8–12 hours
PID	2 grams IV q 8 hours
Life-threatening infections	3–4 grams IV q 8 hours
Uncomplicated gonorrhea	1 gram IM as one dose

 SPECIAL POPULATIONS

RENAL IMPAIRMENT:

Creatinine clearance	Dose (less severe infections)	Severe infections
50–79 mL/min	500 mg q 8 hours	750–1500 mg q 8 hours
5–49 mL/min	250–500 mg q 12 hours	500–1000 mg q 12 hours
<5 mL/min	500 mg q 48 hours or 250 mg q 24 hours	500 mg q 24–48 hours or 1 g q 48 hours
Hemodialysis	Same as <5 mL/min, but after dialysis on dialysis days	
CAPD	0.5–1 gram very 24 hours	
CRRT	250–500 mg q 12 hours	500–1000 mg q 12 hours

HEPATIC DYSFUNCTION: No dose adjustment is necessary.

PEDIATRICS: 6 months and older: 50 mg/kg q 8 hours.
Dosage may be increased to a total daily dose of 200 mg/kg (not to exceed the maximum adult dose for serious infection).

 THE ART OF ANTIMICROBIAL THERAPY

Clinical Pearls

1. Ceftizoxime is dose adjusted for renal dysfunction.
2. Cross allergy with penicillins is <10 % and can be used in life-threatening infections with caution if the allergy is not severe.
3. Because of the serious nature of some urinary tract infections due to *P. aeruginosa* and because many strains of *Pseudomonas* species are only moderately susceptible to ceftizoxime, a higher dosage is recommended. Other therapy should be instituted if the response is not prompt.

BASIC CHARACTERISTICS

Class: Second generation cephalosporin.

Mechanism of Action: Binds penicillin-binding protein, disrupting cell wall synthesis.

Mechanisms of Resistance:

1. The PBP can be altered, with reduced affinity.

2. Production of a beta-lactamase, resulting in hydrolysis of the beta-lactam ring.

3. Decreased ability of the antibiotic to reach the PBP when bacteria decrease porin production, resulting in a decrease of the drug concentration within the cell.

Metabolic Route: Cefotetan is predominantly excreted unchanged in the urine.

 FDA-APPROVED INDICATIONS

Treatment of the following infections when caused by susceptible organisms:

Urinary tract infections

Lower respiratory tract infections

Skin and skin structure infections

Gynecologic infections

Intra-abdominal infections

Bone and joint infections

Prophylaxis of surgical procedures that are classified as clean contaminated or potentially contaminated.

 SIDE EFFECTS/TOXICITY

Cefotetan is **contraindicated** in patients with a known allergy to the cephalosporin group of antibiotics and in those individuals who have experienced a cephalosporin-associated hemolytic anemia. Cefotetan should be used with caution if hypersensitivity exists to penicillin.

Toxicity includes fever, anaphylaxis, rash including Stevens–Johnson syndrome, erythema multiforme and toxic epidermal necrolysis, angioedema, flushing, serum-sickness-like reactions, encephalopathy, seizures, diarrhea, *Clostridium difficile*-associated diarrhea and pseudomembranous colitis, oral candidiasis, anorexia, nausea, vomiting, stomach cramps, flatulence, hepatitis, renal impairment, genital moniliasis, vaginitis, hemorrhage, prolonged prothrombin time, pancytopenia, positive Coombs' test.

There appears to be an increased risk of developing hemolytic anemia on cefotetan relative to other cephalosporins.

 DRUG INTERACTIONS/FOOD INTERACTIONS

If cefotetan and an aminoglycoside are used concomitantly, renal function should be carefully monitored, because nephrotoxicity may be potentiated. As with other cephalosporins, high concentrations of cefotetan may produce false increases in the levels of creatinine reported. Cephalosporins may cause false-positive urine glucose determinations when using cupric sulfate solution (Benedict's solution, *Clinitest®*). Tests utilizing glucose oxidase (*Tes-Tape®*, *Clinistix®*) are not affected by cephalosporins.

Antibiotics Manual: A Guide to Commonly Used Antimicrobials, Second Edition. David Schlossberg and Rafik Samuel.
© 2017 John Wiley & Sons Ltd. Published 2017 by John Wiley & Sons Ltd.

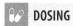 **DOSING**

Disease state	Dose
Urinary tract	500 mg every 12 hours IV or IM
	1 or 2 g every 24 hours IV or IM
	1 or 2 g every 12 hours IV or IM
Skin and soft tissue	2 g every 24 hours IV
	1 g every 12 hours IV or IM
Severe infections	2 grams every 12 hours IV
Life threatening	3 grams every 12 hours IV
Prophylaxis	1 or 2 g 30–60 minutes prior to surgery

In patients undergoing cesarean section, the dose should be administered as soon as the umbilical cord is clamped.

 SPECIAL POPULATIONS

RENAL IMPAIRMENT: The dose of cefotetan can be maintained with the interval adjusted as below:

Creatinine clearance	Dosing interval
>30	Every 12 hours
10–30	Every 24 hours
<10	Every 48 hours
Hemodialysis	After dialysis only
CAPD	Every 24 hours
CRRT	750 mg every 12 hours

or

the dosing interval may remain constant at 12 hour intervals, but the dose reduced to one-half for patients with a creatinine clearance of 10–30 mL/min and one-quarter for patients with a creatinine clearance of less than 10 mL/min.

HEPATIC DYSFUNCTION: No dose adjustment is necessary.

PEDIATRICS: Safety and effectiveness in children have not been established.

 THE ART OF ANTIMICROBIAL THERAPY

Clinical Pearls

1. Cefotetan is dose adjusted for renal dysfunction.
2. Cross allergy with penicillins is <10 %.
3. Cefotetan can be given IM or IV.
4. There is an increased risk of hemolytic anemia with cefotetan, relative to other cephalosporins.

BASIC CHARACTERISTICS

Class: Second generation cephalosporin.

Mechanism of Action: Binds penicillin-binding protein, disrupting cell wall synthesis.

Mechanisms of Resistance:

1. The PBP can be altered, with reduced affinity.
2. Production of a beta-lactamase, resulting in hydrolysis of the beta-lactam ring.
3. Decreased ability of the antibiotic to reach the PBP when bacteria decrease porin production, resulting in a decrease of the drug concentration within the cell.

Metabolic Route: Cefuroxime axetil is an ester that is quickly metabolized into the active cefuroxime. Cefuroxime is excreted unchanged in the urine.

 FDA-APPROVED INDICATIONS

1. **Cefuroxime tablets** are indicated for the treatment of patients with mild to moderate infections caused by susceptible strains of microorganisms in the following diseases:

   Pharyngitis/tonsillitis

   Acute bacterial otitis media

   Acute bacterial maxillary sinusitis

   Acute bacterial exacerbations of chronic bronchitis and secondary bacterial infections of acute bronchitis

   Uncomplicated skin and skin-structure infections

   Uncomplicated urinary tract infections

   Uncomplicated gonorrhea

   Early Lyme disease (erythema migrans)

2. **Cefuroxime oral suspension** is indicated for the treatment of pediatric patients 3 months to 12 years of age with mild to moderate infections caused by susceptible strains of microorganisms in the following diseases:

   Pharyngitis/tonsillitis

   Acute bacterial otitis media

   Impetigo

3. **Cefuroxime for injection** is indicated for the treatment of patients with infections caused by susceptible organisms in the following diseases:

   Lower respiratory tract infections

   Urinary tract infections

   Skin and skin-structure infections

   Septicemia

   Meningitis

Antibiotics Manual: A Guide to Commonly Used Antimicrobials, Second Edition. David Schlossberg and Rafik Samuel.
© 2017 John Wiley & Sons Ltd. Published 2017 by John Wiley & Sons Ltd.

Gonorrhea

Bone and joint

Prevention-preoperative prophylaxis in certain patients

 SIDE EFFECTS/TOXICITY

Cefuroxime is **contraindicated** in patients with known allergy to cephalosporins.

Cefuroxime should be used with caution if hypersensitivity exists to penicillin.

Toxicity includes phlebitis, fever, anaphylaxis, rash including Stevens–Johnson syndrome, erythema multiforme and toxic epidermal necrolysis, angioedema, flushing, serum-sickness-like reactions, encephalopathy, seizures, diarrhea, *Clostridium difficile*-associated diarrhea and pseudomembranous colitis, oral candidiasis, anorexia, taste perversion, nausea, vomiting, stomach cramps, flatulence, hepatitis, renal impairment, genital moniliasis, vaginitis, hemorrhage, prolonged prothrombin time, pancytopenia, hemolytic anemia, positive Coombs' test.

 DRUG INTERACTIONS/FOOD INTERACTIONS

Cefuroxime tablets may be administered with or without food.

Cefuroxime oral suspension must be administered with food.

Concomitant administration of probenecid with cefuroxime axetil tablets increases the serum concentration.

Drugs that reduce gastric acidity may result in a lower bioavailability of cefuroxime. Cephalosporins may cause false-positive urine glucose determinations when using cupric sulfate solution (Benedict's solution, *Clinitest*®). Tests utilizing glucose oxidase (*Tes-Tape*®, *Clinistix*®) are not affected by cephalosporins.

 DOSING

Cefuroxime tablets: 250 mg and 500 mg.

The following dosing is for the tablet. The pediatric section has the dosing for the oral suspension.

Disease state	Dosage	Duration
Pharyngitis/tonsillitis	250 mg q12 hours	10 days
Acute maxillary sinusitis	250 mg q 12 hours	10 days
Acute exacerbation of bronchitis	250–500 mg q 12 hours	10 days
Secondary infections of bronchitis	250–500 mg q 12 hours	5–10 days
Skin and soft tissue infections	250–500 mg q 12 hours	10 days
Urinary tract infections	250 mg q 12 hours	7–10 days
Gonorrhea	1 gram once	One dose
Lyme disease	500 mg q 12 hours	20 days

Cefuroxime for injection

Disease state	Dose
Uncomplicated urinary tract infections	750 mg or 1.5 grams every 8 hours IV or IM
Skin and skin-structure infections	750 mg or 1.5 grams every 8 hours IV or IM
Disseminated gonococcal infections	750 mg or 1.5 grams every 8 hours IV or IM
Uncomplicated pneumonia	750 mg or 1.5 grams every 8 hours IV or IM
Bone and joint infections	1.5 gram dose every 8 hours IV or IM
Life-threatening infections (meningitis)	1.5 grams every 6 hours IV or IM
Preventative during surgery	1.5 grams 30–60 min before incision IV or IM; then 750 mg every 8 hours when the procedure is prolonged
Preventive during open heart surgery	1.5 grams at induction then every 12 hours for a total of 6 grams IV or IM

 ## SPECIAL POPULATIONS

RENAL IMPAIRMENT:

Creatinine clearance	Dose of cefuroxime injection
>20 mL/min	750 mg–1.5 grams q 8 hours
10–20 mL/min	750 mg q 12 hours
<10 mL/min	750 mg daily
Hemodialysis	750 mg daily, administer after dialysis on dialysis days
CAPD	750 mg daily
CRRT	1 gm q 12 hours

The safety and efficacy of cefuroxime tablet and oral suspension have not been established; renal failure can be expected to prolong the half-life.

HEPATIC DYSFUNCTION: No dose adjustment is necessary.

PEDIATRICS: The safety and effectiveness of cefuroxime have been established for pediatric patients aged 3 months to 12 years.

Cefuroxime oral suspension provides the equivalent of 125 mg or 250 mg of cefuroxime per 5 mL.

Disease state	Dosage	Duration
Pharyngitis/tonsillitis	10 mg/kg q 12 hours	10 days
Acute otitis media	15 mg/kg q 12 hours	10 days
Acute maxillary sinusitis	15 mg/kg q 12 hours	10 days
Impetigo	15 mg/kg q 12 hours	10 days

Cefuroxime for injection

Mild to moderate infections	50 to 100 mg/kg/day in divided doses q 6 to 8 hours
Severe infections	100 mg/kg/day in divided doses q 6 to 8 hours
Bone and joint infections	150 mg/kg/day in divided doses q 8 hours
Bacterial meningitis	200 to 240 mg/kg/day in divided doses q 6 to 8 hours

 ## THE ART OF ANTIMICROBIAL THERAPY

Clinical Pearls

1. Cefuroxime must be adjusted for renal dysfunction.
2. Cross allergy with penicillins is <10 % and can be used in life-threatening infections (e.g., meningitis) with caution if the allergy is not severe.
3. Cefuroxime tablets and oral suspension are not bioequivalent and are not interchangeable on a milligram-per-milligram basis.
4. Cefuroxime tablets may be administered with or without food. Cefuroxime oral suspension must be administered with food.

■ CEFZIL (Cefprozil)

 BASIC CHARACTERISTICS

Class: Second generation cephalosporin.

Mechanism of Action: Binds penicillin-binding protein, disrupting cell wall synthesis.

Mechanisms of Resistance:

1. The PBP can be altered, with reduced affinity.

2. Production of a beta-lactamase, resulting in hydrolysis of the beta-lactam ring.

3. Decreased ability of the antibiotic to reach the PBP when bacteria decrease porin production, resulting in a decrease of the drug concentration within the cell.

Metabolic Route: The majority of cefprozil is excreted unchanged in the urine.

 FDA-APPROVED INDICATIONS

Treatment of patients with mild to moderate infections caused by susceptible strains of microorganisms in the conditions listed below:

Pharyngitis/tonsillitis

Otitis media

Acute sinusitis

Secondary bacterial infection of acute bronchitis and acute bacterial exacerbation of chronic bronchitis

Uncomplicated skin and skin-structure infections

 SIDE EFFECTS/TOXICITY

Cefprozil is **contraindicated** in patients with known allergy to cephalosporins.

Cefprozil should be used with caution if hypersensitivity exists to penicillin.

Toxicity includes phlebitis, fever, anaphylaxis, rash including Stevens–Johnson syndrome, erythema multiforme and toxic epidermal necrolysis, angioedema, flushing, serum-sickness-like reactions, encephalopathy, seizures, diarrhea, *Clostridium dif-ficile*-associated diarrhea and pseudomembranous colitis, oral candidiasis, anorexia, taste perversion, nausea, vomiting, stomach cramps, flatulence, hepatitis, renal impairment, genital moniliasis, vaginitis, hemorrhage, prolonged prothrombin time, pancytopenia, hemolytic anemia, and positive Coombs' test.

 DRUG INTERACTIONS/FOOD INTERACTIONS

Drugs that reduce gastric acidity may result in a lower bioavailability of cefprozil. Cephalosporins may cause false-positive urine glucose determinations when using cupric sulfate solution (Benedict's solution, *Clinitest®*). Tests utilizing glucose oxidase (*Tes-Tape®, Clinistix®*) are not affected by cephalosporins.

 DOSING

Cefprozil is supplied in 250 mg and 500 mg tablets.

Antibiotics Manual: A Guide to Commonly Used Antimicrobials, Second Edition. David Schlossberg and Rafik Samuel.
© 2017 John Wiley & Sons Ltd. Published 2017 by John Wiley & Sons Ltd.

It is also available in a cream colored suspension 125 mg/5 mL and 250 mg/5 mL.

Infection	Dose	Duration
Pharyngitis/tonsillitis	500 mg daily	10 days
Acute sinusitis	250–500 q 12 hours	10 days
Acute bronchitis	500 mg q 12 hours	10 days
Uncomplicated skin and soft tissue	250 mg q 12 hours	10 days

SPECIAL POPULATIONS

RENAL IMPAIRMENT:

Creatinine clearance, mL/min	Dose
10–50	Reduce dose by 50 %
<10	Reduce dose by 50 % and give once daily
Hemodialysis	Usual dose, but given after dialysis only
CAPD	Reduce dose by 50 %
CRRT	Reduce dose by 50 %

HEPATIC DYSFUNCTION: No dose adjustment is necessary.

PEDIATRICS: **Children 2–12 years of age**

Infection	Dose	Duration
Pharyngitis/tonsillitis	7.5 mg/kg q 12 hours	10 days
Uncomplicated skin and soft tissue	20 mg/kg daily	10 days

Children 6 months–12 years

Infection	Dose	Duration
Otitis media	15 mg/kg q 12 hours	10 days
Sinusitis	7.5–15 mg/kg q 12 hours	10 days

THE ART OF ANTIMICROBIAL THERAPY

Clinical Pearls

1. Cefprozil must be adjusted for renal dysfunction.
2. Cross-allergy with penicillins is <10 %.
3. Phenylketonurics: cefprozil for oral suspension contains 8.4 mg of phenylalanine per 5 mL (1 teaspoonful) constituted suspension for both the 125 mg/5 mL and 250 mg/5 mL dosage forms.

■ CHLOROMYCETIN (Chloramphenicol)

 BASIC CHARACTERISTICS

Class: Antiribosomal antimicrobial.

Mechanism of Action: Inhibits bacterial protein synthesis by interfering with the transfer of activated amino acids from soluble RNA to ribosomes.

Mechanisms of Resistance: Data incomplete.

Metabolic Route: Chloramphenicol is excreted in the urine, predominantly as metabolically inactive metabolites.

 FDA-APPROVED INDICATIONS

Acute infections caused by *Salmonella typhi*
Serious infections caused by:

Salmonella species

H. influenzae, especially meningeal infections

Rickettsia

Lymphogranuloma-psittacosis group

Various gram-negative bacteria causing bacteremia, meningitis, or other serious gram-negative infections

Other susceptible organisms that have been demonstrated to be resistant to all other appropriate antimicrobial agents.

 SIDE EFFECTS/TOXICITY

> **WARNING:** Serious and fatal blood dyscrasias (aplastic anemia, hypoplastic anemia, thrombocytopenia, and granulocyto-penia) are known to occur after the administration of chloramphenicol. In addition, there have been reports of aplastic anemia attributed to chloramphenicol that later terminated in leukemia. Blood dyscrasias have occurred after both short-term and prolonged therapy with this drug. Chloramphenicol must not be used when less potentially dangerous agents will be effective. *It must not be used in the treatment of trivial infections or where it is not indicated, as in colds, influenza, infections of the throat, or as a prophylactic agent to prevent bacterial infections.*
>
> It is essential that adequate blood studies be made during treatment with the drug. While blood studies may detect early peripheral blood changes, such as leukopenia, reticulocytopenia, or granulocytopenia, before they become irreversible, such studies cannot be relied on to detect bone marrow depression prior to development of aplastic anemia. To facilitate appropriate studies and observation during therapy, it is desirable that patients be hospitalized.

Chloramphenicol is **contraindicated** in individuals with a history of previous hypersensitivity and/or toxic reaction to it.

Other side effects: Hypersensitivity reactions including fever, rash, angioedema, urticaria, and anaphylaxis toxic reactions including fatalities in the premature and neonate, ("gray syndrome"), *Clostridium difficile*-associated diarrhea, paroxysmal nocturnal hemoglobinuria, nausea, vomiting, glossitis, stomatitis, diarrhea, enterocolitis, headache, mild depression, mental confusion, delirium, optic neuritis, and peripheral neuritis.

Antibiotics Manual: A Guide to Commonly Used Antimicrobials, Second Edition. David Schlossberg and Rafik Samuel.
© 2017 John Wiley & Sons Ltd. Published 2017 by John Wiley & Sons Ltd.

DRUG INTERACTIONS/FOOD INTERACTIONS

Concurrent therapy with other drugs that may cause bone marrow depression should be avoided.

DOSING

Adults should receive 50 mg/kg/day intravenously in divided doses at 6-hour intervals.

SPECIAL POPULATIONS

RENAL IMPAIRMENT: No change.

HEPATIC DYSFUNCTION: No clear recommendations, but dose should be decreased.

PEDIATRICS: Dosage of 50 mg/kg/day divided into 4 doses at 6-hour intervals.

Neonates

A total of 25 mg/kg/day in 4 equal doses at 6-hour intervals.

After the first two weeks of life, full-term neonates ordinarily may receive up to a total of 50 mg/kg/day equally divided into 4 doses at 6-hour intervals.

In young infants and other pediatric patients in whom immature metabolic functions are suspected, a dose of 25 mg/kg/day.

THE ART OF ANTIMICROBIAL THERAPY

Clinical Pearls

1. Chloramphenicol must be used only in those serious infections for which less potentially dangerous drugs are ineffective or contraindicated.
2. Baseline blood studies should be followed by blood studies every two days during therapy. The drug should be discontinued upon appearance of leukopenia, thrombocytopenia, anemia, or any other blood study findings attributable to chloramphenicol.
3. Patients started on intravenous chloramphenicol should be changed to the oral form of another appropriate antibiotic as soon as possible.
4. Repeated courses of chloramphenicol treatment should be avoided if at all possible.

■ CHLOROQUINE PHOSPHATE (Aralen), HYDROXYCHLOROQUINE

 BASIC CHARACTERISTICS

Class: 4-Aminoquinolone.

Mechanism of Action: Forms toxic complexes with heme molecules, depriving the parasite of hemoglobin.

Mechanism of Resistance: Mutation in transport molecule of digestive vacuole membrane (PfCRT), reducing the amount of drug that accumulates in the digestive vacuoles.

Metabolic Route: Half is excreted in the urine and the rest is degraded to multiple metabolic products.

 FDA-APPROVED INDICATIONS

Chloroquine: Suppressive treatment and acute attacks of malaria due to *P. vivax, P. malariae, P. ovale,* and susceptible strains of *P. falciparum.*

Treatment of extraintestinal amebiasis.

Hydroxychloroquine: Suppressive treatment and treatment of acute attacks of malaria due to *Plasmodium vivax, P. malariae, P. ovale,* and susceptible strains of *P. falciparum.*

 SIDE EFFECTS/TOXICITY

> **WARNING:** For malaria and extraintestinal amebiasis.

Other toxicities: psoriasis, porphyria, hypotension, tachycardia, bradycardia, A-V block or other transient conduction altera-tions, rash including Stevens–Johnson syndrome and toxic epidermal necrolysis, psychiatric symptoms including anxiety, paranoia, depression, hallucinations and psychosis, nausea, vomiting, diarrhea, hepatitis, seizures, nerve deafness, tinnitus, visual disturbances, myopathy, retinopathy, anemia, leucopenia, and thrombocytopenia.

 DRUG INTERACTIONS/FOOD INTERACTIONS

Antacids and kaolin can reduce the absorption of chloroquine; separate by 4 hours.

Concomitant use of cimetidine should be avoided.

An interval of at least two hours between intake of ampicillin and chloroquine should be observed.

May increase cyclosporine levels; close monitoring of serum cyclosporine level is recommended.

 DOSING

Chloroquine phosphate is calculated as the base. Each 250 mg tablet of chloroquine phosphate is equivalent to 150 mg base and each 500 mg tablet of chloroquine phosphate is equivalent to 300 mg base.

Malaria prophylaxis: 500 mg (=300 mg base) on exactly the same day of each week. Prophylactic therapy should begin two weeks prior to exposure and continue for eight weeks after leaving the endemic area.

Antibiotics Manual: A Guide to Commonly Used Antimicrobials, Second Edition. David Schlossberg and Rafik Samuel.
© 2017 John Wiley & Sons Ltd. Published 2017 by John Wiley & Sons Ltd.

Malaria treatment: An initial dose of 1 g (=600 mg base) followed by an additional 500 mg (=300 mg base) after six to eight hours and a single dose of 500 mg (=300 mg base) on each of two consecutive days. This represents a total dose of 2.5 g chloroquine phosphate or 1.5 g base in three days.

Extraintestinal amebiasis: 1 g (600 mg base) daily for two days, followed by 500 mg (300 mg base) daily for at least two to three weeks.

Hydroxychloroquine: One tablet of 200 mg of hydroxychloroquine is equivalent to 155 mg base.

Malaria prophylaxis: *In adults*, 400 mg (=310 mg base) on exactly the same day of each week. If circumstances permit, suppressive therapy should begin two weeks prior to exposure. The suppressive therapy should be continued for eight weeks after leaving the endemic area.

Treatment: An initial dose of 800 mg (=620 mg base) followed by 400 mg (=310 mg base) in six to eight hours and 400 mg (=310 mg base) on each of two consecutive days (total 2 g hydroxychloroquine sulfate or 1.55 g base). An alternative method, employing a single dose of 800 mg (=620 mg base), has also proved effective.

 SPECIAL POPULATIONS

RENAL IMPAIRMENT: There is no adjustment needed.

HEPATIC DYSFUNCTION: Use with caution.

PEDIATRICS:

Chloroquine phosphate

The weekly **prophylactic** dosage is 5 mg calculated as base, per kg of body weight, but should not exceed the adult dose regardless of weight.

For treatment:

First dose: 10 mg base per kg (but not exceeding a single dose of 600 mg base).

Second dose (6 hours after first dose): 5 mg base per kg (but not exceeding a single dose of 300 mg base).

Third dose (24 hours after first dose): 5 mg base per kg.

Fourth dose (36 hours after first dose): 5 mg base per kg.

Hydroxychloroquine

The weekly **prophylactic dosage** is 5 mg, calculated as base, per kg of body weight, but should not exceed the adult dose regardless of weight.

Treatment:

First dose: 10 mg base per kg (but not exceeding a single dose of 620 mg base).

Second dose: 5 mg base per kg (but not exceeding a single dose of 310 mg base) 6 hours after first dose.

Third dose: 5 mg base per kg 18 hours after second dose.

Fourth dose: 5 mg base per kg 24 hours after third dose.

THE ART OF ANTIMICROBIAL THERAPY

Clinical Pearls

1. *P. falcipirum* is usually resistant to chloroquine in all regions of the world except the Caribbean and the Middle East.

2. Chloroquine does not eliminate hepatic phase parasites, and patients with acute *P. vivax* malaria are at high risk of relapse; to avoid relapse, after initial treatment of the acute infection, patients should subsequently be treated with an 8-aminoquinoline derivative (e.g., primaquine).

3. Chloroquine can induce hemolysis in patients with G6PD deficiency.

4. Caution is urged when using chloroquine in patients with a history of epilepsy, auditory damage, liver disease, and alcoholism.

5. Since irreversible retinal damage may occur with prolonged or high dose therapy, ophthalmologic monitoring is advisable.

6. Concomitant use with mefloquine may increase the risk of seizures.

7. Complete blood cell counts should be made periodically if patients are given prolonged therapy.

BASIC CHARACTERISTICS

Class: Fluoroquinolone.

Mechanism of Action: Inhibition of bacterial topoisomerase IV and DNA gyrase.

Mechanisms of Resistance: Mutations in DNA gyrase and/or topoisomerase IV or through altered efflux,

Metabolic Route: Ciprofloxacin is predominantly excreted in the urine.

 FDA-APPROVED INDICATIONS

Ciprofloxacin is indicated for the treatment of serious infections caused by susceptible strains of microorganisms in the diseases listed below:

Urinary tract infections

Acute uncomplicated cystitis in females

Chronic bacterial prostatitis

Lower respiratory tract infections

Acute sinusitis

Skin and skin structure infections

Bone and joint infections

Complicated intra-abdominal infections

Infectious diarrhea

Typhoid fever (enteric fever)

Uncomplicated cervical and urethral gonorrhea

Inhalational anthrax prophylaxis

Also Used for: inhalational and cutaneous anthrax, plague, tularemia, traveler's diarrhea.

Cipro XR is indicated only for the treatment of urinary tract infections, including acute uncomplicated pyelonephritis, caused by susceptible strains of the designated microorganisms as listed below:

    Uncomplicated urinary tract infections (acute cystitis)

    Complicated urinary tract infections

    Acute uncomplicated pyelonephritis

 SIDE EFFECTS/TOXICITY

> **WARNING:** Serious adverse reactions including tendinitis, tendon rupture, peripheral neuropathy, central nervous system effects, and exacerbation of myasthenia gravis. Fluoroquinolones, including ciprofloxacin, have been associated with disabling and potentially irreversible serious adverse reactions that have occurred together, including tendinitis and tendon rupture, peripheral neuropathy, and central nervous system effects.

Discontinue ciprofloxacin immediately and avoid the use of fluoroquinolones, including ciprofloxacin, in patients who experience any of these serious adverse reactions. Fluoroquinolones, including ciprofloxacin, may exacerbate muscle weakness in patients with myasthenia gravis. Avoid ciprofloxacin in patients with a known history of myasthenia gravis.

Because fluoroquinolones, including ciprofloxacin, have been associated with serious adverse reactions, reserve ciprofloxacin for use in patients who have no alternative treatment options for the following indications: acute exacerbation of chronic bronchitis, acute uncomplicated cystitis, and acute sinusitis.

Ciprofloxacin is **contraindicated** in persons with a history of hypersensitivity associated with the use of ciprofloxacin or any quinolone.

Other adverse effects: hypersensitivity, angioedema, headache, **seizures**, increased intracranial pressure, psychosis, tremors, agitation, lightheadedness, confusion, hallucinations, paranoia, depression, nightmares, insomnia, and suicidal thoughts or acts; **tendon** ruptures of the shoulder, hand, Achilles tendon, **photosensitivity**, **prolongation of the QT** interval and arrhythmia, rare cases of torsades de pointes, renal failure, peripheral neuropathy, *Clostridium difficile*-associated diarrhea, nausea, vomiting, elevations in ALT and AST, blurred vision, and pancytopenia.

 DRUG INTERACTIONS/FOOD INTERACTIONS

1. Ciprofloxacin absorption may be decreased by **antacids** containing calcium, magnesium, or aluminum; sucralfate; divalent or trivalent cations such as iron; or multivitamins containing zinc. Ciprofloxacin should be taken 2 hours before or 6 hours after these products.

2. Concomitant administration with tizanidine is contraindicated.

3. Cimetidine results in significant increases in the half-life of some quinolones.

4. Ciprofloxacin inhibits cytochrome P450 enzyme activity. This may result in a **prolonged half-life** for some drugs that are also metabolized by this system, such as theophylline, caffeine, cyclosporine, theophylline/methylxanthines, and warfarin when coadministered with quinolones.

5. The concomitant administration of a nonsteroidal anti-inflammatory drug with a quinolone may increase the risk of CNS stimulation and seizures.

6. The concomitant use of probenecid decreases renal tubular secretion.

7. Disturbances of blood glucose, including hyperglycemia and hypoglycemia, may be seen in patients treated concurrently with antidiabetic agents.

8. Ciprofloxacin may produce false-positive urine screening results for opiates.

 DOSING

Cipro

Ciprofloxacin is available as 250 mg, 500 mg, and 750 mg tablets, as a suspension that is 5 % (250 mg/5 mL) and 10 % (500 mg/5 mL), and in an intravenous formulation.

Usual adult dosage: 500 mg–750 mg PO bid or 400 mg IV q 8–12 h.

Usual duration: 7–14 days.

Exceptions:

UTI: 250 mg q 12 h × 3 days (uncomplicated) or 250 mg q 12 h × 7–14 days (mild to moderate).

Traveler's diarrhea; 750 mg × 1 (mild) or 500 mg bid × 3 days (severe).

Duration for chronic prostatitis and bone/joint infections: >4 weeks.

Duration for anthrax: 60 days.

Cipro XR

Cipro XR is supplied as 500 mg and 1000 mg extended release capsules.

Indication	Dose		Usual duration
Uncomplicated urinary tract infection (acute cystitis)	500 mg		q 24 h 3 days
Complicated urinary tract infection	1000 mg	q 24 h	7–14 days
Acute uncomplicated pyelonephritis	1000 mg	q 24 h	7–14 days

⊕ SPECIAL POPULATIONS

RENAL IMPAIRMENT:

Ciprofloxacin oral tablet or suspension:

Creatinine clearance, mL/min	Dose
>50	Usual dosage
30–50	250–500 mg q 12 h
5–29	250–500 mg q 18 h
Hemodialysis	250–500 mg q 24 h (after dialysis)
CAPD	250 mg q 8 h
CRRT	250–500 mg q 12 h

Cipro XR

Creatinine clearance, mL/min	Dose
<30	500 mg daily
Hemodialysis	500 mg daily, administer after dialysis on dialysis days
CAPD	500 mg daily
CRRT	N/A

HEPATIC DYSFUNCTION: A maximum dose of 400 mg of ciprofloxacin per day should not be exceeded.

PEDIATRICS: Safety and efficacy in pediatric patients less than 18 years of age have not yet been established. However, it is approved as an alternative agent for complicated urinary tract infections and pyelonephritis and prophylaxis for inhaled anthrax.

Infection	Route of administration	Dose, mg/kg	Frequency	Total duration
Complicated urinary tract or pyelonephritis	Intravenous	6 to 10 mg/kg	q 8 h	10–21 days
	Oral	10 mg/kg to 20 mg/kg	q 12 h	
Inhalational anthrax (post-exposure, cutaneous)	Intravenous	10 mg/kg	Every 12 hours	60 days
	Oral	15 mg/kg	Every 12 hours	

THE ART OF ANTIMICROBIAL THERAPY

Clinical Pearls

1. Ciprofloxacin should be given at least 2 hours before cations or 6 hours after.
2. Cipro XR and Cipro are not interchangeable.
3. The oral Cipro and IV Cipro doses are not the same. For every 250 mg oral, the equivalent is 200 mg intravenously.
4. All fluoroquinolones can cause tendon rupture, especially in patients over 60 years of age.
5. All fluoroquinolones can prolong QT intervals and caution should be used when given with medications that affect QT intervals.
6. All fluoroquinolones can cause phototoxicity.
7. All fluoroquinolones can lower the seizure threshold and cause other CNS side effects.
8. Ciprofloxacin should be avoided if possible in children, pregnant women, and nursing mothers, because of concern for cartilage developmental problems.
9. Ciprofloxacin has activity against Mycobacteria; therefore ciprofloxacin monotherapy should be avoided if mycobacterial infection is possible.
10. Treatment of gonorrhea with fluoroquinolones should be undertaken with caution because of rising resistance.
11. In 2016, an FDA Safety Communication advised that the serious side effects associated with fluoroquinolones generally outweigh the benefits for patients with sinusitis, bronchitis, and uncomplicated urinary tract infections, who have other treatment options.

BASIC CHARACTERISTICS

Class: Third generation cephalosporin.

Mechanism of Action: Binds penicillin-binding protein, disrupting cell wall synthesis.

Mechanisms of Resistance:

1. The PBP can be altered, with reduced affinity.
2. Production of a beta-lactamase resulting in hydrolysis of the beta-lactam ring.
3. Decreased ability of the antibiotic to reach the PBP when bacteria decrease porin production, resulting in a decrease of the drug concentration within the cell.

Metabolic Route: Predominantly excreted in the urine, as unchanged drug and metabolites.

 ## FDA-APPROVED INDICATIONS

Treatment of patients with serious infections caused by susceptible strains of microorganisms in the diseases listed below:

Lower respiratory tract infections

Genitourinary infections

Gynecologic infections: pelvic inflammatory disease, endometritis, and pelvic cellulitis

Bacteremia/septicemia

Skin and skin structure infections

Intra-abdominal infections

Bone and/or joint infections

Central nervous system infections, e.g., meningitis and ventriculitis

Prevention of certain infections perioperatively

 ## SIDE EFFECTS/TOXICITY

Cefotaxime is **contraindicated** in patients who have shown hypersensitivity to any cephalosporin and should be used with caution if hypersensitivity exists to penicillin.

Toxicity includes fever, anaphylaxis, rash including Stevens–Johnson syndrome, erythema multiforme and toxic epidermal necrolysis, angioedema, flushing, serum-sickness-like reactions, encephalopathy, seizures, diarrhea, *Clostridium difficile*-associated diarrhea and pseudomembranous colitis, oral candidiasis, anorexia, nausea, vomiting, stomach cramps, flatulence, hepatitis, renal impairment, genital moniliasis, vaginitis, hemorrhage, prolonged prothrombin time, pancytopenia, hemolytic anemia, positive Coombs' test, and potentially life-threatening arrhythmias following rapid (less than 60 seconds) bolus administration via central venous catheter.

 ## DRUG INTERACTIONS/FOOD INTERACTIONS

Increased nephrotoxicity has been reported following concomitant administration of cephalosporins and aminoglycoside antibiotics. Cephalosporins may cause false-positive urine glucose determinations when using cupric sulfate solution (Benedict's solution, *Clinitest®*). Tests utilizing glucose oxidase (*Tes-Tape®*, *Clinistix®*) are not affected by cephalosporins.

Antibiotics Manual: A Guide to Commonly Used Antimicrobials, Second Edition. David Schlossberg and Rafik Samuel.
© 2017 John Wiley & Sons Ltd. Published 2017 by John Wiley & Sons Ltd.

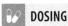 **DOSING**

Severity of infection	Dose
Uncomplicated	1 g every 12 hours IM or IV
Moderate to complicated	1–2 grams every 8 hours IM or IV
Life threatening	2 grams every 4 hours IM or IV
Prevention	1 gram 30–90 minutes prior to start of surgery
Gonococcal urethritis/cervicitis	0.5 gram IM (single dose)
Rectal gonorrhea in females	0.5 gram IM (single dose)
Rectal gonorrhea in males	1.0 gram IM (single dose)

 SPECIAL POPULATIONS

RENAL IMPAIRMENT:

Creatinine clearance, mL/min	Dose
10–50	Usual dose every 8–12 hours
<10	Usual dose once daily
Hemodialysis	1 gram after dialysis
CAPD	1 gram daily
CRRT	1 gram every 12 hours

HEPATIC DYSFUNCTION: No dose adjustment is necessary.

PEDIATRICS: For body weights less than 50 kg, the recommended daily dose is 50 to 180 mg/kg body weight divided into four to six equal doses. The higher dosages should be used for more severe or serious infections, including meningitis. For body weights 50 kg or more, the usual adult dosage should be used; the maximum daily dosage should not exceed 12 grams.

 THE ART OF ANTIMICROBIAL THERAPY

Clinical Pearls
1. Cefotaxime is dose-adjusted for renal dysfunction.
2. Cross allergy with penicillins is <10 % and can be used in life-threatening infections (e.g., meningitis) with caution if the allergy is not severe.
3. Cefotaxime may be administered IM or IV.

BASIC CHARACTERISTICS

Class: Lincosamide.

Mechanism of Action: Clindamycin inhibits bacterial protein synthesis by binding to the 50S subunit of the ribosome.

Mechanisms of Resistance:

1. Alteration of the 50S ribosomal protein by an amino acid substitution.
2. Alteration in the 23S ribosomal RNA subunit by methylation (MLS gene).
3. Nucleotidylation of the hydroxyl group of clindamycin.

Metabolic Route: Metabolized and excreted in the urine and feces.

 FDA-APPROVED INDICATIONS

Clindamycin capsules and granules for suspension are indicated in the treatment of serious infections caused by susceptible anaerobic bacteria, streptococci, pneumococci, and staphylococci.

Clindamycin for injection is indicated in the treatment of serious infections caused by susceptible strains of the designated organisms in the conditions listed below. Its use should be reserved for penicillin-allergic patients or other patients for whom, in the judgment of the physician, a penicillin is inappropriate. Because of the risk of antibiotic-associated pseudomembranous colitis, before selecting clindamycin the physician should consider the nature of the infection and the suitability of less toxic alternatives.

1. Lower respiratory tract infections including pneumonia, empyema, and lung abscess.
2. Skin and skin structure infections.
3. Gynecological infections including endometritis, nongonococcal tubo-ovarian abscess, pelvic cellulitis, and postsurgical vaginal cuff infection.
4. Intra-abdominal infections including peritonitis and intra-abdominal abscess caused by susceptible anaerobic organisms.
5. Septicemia.
6. Bone and joint infections.

Also Used for: Clindamycin in combination with primaquine has been used to treat *Pneumocystis jirovecii* pneumonia (PCP).

Clindamycin in combination with pyrimethamine has been used to treat *Toxoplasma gondii* infections in HIV infected patients.

Clindamycin in combination with primaquine has been used to treat *Plasmodium falcipirum* malaria.

Clindamycin in combination with quinine has been used to treat babesiosis.

 SIDE EFFECTS/TOXICITY

WARNING: *Clostridium difficile*-**associated diarrhea (CDAD)** has been reported with use of nearly all antibacterial agents, including clindamycin in 5 % dextrose injection and may range in severity from mild diarrhea to fatal colitis. Treatment with antibacterial agents alters the normal flora of the colon leading to overgrowth of *C. difficile*.

Antibiotics Manual: A Guide to Commonly Used Antimicrobials, Second Edition. David Schlossberg and Rafik Samuel.
© 2017 John Wiley & Sons Ltd. Published 2017 by John Wiley & Sons Ltd.

Because clindamycin in 5 % dextrose injection therapy has been associated with severe colitis, which may end fatally, it should be reserved for serious infections where less toxic antimicrobial agents are inappropriate. It should not be used in patients with nonbacterial infections such as most upper respiratory tract infections. *C. difficile* produces toxins A and B which contribute to the development of CDAD. Hypertoxin producing strains of *C. difficile* cause increased morbidity and mortality, as these infections can be refractory to antimicrobial therapy and may require colectomy. CDAD must be considered in all patients who present with diarrhea following antibiotic use. Careful medical history is necessary since CDAD has been reported to occur over two months after the administration of antibacterial agents.

If CDAD is suspected or confirmed, ongoing antibiotic use not directed against *C. difficile* may need to be discontinued. Appropriate fluid and electrolyte management, protein supplementation, antibiotic treatment of *C. difficile*, and surgical evaluation should be instituted as clinically indicated.

Contraindicated in individuals with a history of hypersensitivity to preparations containing clindamycin or lincomycin.

Side effects include *Clostridium difficile*-associated diarrhea (CDAD), esophagitis, abdominal pain, nausea, vomiting, diarrhea, morbilliform and vesiculobullous rash, urticaria, erythema multiforme, Stevens–Johnson syndrome, pruritus, vaginitis, abnormal liver function tests, neutropenia, eosinophilia, polyarthritis, neuromuscular blockade.

 ## DRUG INTERACTIONS/FOOD INTERACTIONS

Clindamycin capsules and granules can be taken without regard to food.

Use with caution in patients receiving musculoskeletal blocking agents.

Antagonism has been demonstrated between clindamycin and erythromycin *in vitro*.

 ## DOSING

Clindamycin is supplied as 75 mg, 150 mg, and 300 mg capsules.

Clindamycin flavored granules for oral solution in a concentration of 75 mg/5 mL.

Clindamycin can also be administered intravenously.

Clindamycin capsules

Serious infections: 150 to 300 mg every 6 hours.

More severe infections: 300 to 450 mg every 6 hours.

Clindamycin for injection

Serious infections: 600–1200 mg/day in 2, 3, or 4 equal doses.

More severe infections: 1200–2700 mg/day in 2, 3, or 4 equal doses.

In life-threatening situations, doses of as much as 4800 mg daily have been given intravenously.

 ## SPECIAL POPULATIONS

RENAL IMPAIRMENT: No dosage adjustment is necessary.

HEPATIC DYSFUNCTION: No dose adjustment is necessary.

Clindamycin capsules or IV

Serious infections: 8 to 16 mg/kg/day divided into 3 or 4 equal doses.

More severe infections: 16 to 20 mg/kg/day divided into 3 or 4 equal doses.

Clindamycin granules

Serious infections: 8–12 mg/kg/day divided into 3 or 4 equal doses.

Severe infections: 13–16 mg/kg/day divided into 3 or 4 equal doses.

More severe infections: 17–25 mg/kg/day divided into 3 or 4 equal doses.

In pediatric patients weighing 10 kg or less, 37.5 mg three times a day should be considered the minimum recommended dose.

 THE ART OF ANTIMICROBIAL THERAPY

Clinical Pearls

1. To avoid the possibility of esophageal irritation, clindamycin capsules should be taken with a full glass of water.
2. Clindamycin in combination with other agents has been effective in treating PCP, toxoplasmosis, and falciparum malaria.
3. When treating staphylococcal infections, be sure to assess for inducible resistance (D-Test) to clindamycin in organisms demonstrating erythromycin resistance and clindamycin susceptibility.
4. The 75 mg and 150 mg capsules contain tartrazine, which may cause allergic reactions (including bronchospasm). Tartrazine allergy is frequently seen in patients who also have aspirin hypersensitivity.

COARTEM (Artemether/Lumefantrine)

 ## BASIC CHARACTERISTICS

Class: Fixed dose combination of artemether and lumefantrine in the ratio of 1:6 is an antimalarial agent.

Mechanism of Action: Artemether is metabolized into dihydroartemisinin (DHA).

1. Lumefantrine inhibits the formation of β-hematin by forming a complex with hemin.
2. Both artemether and lumefantrine inhibit nucleic acid and protein synthesis.

Metabolic Route: Lumefantrine is excreted unchanged in feces and with traces only in urine. Metabolites of both drug components were eliminated in bile/feces and urine.

 ## FDA-APPROVED INDICATIONS

Treatment of acute, uncomplicated malaria infections due to *Plasmodium falciparum* in patients of 5 kg bodyweight and above.

 ## SIDE EFFECTS/TOXICITY

Contraindicated in:

1. Patients hypersensitive to artemether, lumefantrine, or to any of the excipients of artemether/lumefantrine.
2. Patients with congenital prolongation of the QT interval (e.g., long QT syndrome) or any other clinical condition known to prolong the QTc interval, such as patients with a history of symptomatic cardiac arrhythmias, with clinically relevant bradycardia, or with severe cardiac disease.
3. Patients with a family history of congenital prolongation of the QT interval or sudden death.
4. Patients with known disturbances of electrolyte balance, e.g., hypokalemia or hypomagnesemia.

Frequently reported adverse reactions were headache, anorexia, dizziness, asthenia, pyrexia, cough, vomiting, and headache.

Other reported events include eosinophilia, tinnitus, conjunctivitis, constipation, dyspepsia, dysphagia, peptic ulcer, hepatitis, gait disturbance, hypokalemia, back pain, ataxia, clonus, fine motor delay, hyperreflexia, hypoaesthesia, nystagmus, tremor, agitation, mood swings, hematuria, proteinuria, asthma, pharyngolaryngeal pain, urticaria, and angioedema.

DRUG INTERACTIONS/FOOD INTERACTIONS

Artemether/lumefantrine tablets should be taken with food.

Contraindicated to administer artemether/lumefantrine with:

1. Patients receiving other medications that prolong the QT interval, such as class IA (quinidine, procainamide, disopyramide) or class III (amiodarone, sotalol) antiarrhythmic agents; antipsychotics (pimozide, ziprasidone); antidepressants; certain antibiotics (macrolide antibiotics, fluoroquinolone antibiotics, imidazole, and triazole antifungal agents); certain non-sedating antihistaminics (terfenadine, astemizole); or cisapride.
2. Patients receiving medications that are metabolized by the cytochrome enzyme CYP2D6, which also have cardiac effects (e.g., flecainide, imipramine, amitriptyline, clomipramine).

Antibiotics Manual: A Guide to Commonly Used Antimicrobials, Second Edition. David Schlossberg and Rafik Samuel.
© 2017 John Wiley & Sons Ltd. Published 2017 by John Wiley & Sons Ltd.

When artemether/lumefantrine is coadministered with an inhibitor of CYP3A4, including grapefruit juice, it may result in increased concentrations of artemether and/or lumefantrine and potentiate QT prolongation.

When artemether/lumefantrine is coadministered with inducers of CYP3A4 it may result in decreased concentrations of artemether and/or lumefantrine and loss of antimalarial efficacy.

Drugs that have a mixed effect on CYP3A4, especially antiretroviral drugs, and those that have an effect on the QT interval should be used with caution in patients taking artemether/lumefantrine; the result may be an increase in lumefantrine concentrations causing QT prolongation or a decrease in concentrations of the ART resulting in loss of efficacy, or a decrease in artemether and/or lumefantrine concentrations resulting in loss of antimalarial efficacy of artemether/lumefantrine. Artemether/lumefantrine may reduce the effectiveness of hormonal contraceptives. Therefore, patients using oral, transdermal patch, or other systemic hormonal contraceptives should be advised to use an additional nonhormonal method of birth control.

 ## DOSING

Coartem tablets contain 20 mg of artemether and 120 mg of lumefantrine.

Four tablets as a single initial dose, 4 tablets again after 8 hours and then 4 tablets twice daily (morning and evening) for the following two days (total course of 24 tablets).

 ## SPECIAL POPULATIONS

RENAL IMPAIRMENT: There is no dose adjustment for renal insufficiency.

HEPATIC DYSFUNCTION: No dose adjustment for mild to moderate hepatic dysfunction.

PEDIATRICS: The safety and efficacy have not been established in pediatric patients who weigh less than 5 kg.

A 3-day treatment schedule with a total of 6 doses is recommended as below:

Weight	Regimen
5–15 kg	1 tablet, then 1 tablet 8 hours later, then 1 tablet bid for 2 days
15–25 kg	2 tablets, then 2 tablets 8 hours later, then 2 tablets bid for 2 days
25–35 kg	3 tablets, then 3 tablets 8 hours later, then 3 tablets bid for 2 days
>35 kg	4 tablets, then 4 tablets 8 hours later, then 4 tablets bid for 2 days

 ## THE ART OF ANTIMICROBIAL THERAPY

Clinical Pearls

1. Artemether/lumefantrine have been shown to be effective in geographical regions where resistance to chloroquine has been reported.
2. Artemether/lumefantrine is not approved for patients with severe or complicated *P. falciparum* malaria.
3. Artemether/lumefantrine is not approved for the prevention of malaria.
4. Coartem tablets may be crushed and mixed with a small amount of water.

■ COLY-MYCIN® M PARENTERAL (Colistimethate for Injection)

 BASIC CHARACTERISTICS

Class: Polypeptide.
Mechanism of Action: Disrupts the bacterial cell membrane.
Metabolic Route: Primarily excreted by the kidneys.

 FDA-APPROVED INDICATIONS

Treatment of acute or chronic infections due to sensitive strains of certain gram-negative bacilli. It is particularly indicated when the infection is caused by sensitive strains of *Pseudomonas aeruginosa*. This antibiotic is not indicated for infections due to *Proteus* or *Neisseria*. Colistimethate has proven clinically effective in treatment of infections due to the following gram-negative organisms: *Enterobacter aerogenes*, *Escherichia coli*, *Klebsiella pneumoniae*, and *Pseudomonas aeruginosa*.

 SIDE EFFECTS/TOXICITY

Nephrotoxicity, transient neurological disturbances (circumoral paresthesia or numbness, tingling or formication of the extremities, generalized pruritus, vertigo, dizziness, and slurring of speech), neuromuscular blockade, CDAD, fever, apnea, and nausea.

 DRUG INTERACTIONS/FOOD INTERACTIONS

Avoid drugs that interfere with nerve transmission, for example, aminoglycosides and polymyxin; curareform muscle relaxants potentiate the meuromuscular blocking effect; some cephalosporins may enhance the nephrotoxicity.

 DOSING

(1 mg = 12500 units)
Adults and pediatric patients – intravenous or intramuscular administration: Colistimethate should be given in 2 to 4 divided doses at dose levels of 2.5 to 5 mg/kg per day for patients with normal renal function, depending on the severity of the infection.
Intrathecal: 10 mg/day.
Inhalation: 50–75 mg in 3–4 ml saline via nebulizer q 8 h.

Antibiotics Manual: A Guide to Commonly Used Antimicrobials, Second Edition. David Schlossberg and Rafik Samuel.
© 2017 John Wiley & Sons Ltd. Published 2017 by John Wiley & Sons Ltd.

SPECIAL POPULATIONS

RENAL IMPAIRMENT:

Renal function	Normal	Degree of impairment		
		Mild	Moderate	Considerable
Plasma creatinine, mg/100 mL	0.7–1.2	1.3–1.5	1.6–2.5	2.6–4.0
Urea clearance, % of normal	80–100	40–70	25–40	10–25
Dosage: unit dose of Coly-Mycin M, mg	100–150	75–115	66–150	100–150
Frequency, times/day	4 to 2	2	2 or 1	Every 36 hours
Total daily dose, mg	300	150–230	133–150	100
Approximate daily dose, mg/kg/day	5.0	2.5–3.8	2.5	1.5

Postdialysis dose: None.

HEPATIC DYSFUNCTION: Probably no dose adjustment necessary.

 THE ART OF ANTIMICROBIAL THERAPY

Clinical Pearls

1. Many gram-negative bacilli are resistant, including *Proteus*, *Serratia*, *Providentia*, *Burkholderia*, *Moraxella*, *Vibrio*, *Morganella*, *Helicobacter*, and *Edwardsiella*.
2. Monitor for nephrotoxicity, neurotoxicity, CDAD, respiratory paralysis.

■ COLY-MYCIN (Colistimethate Sodium)

 BASIC CHARACTERISTICS

Class: Cell membrane altering antibiotic.

Mechanism of Action: Colistimethate sodium is a surface active agent that penetrates into and disrupts the bacterial cell membrane.

Mechanisms of Resistance: Data incomplete.

Metabolic Route: Colistimethate is excreted in the urine.

 FDA-APPROVED INDICATIONS

Treatment of acute or chronic infections due to sensitive strains of gram-negative bacilli. It is particularly indicated when the infection is caused by sensitive strains of *Pseudomonas aeruginosa*.

 SIDE EFFECTS/TOXICITY

Nephrotoxicity

Transient neurological disturbances including circumoral paresthesia or numbness, tingling of the extremities, generalized pruritus, vertigo, dizziness, and slurring of speech.

Also seen: Gastrointestinal upset, generalized itching, urticaria, rash, fever, respiratory arrest (after intramuscular administration), and *Clostridium difficile*-associated diarrhea.

 DRUG INTERACTIONS/FOOD INTERACTIONS

Aminoglycosides, curariform muscle relaxants, ether, succinylcholine, gallamine, decamethonium, sodium citrate, and polymyxin interfere with nerve transmission at the neuromuscular junction and should not be given concomitantly with colistin except with the greatest caution.

Cephalothin may enhance the nephrotoxicity.

 DOSING

Colistimethate should be given in 2 to 4 divided doses of 2.5 to 5 mg/kg per day for patients with normal renal function, depending on the severity of the infection.

In obese individuals, dosage should be based on ideal body weight.

 SPECIAL POPULATIONS

RENAL IMPAIRMENT:

Creatinine clearance, mL/min	Dose
40–60	2.5 mg/kg q 12 h
10–39	2.5 mg/kg q 24 h
<10	1.5 mg/kg q 36 h
After HD or PD	1.5 mg/kg q 36 h; no extra dose
CRRT	2.5 mg/kg q 24 h

Antibiotics Manual: A Guide to Commonly Used Antimicrobials, Second Edition. David Schlossberg and Rafik Samuel.
© 2017 John Wiley & Sons Ltd. Published 2017 by John Wiley & Sons Ltd.

HEPATIC DYSFUNCTION: No dose adjustment is necessary

PEDIATRICS: As for adults. Close clinical monitoring of pediatric patients is recommended.

 THE ART OF ANTIMICROBIAL THERAPY

Clinical Pearls

1. Colistimethate is not indicated for infections due to *Proteus* or *Neisseria*.
2. Overdosage can result in renal insufficiency, muscle weakness, and apnea.
3. Avoid the coadministration of nephrotoxic agents or neuromuscular blocking agents when administering colistimethate.

BASIC CHARACTERISTICS

Class: Nucleoside reverse transcriptase inhibitor (NRTI) with activity against HIV.

Mechanism of Action: Converted by cellular enzymes to its active drugs lamivudine triphosphate (a cytosine analog and zidovudine triphosphate (a thymadine analog). These triphosphate analogs compete with the naturally occurring nucleotides for incorporation in newly forming HIV DNA. Since the triphosphate analogs do not have terminal hydroxyl groups, they halt transcription and replication of the virus.

Mechanism of Resistance: Zidovudine mutations change the structure of HIV reverse transcriptase, leading to pyrophospho-rolysis of the nucleoside analogs, which allows transcription of DNA to continue. Resistance mutations include the "TAMS": 41L, 67N, 70R, 210W, 215F, and 219E.

Lamivudine mutations change the structure of HIV reverse transcriptase, leading to preferred incorporation of cytosine triphos-phate and decreased incorporation of lamivudine triphosphate, which allows transcription of DNA to continue. Resistance mutations include M184V.

Metabolic Route: Zidovudine is primarily eliminated by hepatic metabolism. The major metabolite of zidovudine is 3′-azido-3′-deoxy-5′-O-β-D-glucopyranuronosylthymidine (GZDV).

The majority of lamivudine is eliminated unchanged in urine by active organic cationic secretion.

 FDA-APROVED INDICATIONS

Treatment of HIV infection, in combination with other antiretrovirals.

 SIDE EFFECTS/TOXICITY

> **WARNING:** Zidovudine, a component of Combivir, has been associated with **hematologic toxicity** including neutropenia and severe anemia, particularly in patients with advanced human immunodeficiency virus (HIV-1) disease.

Myopathy: Prolonged use of zidovudine has been associated with symptomatic myopathy.

Lactic acidosis and severe hepatomegaly with steatosis: Lactic acidosis and severe hepatomegaly with steatosis, including fatal cases, have been reported with the use of nucleoside analogs alone or in combination, including lamivudine, zidovudine, and other antiretrovirals. Discontinue Combivir if clinical or laboratory findings suggestive of lactic acidosis or pronounced hepatotoxicity occur.

Exacerbations of hepatitis B: Severe acute exacerbations of hepatitis B have been reported in patients who are coinfected with hepatitis B virus (HBV) and HIV-1 and have discontinued lamivudine, which is one component of Combivir. Hepatic function should be monitored closely with both clinical and laboratory follow-up for at least several months in patients who discontinue Combivir and are coinfected with HIV-1 and HBV. If appropriate, initiation of antihepatitis B therapy may be warranted.

Other side effects: Immune reconstitution inflammatory syndrome, fat redistribution including central obesity and dorsocer-vical fat enlargement, peripheral wasting, facial wasting, breast enlargement, headache, nausea, malaise and fatigue, nasal symptoms, diarrhea, and cough.

Antibiotics Manual: A Guide to Commonly Used Antimicrobials, Second Edition. David Schlossberg and Rafik Samuel.
© 2017 John Wiley & Sons Ltd. Published 2017 by John Wiley & Sons Ltd.

DRUG INTERACTIONS/FOOD INTERACTIONS

Combivir can be taken with or without food and is unaffected by pH.

Combivir should not be used with stavudine, since zidovudine and stavudine are both thymidine analogues and may be antagonistic.

Combivir should not be used with doxorubicin.

Combivir should not be administered with ribavirin because of additive effects on anemia.

Combivir should not be used with emtricitabine or any medications containing emtricitabine because both lamivudine and emtricitabine are cytosine analogs and may be antagonistic. These include Emtriva, Truvada, Descovy, Atripla, Stribild, Genvoya, Complera, and Odefsey.

Combivir should not be given with other antiretrovirals containing lamivudine or zidovudine. These include Epivir, Trizivir, Epzicom, Triumeq, and Retrovir.

 DOSING

Combivir is administered in a fixed dose combination of zidovudine 300 mg and lamivudine 150 mg. The recommended adult dose is one tablet twice daily.

 SPECIAL POPULATIONS

RENAL IMPAIRMENT: This formulation should not be used in patients with a creatinine clearance less than 50 ml/min.

HEPATIC DYSFUNCTION: No dose adjustment necessary.

PEDIATRICS: The recommended dosage for pediatric patients who weigh greater than or equal to 30 kg is 1 tablet administered orally twice daily.

 THE ART OF ANTIMICROBIAL THERAPY

Clinical Pearls

1. Combivir should be used in combination with other antiretroviral agents.
2. Combivir contains both lamivudine and zidovudine and should not be used with medications containing these components including Retrovir, Trizivir, Epzicom, Triumeq, and Epivir.
3. Unlike other NRTIs, pharmacokinetic studies do not support once daily dosing of Combivir.
4. Since Combivir or any medication containing lamivudine has activity against hepatitis B it is important to check for hepatitis B since using Combivir or any medication containing lamivudine alone in hepatitis B infected individuals leads to rapid resistance to lamivudine.

COMPLERA (Tenofovir + Emtricitabine + Rilpivirine)

BASIC CHACTERISTICS

Class: Nucleotide reverse transcriptase inhibitor, nucleoside reverse transcriptase inhibitor, and nonnucleoside reverse transcriptase inhibitor.

Mechanism of action: Tenofovir and emtricitabine are converted by cellular enzymes to their active drugs tenofovir biphosphate (an analog of adenosine triphosphate) and emtricitabine triphosphate (an analog of cytosine triphosphate). These drugs compete with the naturally occurring nucleotides for incorporation in newly forming HIV DNA. Since they do not have a terminal hydroxyl group, they halt transcription and replication of the virus.

Rilpivirine inhibits reverse transcriptase activity by binding the enzyme.

Mechanism of Resistance: Changes in the structure of HIV reverse transcriptase leads to preferred incorporation of adenosine triphosphate and decreased incorporation of tenofovir biphosphate, which allows transcription of DNA to continue. Resistance mutations include K65R, M184V and "TAMS": 41L, 67N, 70R, 210W, 215F, and 219E.

Changes in the structure of reverse transcriptase prevents rilpivirine from binding the enzyme and allowing transcription to continue. The most frequent resistance mutation is E138K.

Metabolic Route: Tenofovir and emtricitabine are excreted in the urine unchanged.

Rilpivirine primarily undergoes oxidative metabolism mediated by the cytochrome P450 CYP 3A.

FDA-APPROVED INDICATIONS

Treatment of HIV-1 in combination with other antiretroviral agents.

SIDE EFFECTS/TOXICITY:

> **WARNING: Severe acute exacerbations of hepatitis** have been reported in hepatitis B-infected patients who have discontinued antihepatitis B therapy, including Complera or any medications containing either tenofovir or emtricitabine. Hepatic function should be monitored closely with both clinical and laboratory follow-up for at least several months in patients who discontinue antihepatitis B therapy, including Complera. If appropriate, resumption of antihepatitis B therapy may be warranted.
>
> **Lactic acidosis** and hepatomegaly with steatosis have been reported with nucleoside analogs, including tenofovir. If this syndrome occurs, the drug should be discontinued.

Other adverse events: Immune reconstitution inflammatory syndrome, fat redistribution including central obesity and dorsocervical fat enlargement, peripheral wasting, facial wasting, breast enlargement, diarrhea, nausea, fatigue, headache, dizziness, depression, insomnia, abnormal dreams, rash, renal impairment, including acute renal failure and Fanconi syndrome, decreased bone mineral density, abdominal discomfort, cholecystitis, cholelithiasis, decreased appetite, sleep disorders, anxiety, glomerulonephritis, and nephrolithiasis.

DRUG INTERACTIONS/FOOD INTERACTIONS

Complera should be administered with at least a 533 calorie meal.

Antibiotics Manual: A Guide to Commonly Used Antimicrobials, Second Edition. David Schlossberg and Rafik Samuel.
© 2017 John Wiley & Sons Ltd. Published 2017 by John Wiley & Sons Ltd.

Rilpivirine is primarily metabolized by cytochrome P450 (CYP)3A, and drugs that induce or inhibit CYP3A may affect the clearance of rilpivirine.

Complera should not be administered with delavirdine, efavirenz, etravirine, nevirapine, carbamazepine, oxcarbazepine, phenobarbital, phenytoin, rifampin, rifapentine, proton pump inhibitors, dexamethasone, or St John's wort.

Complera should not be given with didanosine because of decreased CD4 counts in patients maintained on this regimen. If didanosine is given with Complera or any medication containing tenofovir, the didanosine should be decreased to 250 mg daily.

Complera or any medication containing tenofovir decreases the levels of atazanavir. If given together, atazanavir must be given with ritonavir.

Complera should not be administered with any medication containing lamivudine because lamivudine and emtricitabine are both cytosine analogs and may be antagonistic.

Complera should not be administered with any medications that contain tenofovir, emtricitabine, or rilpivirine: Viread, Emtriva, Atripla, Descovy, Stribild, Genvoya, Edurant, or Odefsey.

If administered with antacids, Complera should be given 4 hours before or 2 hours after.

If administered with H2 blockers, they should be given 12 hours apart.

If Complera is coadministered with rifabutin, an additional 25 mg tablet of rilpivirine (Edurant) once per day is recommended.

 ## DOSING

Fixed dose combination of tenofovir DF 300 mg + emtricitabine 200 mg + rilpivirine 25 mg given once daily.

 ## SPECIAL POPULATIONS

RENAL IMPAIRMENT: Do not administer for estimated creatinine clearance below 50 mL per minute).

HEPATIC DYSFUNCTION: Not studied in those with child Pugh class C hepatic impairment.

PEDIATRICS: **for treatment:** Recommended for those over 12 years of age

 ## THE ART OF ANTIMICROBIAL THERAPY

Clinical Pearls

1. Complera should not be used with other agents containing tenofovir, emtricitabine, or rilpivirine: Viread, Emtriva, Atripla, Descovy, Stribild, Genvoya, Edurant, or Odefsey.
2. Complera should not be used with other nonnucleoside reverse transcriptase inhibitors, such as efavirenz, nevirapine, etravirine, or delavirdine.
3. Complera must be given with a meal of at least 533 calories.
4. Protein supplement drinks are not sufficient to ensure adequate levels of rilpivirine.
5. Do not initiate Complera in patients who have a viral load of > 100 000 copies.
6. Do not administer Complera with a proton pump inhibitor.

■ COPEGUS, REBETOL, RIBASPHERE (Ribavirin Oral)

 ## BASIC CHARACTERISTICS

Class: Nucleoside analog.

Mechanism of Action: Not known.

Mechanism of Resistance: Not known.

Metabolic Route: Ribavirin is metabolized by phosphorylation or deribosylation/hydrolysis to yield a triazole carboxylic acid metabolite and is excreted renally.

 ## FDA-APPROVED INDICATIONS

For treatment of HCV and RSV as follows:

Adult use

Copegus in combination with peginterferon alfa-2a is indicated for the treatment of adults with chronic hepatitis C virus infection who have compensated liver disease and have not been previously treated with interferon alpha.

Rebetol and **Ribasphere** are indicated in combination with interferon alfa-2b, recombinant and peginterferon alfa-2b for the treatment of chronic hepatitis C in patients 18 years of age and older with compensated liver disease.

Pediatric use

Rebetol (ribavirin, USP) capsules are indicated in combination with interferon alfa-2b for injection for the treatment of chronic hepatitis C in patients 3 years of age and older with compensated liver disease.

Also used for: Some authorities recommend consideration of ribavirin therapy for any patient with viral hemorrhagic fever caused by arenavirus (Lassa fever, New World hemorrhagic fevers) or bunyavirus (hantavirus, Rift Valley fever, Crimean–Congo hemorrhagic fever), or for suspected VHF if the etiology is unknown.

 ## SIDE EFFECTS/TOXICITY

> **WARNING:** Oral ribavirin monotherapy is not effective for the treatment of chronic hepatitis C virus infection and should not be used alone for this indication. The primary clinical toxicity of ribavirin is hemolytic anemia. The anemia associated with ribavirin therapy may result in worsening of cardiac disease that has led to fatal and nonfatal myocardial infarctions. Patients with a history of significant or unstable cardiac disease should not be treated with ribavirin.
>
> Significant teratogenic and/or embryocidal effects have been demonstrated in all animal species exposed to ribavirin. In addition, ribavirin has a multiple dose half-life of 12 days, and it may persist in nonplasma compartments for as long as 6 months. Ribavirin therapy is contraindicated in women who are pregnant and in the male partners of women who are pregnant. Extreme care must be taken to avoid pregnancy during therapy and for 6 months after completion of therapy in both female patients and in female partners of male patients who are taking ribavirin therapy. At least two reliable forms of effective contraception must be utilized during treatment and during the 6-month posttreatment follow-up period.

Ribavirin is **contraindicated** in patients with a history of hypersensitivity, autoimmune hepatitis, hemoglobinopathies (e.g., thalassemia major, sickle-cell anemia).

Other toxicities of oral ribavirin include hemolytic anemia, which may result in worsening of cardiac disease and myocardial infarctions. Patients with a history of significant or unstable cardiac disease should not be treated with ribavirin. Also seen are pancreatitis, pneumonia, dental, and periodontal disorders.

DRUG INTERACTIONS/FOOD INTERACTIONS

It is recommended to take ribavirin with food.

Coadministration of ribavirin capsules or solution and didanosine is not recommended. Use of ribavirin with zidovudine or stavudine should be used with caution.

 DOSING

Oral ribavirin is supplied in 200 mg capsules, tablets of 200, 400, and 600 mg, and a clear, colorless to pale or light yellow bubble gum-flavored liquid (40 mg/mL).

The recommended daily dose of **Rebetol** is based on body weight as follows:

Body weight	Dosing
>75 kg	600 mg twice daily
<75 kg	400 mg in the am and 600 mg in the pm

The recommended daily dose of **Ribasphere** is based on body weight as follows:

Body weight	Dosing
<66 kg	400 mg twice daily
66–80 kg	400 mg in the am and 600 mg in the pm
81–105 kg	600 mg twice daily
>105 kg	600 mg in the am and 800 mg in the pm

The recommended daily dose of **Copegus** is based on body weight and genotype:

Body weight	Genotype	Dosing
>75 kg	1, 4	600 mg twice daily
<75 kg	1, 4	400 mg in the am and 600 mg in the pm
Any weight	2, 3	400 mg twice daily
HIV coinfection	Any	400 mg twice daily

Recommended combinations with other hepatitis C virus antivirals. Please review the other medication's chapter for dose and duration of treatment:

HCV genotype or other category	Medication in addition to ribavirin
Genotype 1	Daclatasvir + sofosbuvir
	Harvoni
	Simeprevir + peg-IFN-alfa
	Sofosbuvir + peg-IFN-alfa
	Viekira pak
	Zepatier

HCV genotype or other category	Medication in addition to ribavirin
Genotype 2	Sofosbuvir
Genotype 3	Daclatasvir + sofosbuvir
	Sofosbuvir
Genotype 4	Simeprevir + peg-IFN-alfa
	Sofosbuvir + peg-IFN-alfa
	Technivie
	Zepatier
Transplant recipient	Daclatasvir + sofosbuvir (genotype 3)
	Harvoni (genotype 1 or 4)
	Viekira pak (genotype 1)
Decompensated cirrhosis	Epclusa

 ## SPECIAL POPULATIONS

RENAL IMPAIRMENT: Patients with creatinine clearance <50 mL/min should not be treated with ribavirin.

HEPATIC DYSFUNCTION: Caution should be used when administered to patients with hepatic impairment.

PEDIATRICS: Oral ribavirin is administered as follows in children 3 years and older:

Weight	Rebetol and Ribasphere	Copegus
23–33 kg	N/A	200 mg twice daily
34–46 kg	N/A	200 mg in am then 400 mg in pm
<47 kg	15 mg/kg/day	N/A
47–59 kg	400 mg twice daily	400 mg twice daily
60–73 kg	400 mg in am then 600 mg in pm	400 mg in am then 600 mg in pm
>73 kg	600 mg twice daily	600 mg twice daily

 ## THE ART OF ANTIMICROBIAL THERAPY

Clinical Pearls

1. Use caution when dosing oral ribavirin because the dose varies by brand
2. Ribavirin is pregnancy category X; women should use 2 forms of contraception for birth control. This caution extends to **men as well**.
3. Routine monitoring during therapy should include CBC, liver function tests and TSH, pregnancy tests, and ECG.
4. Many options with better tolerability exist to treat hepatitis C. Please review the most updated guidelines for current recommendations.

BASIC CHARACTERISTICS

Class: Azole.

Mechanism of Action: Inhibits the synthesis of ergosterol, a key component of the fungal cell membrane, through the inhibition of cytochrome P-450-dependent enzyme lanosterol 14-alpha-demethylase.

Mechanism of Resistance:

1. Substitutions in the target gene CYP51.
2. Changes in sterol profile.
3. Elevated efflux pump activity.

Metabolic Route: Excreted by the kidneys and in the feces.

 FDA-APPROVED INDICATIONS

Invasive aspergillosis in patients 18 years of age and older.

Invasive mucormycosis in patients 18 years of age and older.

 SIDE EFFECTS/TOXICITY

Nausea, vomiting, diarrhea, headache, hepatotoxicity, hypokalemia, constipation, dyspnea, cough, peripheral edema, and back pain. Shortened QTc interval in a concentration-related manner.

Other toxicities: infusion-related reactions, pancytopenia, atrial fibrillation, atrial flutter, bradycardia, palpitations, supraventricular extrasystoles, supraventricular tachycardia, ventricular extrasystoles, cardiac arrest, tinnitus, vertigo, optic neuropathy, abdominal distension, gastritis, gingivitis, stomatitis, catheter thrombosis, malaise, chills, cholecystitis, cholelithiasis, hepatomegaly, hepatic failure, renal failure, acute respiratory failure, hypersensitivity, hypoalbuminemia, hypoglycemia, hyponatremia, myositis, bone pain, neck pain, convulsion, dysgeusia, encephalopathy, hypoesthesia, migraine, peripheral neuropathy, paraesthesia, somnolence, stupor, syncope, tremor, confusion, hallucination, depression, hematuria, proteinuria, bronchospasm, tachypnea, alopecia, dermatitis, exfoliative dermatitis, erythema, petechiae, urticaria, thrombophlebitis.

 DRUG INTERACTIONS/FOOD INTERACTIONS

Coadministration of isavuconazole with strong CYP3A4 inhibitors such as ketoconazole or high-dose ritonavir and strong CYP3A4 inducers such as rifampin, carbamazepine, St John's wort, or long-acting barbiturates is **contraindicated**.

May be given with or without food.

 DOSING

IV: Loading dose of 1 reconstituted vial (372 mg) q 8 h for 6 doses.
   Maintenance dose: 1 reconstituted vial (372 mg) once daily.

PO: Loading dose of 2 capsules (186 mg each) q 8 h for 6 doses.
   Maintenance dose: 2 capsules (186 mg each) once daily.

Antibiotics Manual: A Guide to Commonly Used Antimicrobials, Second Edition. David Schlossberg and Rafik Samuel.
© 2017 John Wiley & Sons Ltd. Published 2017 by John Wiley & Sons Ltd.

SPECIAL POPULATIONS

RENAL IMPAIRMENT: No dose adjustment is needed.

HEPATIC DYSFUNCTION: Isavuconazole has not been studied in patients with severe hepatic dysfunction and should be used in these patients only when the benefits outweigh the risks.

PEDIATRIC: Safety and effectiveness in pediatric patients younger than 18 years has not been established.

 THE ART OF ANTIMICROBIAL THERAPY

Clinical Pearls

1. There is no information regarding cross-sensitivity between isavuconazole and other azole antifungal agents.
2. *In vitro* and animal studies suggest cross-resistance between isavuconazole and other azoles. The relevance of cross-resistance to clinical outcome has not been fully characterized. However, patients failing prior azole therapy may require alternative antifungal therapy.
3. Isavuconazole is **contraindicated** in people with familial shortened QT.

BASIC CHARACTERISTICS

Class: Cyclic lipopeptide.

Mechanism of Action: Binds to bacterial membranes and causes a rapid depolarization of membrane potential resulting in bacterial cell death.

Mechanisms of Resistance: Not fully understood. However, increasing MICs in *S. aureus* have been reported while receiving daptomycin.

Metabolic Route: Excreted unchanged in the urine.

 ## FDA-APPROVED INDICATIONS

Complicated skin and skin structure infections (cSSSIs) caused by susceptible gram-positive organisms.

Staphylococcus aureus **bloodstream infections** (bacteremia), including those with right-sided infective endocarditis.

 ## SIDE EFFECTS/TOXICITY

Anaphylaxis, rash, rhabdomyolysis, arrhythmias, blurred vision, oral and vaginal candidiasis, gram-negative infections, *Clostridium difficile*-associated diarrhea (CDAD), abnormal liver function tests, elevated CPK (daptomycin should be discontinued in symptomatic patients with CPK elevation >1000 U/L or in patients without reported symptoms who have marked elevations in CPK >2000 U/L), peripheral neuropathy, and thrombocytopenia.

 ## DRUG INTERACTIONS/FOOD INTERACTIONS

Caution is warranted when daptomycin is coadministered with tobramycin.

Daptomycin can cause a false prolongation of prothrombin time (PT) and elevation of the international normalized ratio (INR); it is recommended that the PT/INR be repeated with blood drawn just prior to the next dose of daptomycin. If still elevated, PT should be evaluated with an alternative method if possible and other causes of prolonged PT should be sought.

Consideration should be given to temporarily suspending use of HMG-CoA reductase inhibitors.

 ## DOSING

Disease state	Dose
Complicated skin and skin structure infections	4 mg/kg IV daily for 7 to 14 days
Staphylococcus aureus bloodstream infections	6 mg/kg IV daily for 2 to 6 weeks

 ## SPECIAL POPULATIONS

RENAL IMPAIRMENT: The same dose is administered to those with a creatinine clearance <30 mL/min but is given every 48 hours. This includes those on hemodialysis, CAPD, and CRRT.

Antibiotics Manual: A Guide to Commonly Used Antimicrobials, Second Edition. David Schlossberg and Rafik Samuel.
© 2017 John Wiley & Sons Ltd. Published 2017 by John Wiley & Sons Ltd.

HEPATIC DYSFUNCTION: No dose adjustment is necessary.

PEDIATRICS: Safety and efficacy in patients under the age of 18 have not been established.

 ## THE ART OF ANTIMICROBIAL THERAPY

Clinical Pearls
1. Daptomycin should be renally adjusted.
2. CPK should be monitored while receiving daptomycin.
3. Daptomycin may cause false elevation of PT/INR results.
4. Increased MIC in *S. aureus* may develop while on daptomycin therapy.
5. Daptomycin should not be used to treat pneumonia in view of the high failure rate.
6. Daptomycin is not indicated for the treatment of left-sided endocarditis.

BASIC CHARACTERISTICS

Class: Nucleoside analog.

Mechanism of Action: Ganciclovir is a synthetic guanine nucleoside analog of 2'-deoxyguanosine that inhibits replication of herpes viruses. Ganciclovir is active against CMV and HSV. Ganciclovir is phosphorylated and it inhibits viral DNA synthesis by (1) competitive inhibition of viral DNA polymerases and (2) incorporation into viral DNA, resulting in eventual termination of viral DNA elongation.

Mechanism of Resistance: Resistance to ganciclovir in CMV is due to decreased ability to form the active triphosphate moiety; resistant viruses have been described that contain mutations in the UL97 gene of CMV that controls phosphorylation of ganciclovir. Mutations in the viral DNA polymerase have also been reported to confer viral resistance to ganciclovir.

Metabolic Route: Ganciclovir is excreted in the urine.

 FDA-APPROVED INDICATIONS

Ganciclovir IV is indicated for the treatment of CMV retinitis in immunocompromised patients and the prevention of CMV disease in transplant recipients.

Also used for: Ganciclovir has routinely been used for the treatment of CMV pneumonia, gastroenteritis, and disseminated disease in transplant recipients.

Ganciclovir capsules are indicated for prevention of CMV disease in transplant recipients and HIV infected patients. It is also considered an alternative agent for treatment of stable CMV retinitis.

 SIDE EFFECTS/TOXICITY

> **WARNING:** The clinical toxicity of ganciclovir includes granulocytopenia, anemia, and thrombocytopenia. In animal studies ganciclovir was carcinogenic, teratogenic, and caused aspermogenesis.
>
> Ganciclovir for injection is indicated for use only in the treatment of CMV retinitis in immunocompromised patients and for the prevention of CMV disease in transplant patients at risk for CMV disease.
>
> Ganciclovir capsules are indicated only for prevention of CMV disease in patients with advanced HIV infection at risk for CMV disease, for maintenance treatment of CMV retinitis in immunocompromised patients, and for prevention of CMV disease in solid organ transplant recipients.
>
> Because ganciclovir capsules are associated with a risk of more rapid rate of CMV retinitis progression, they should be used as maintenance treatment only in those patients for whom this risk is balanced by benefit associated with avoiding daily intravenous infusions.

Other adverse events include fever, hepatic and renal dysfunction, stomatitis, diarrhea, vomiting, intestinal perforation, pancreatitis, pulmonary fibrosis, seizures, neuropathy, tinnitus, torsades de pointes, sweating, and pruritus.

 DRUG INTERACTIONS/FOOD INTERACTIONS

Ganciclovir capsules are poorly absorbed and should be administered with food.

Antibiotics Manual: A Guide to Commonly Used Antimicrobials, Second Edition. David Schlossberg and Rafik Samuel.
© 2017 John Wiley & Sons Ltd. Published 2017 by John Wiley & Sons Ltd.

Drug interactions: Both zidovudine and ganciclovir have the potential to cause neutropenia and anemia; some patients may not tolerate concomitant therapy with these drugs at full dosage. Generalized seizures have been reported in patients who received ganciclovir and imipenem-cilastatin. These drugs should not be used concomitantly unless the potential benefits outweigh the risks.

Because of the possibility of additive toxicity, drugs such as dapsone, pentamidine, flucytosine, vincristine, vinblastine, adriamycin, amphotericin B, trimethoprim/sulfamethoxazole combinations, or other nucleoside analogs, should be considered for concomitant use with ganciclovir only if the potential benefits are judged to outweigh the risks.

Increases in serum creatinine were observed in patients treated with ganciclovir plus either cyclosporine or amphotericin B, drugs with known potential for nephrotoxicity.

DOSING

Ganciclovir IV

For freatment of CMV retinitis in patients with normal renal function:

Induction treatment: The drug is given as a constant rate infusion over one hour.

The recommended initial dosage for patients with normal renal function is 5 mg/kg intravenously every 12 hours for 14 to 21 days.

Maintenance treatment: Following induction treatment, the recommended maintenance dosage of ganciclovir is 5 mg/kg intravenously given once daily, 7 days per week, or 6 mg/kg once daily, 5 days per week.

For the prevention of CMV disease in transplant recipients with normal renal function:

The recommended initial dosage of ganciclovir for patients with normal renal function is 5 mg/kg intravenously every 12 hours for 7 to 14 days, followed by 5 mg/kg once daily, 7 days per week or 6 mg/kg once daily, 5 days per week.

The duration of treatment with in transplant recipients is dependent upon the duration and degree of immunosuppression.

Ganciclovir capsules

Ganciclovir is supplied as 250 mg and 500 mg capsules. The usual dose is 1000 mg tid.

SPECIAL POPULATIONS

RENAL IMPAIRMENT:

Ganciclovir IV

Creatinine Clearance, mL/min	Induction dose, mg/kg	Maintenance dose, mg/kg
≥70	5 mg/kg q 12 hours	5 mg/kg q day
50–69	2.5 mg/kg q 12 hours	2.5 mg/kg q day
25–49	2.5 mg/kg/day	1.25 mg/kg q day
10–24	1.25 mg/kg/day	0.625 mg/kg q day
Hemodialysis	1.25 mg/kg/after HD	0.625 mg/kg after hemodialysis
CRRT dose	2.5 mg/kg q 12 hours	2.5 mg/kg q day

Ganciclovir capsules

Creatinine Clearance, mL/min	Dose
≥80	1000 mg TID
50–79	500 mg TID
25–49	500 mg BID
10–24	500 mg daily
Hemodialysis	500 mg three times a week administered after dialysis

HEPATIC DYSFUNCTION: No dose adjustment is needed.

PEDIATRICS: Ganciclovir has not been studied in pediatric patients.

 THE ART OF ANTIMICROBIAL THERAPY

Clinical Pearls

1. Ganciclovir should not be administered if the absolute neutrophil count is less than 500 cells/μL or the platelet count is less than 25 000 cells/μL.
2. Ganciclovir is effective against HSV, VZV, and CMV. It may also have activity against EBV and HHV8, although its FDA-approved indications are for specific HSV and CMV infections, as detailed above.
3. Oral ganciclovir is not well absorbed; if using an oral therapy, valganciclovir is more reliable.
4. For those with CMV resistance or if ganciclovir is contraindicated, foscarnet is recommended for treatment.

DAKLINZA (Daclatasvir)

BASIC CHARACTERISTICS

Class: Inhibitor of HCV nonstructural protein 5A (NS5A).

Mechanism of Action: Daclatasvir binds to the N-terminus of NS5A and inhibits both viral RNA replication and virion assembly.

Mechanism of Resistance: Alterations in the structure of the NS5A protein allows replication to continue in the presence of daclatasvir. The mutations leading to resistance include the M28T, Q30E, Q30H, Q30R, L31V, Y93C, Y93H, and Y93N substitutions.

Metabolic Route: Metabolized by CYP3A4 enzymes in the liver.

FDA-APPROVED INDICATIONS

Daclatasvir is indicated for use with sofosbuvir, with or without ribavirin, for the treatment of patients with chronic hepatitis C virus (HCV) genotype 1 or genotype 3 infection.

SIDE EFFECTS/TOXICITY

Patients taking daclatasvir in combination with sofosbuvir and amiodarone are at high risk for symptomatic bradycardia.

Other side effects include: fatigue, headache, nausea, diarrhea, rash, and somnolence.

DRUG INTERACTIONS/FOOD INTERACTIONS

Daclatasvir may be taken without regard to food.

When daclatasvir is used in combination with other agents, the contraindications applicable to those agents are applicable to combination therapies.

Do not coadminister daclatasvir with rifampin, St John's wort, carbamazepine, phenytoin, or amiodarone.

Decrease the dose of daclatasvir to 30 mg daily if combined with: clarithromycin, itraconazole, ketoconazole, nefazodone, posaconazole, telithromycin, voriconazole, atazanavir + ritonavir, indinavir, nelfinavir, saquinavir, or cobicistat.

Increase the dose of daclatasvir to 90 mg daily if combined with: efavirenz, etravirine, nevirapine, bosentan, dexamethasone, modafinil, nafcillin, rifabutin, or rifapentine.

DOSING

Daclatasvir comes in 30 mg, 60 mg, and 90 mg tablets. The usual dose is 60 mg, taken orally, once daily, with or without food.

Patient population	Medication	Duration
Genotype 1 without cirrhosis or with compensated cirrhosis	Daclatasvir + sofosbuvir	12 weeks
Genotype 1 with decompensated cirrhosis or post-transplant	Daclatasvir + sofosbuvir + ribavirin	12 weeks
Genotype 3 without cirrhosis	Daclatasvir + sofosbuvir	12 weeks
Genotype 3 with compensated or decompensated cirrhosis or post-transplant	Daclatasvir + Sofosbuvir + ribavirin	12 weeks

Antibiotics Manual: A Guide to Commonly Used Antimicrobials, Second Edition. David Schlossberg and Rafik Samuel.
© 2017 John Wiley & Sons Ltd. Published 2017 by John Wiley & Sons Ltd.

SPECIAL POPULATIONS

RENAL IMPAIRMENT: No dose adjustment necessary.

HEPATIC DYSFUNCTION: No dose adjustment necessary.

PEDIATRICS: Do not use in patients under 18 years of age.

 THE ART OF ANTIMICROBIAL THERAPY

Clinical Pearls

1. Daclatasvir is active against HCV genotypes 1 and 3 only.
2. Screen for the presence of NS5A polymorphisms in patients **with cirrhosis** who are infected with HCV genotype 1a prior to the initiation of treatment with daclatasvir and sofosbuvir with or without ribavirin.
3. Screen for the presence of NS5A polymorphisms in **all** patients infected with HCV genotype 3 prior to the initiation of treatment with daclatasvir and sofosbuvir with or without ribavirin.
4. Response to treatment is reduced in HCV genotype 3-infected patients with cirrhosis receiving daclatasvir in combination with sofosbuvir for 12 weeks
5. Significant bradycardia has been reported if daclatasvir is administered with sofosbuvir and amiodarone.
6. Review the most current hepatitis C treatment guidelines because they are changing rapidly: http://www.cdc.gov/hepatitis/HCV/index.hcm

■ DALVANCE (Dalbavancin)

 BASIC CHARACTERISTICS

Class: Glycopeptide.

Mechanism of Action: Inhibits bacterial cell-wall formation by blocking the transglycosylation step in peptidoglycan biosynthesis by direct interaction with the terminal D-Ala–D-Ala dipeptidyl residues of peptidoglycan precursors.

Mechanisms of Resistance: Resistance has not been observed at this time.

Metabolic Route: 20 % excreted in feces, 33 % excreted in urine unchanged.

 FDA-APPROVED INDICATIONS

Acute bacterial skin and skin structure infections (ABSSSI) caused by susceptible staphylococci (including MRSA) and streptococci.

 SIDE EFFECTS/TOXICITY

Contraindicated in patients with hypersensitivity to dalbavancin. Possible cross-allergenicity with other glycopeptides, including vancomycin.

Rapid infusions can cause Red Man syndrome.

Clostridium difficile-associated diarrhea, nausea, headache, diarrhea, rash, anemia, leucopenia, thrombocytopenia, petechiae, eosinophilia, thrombocytosis, gastrointestinal hemorrhage, melena, hematochezia, abdominal pain, hepatotoxicity, anaphylactoid reaction, oral candidiasis, vulvovaginal mycotic infection, hypoglycemia, dizziness, bronchospasm, urticaria, flushing, phlebitis, wound hemorrhage, spontaneous hematoma.

 DRUG INTERACTIONS/FOOD INTERACTIONS

Minimal potential for drug–drug interactions with cytochrome P450 (CYP450) substrates, inhibitors, or inducers. Dalbavancin at therapeutic concentrations does not artificially prolong prothrombin time (PT) or activated partial thromboplastin time (aPTT).

 DOSING

1000 mg followed one week later by 500 mg IV or 1500 mg as a single dose.

Administration should be by intravenous infusion over 30 minutes.

 SPECIAL POPULATIONS

RENAL IMPAIRMENT:

Creatine clearance	Doses
<30 mL/min	750 mg followed one week later by 375 mg (2-dose regimen) or 1125 mg (single-dose regimen)
Hemodialysis patients	Usual doses, without regard for timing of hemodialysis

Antibiotics Manual: A Guide to Commonly Used Antimicrobials, Second Edition. David Schlossberg and Rafik Samuel.
© 2017 John Wiley & Sons Ltd. Published 2017 by John Wiley & Sons Ltd.

HEPATIC DYSFUNCTION: No dose adjustment is necessary for mild impairment; use caution for moderate or severe hepatic impairment (Child Pugh class B or C).

PEDIATRICS: Safety and effectiveness in pediatric patients have not been established.

 ## THE ART OF ANTIMICROBIAL THERAPY

Clinical Pearls

1. Infrequent dosing possible due to long half-life: 8.5 days.
2. Cross-hypersensitivity with other glycopeptides possible.
3. 30 minute infusion time minimizes risk of Red Man syndrome.

BASIC CHARACTERISTICS

Class: Sulfone.

Mechanism of Action: Inhibits bacterial dihydropteroate synthase.

Mechanisms of Resistance:

1. Overproduction of PABA.
2. Production of drug-resistant dihydropteroate synthase.
3. Decrease in cell permeability of Dapsone.

Metabolic Route: Dapsone is excreted in the urine.

 FDA-APPROVED INDICATIONS

Dermatitis herpetiformis.

Leprosy: all forms except for cases of proven Dapsone resistance.

Also Used for:

Alternative prophylaxis for *Pneumocystis jirovecii*.

Alternate treatment of PCP (with trimethoprim).

Alternative prophylaxis for toxoplasmosis (with pyrimethamine and leucovorin).

 SIDE EFFECTS/TOXICITY

Hemolysis (especially in those with G6PD deficiency), peripheral neuropathy, nausea, vomiting, abdominal pains, pancreatitis, vertigo, blurred vision, tinnitus, insomnia, fever, headache, psychosis, phototoxicity, pulmonary eosinophilia, tachycardia, albuminuria, nephrotic syndrome, hypoalbuminemia, renal papillary necrosis, male infertility, drug-induced lupus erythematosus, cutaneous reactions, hepatitis, cholestatic jaundice, agranulocytosis, aplastic anemia, methemoglobinemia.

 DRUG INTERACTIONS/FOOD INTERACTIONS

Dapsone can be taken with or without food.

Rifampin lowers dapsone levels but (in leprosy) no adjustment is necessary.

Folic acid antagonists such as pyrimethamine may increase the likelihood of hematologic reactions.

 DOSING

PCP prophylaxis: 100 mg daily.

PCP treatment: 100 mg daily (plus trimethoprim 15 mg/kg/day).

Toxoplasmosis prophylaxis: 50 mg daily (plus pyrimethamine 50 mg weekly and leucovorin 25 mg weekly).

Antibiotics Manual: A Guide to Commonly Used Antimicrobials, Second Edition. David Schlossberg and Rafik Samuel.
© 2017 John Wiley & Sons Ltd. Published 2017 by John Wiley & Sons Ltd.

For leprosy: In bacteriologically negative **tuberculoid** and indeterminate disease, the recommendation is the coadministration of Dapsone 100 mg daily with six months of rifampin 600 mg daily. Then dapsone should be continued for an additional three years for tuberculoid and indeterminate patients and for five years for borderline tuberculoid patients.

In **lepromatous** and borderline lepromatous patients, the recommendation is the coadministration of Dapsone 100 mg daily with two years of rifampin 600 mg daily. Dapsone 100 mg daily is continued for 3–10 years until all signs of clinical activity are controlled with skin scrapings and biopsies negative for one year. Dapsone should then be continued for an additional 10 years for borderline patients and for life for lepromatous patients.

 ## SPECIAL POPULATIONS

RENAL IMPAIRMENT: No adjustment is necessary.

HEPATIC DYSFUNCTION: No dose adjustment is necessary.

PEDIATRICS:

PCP prophylaxis: 2 mg/kg (maximum 100 mg).

Toxoplasma prophylaxis: 2 mg/kg with pyrimethamine 1 mg/kg daily, plus leucovorin 5 mg q 3 days.

 ## THE ART OF ANTIMICROBIAL THERAPY

Clinical Pearls

1. Dapsone should be used in combination with one or more antileprosy drugs when treating leprosy.
2. Dapsone should not be used in patients who are G6PD deficient.

BASIC CHARACTERISTICS

Class: Folic acid antagonist.

Mechanism of Action: Folic acid antagonist.

Metabolic Route: Data incomplete.

 ## FDA-APPROVED INDICATIONS

Treatment of toxoplasmosis when used conjointly with a sulfonamide.

An alternative treatment of acute malaria with a sulfonamide.

Indicated for the chemoprophylaxis of malaria due to susceptible strains of plasmodia.

Also Used for: Prophylaxis of toxoplasmosis (with dapsone) in patients with HIV who cannot tolerate trimethoprim/sulfamethoxazole.

 ## SIDE EFFECTS/TOXICITY

Contraindicated in patients with known hypersensitivity to pyrimethamine or in patients with documented megaloblastic anemia due to folate deficiency. Hypersensitivity reactions, occasionally severe (such as Stevens–Johnson syndrome, toxic epidermal necrolysis, erythema multiforme, and anaphylaxis), hyperphenylalaninemia, anorexia, vomiting, atrophic glossitis, hematuria, arrhythmias, pulmonary eosinophilia, megaloblastic anemia, leukopenia, thrombocytopenia, and pancytopenia.

 ## DRUG INTERACTIONS/FOOD INTERACTIONS

Pyrimethamine should be taken with food to decrease side effects.

The concomitant use of other antifolic drugs including sulfonamides or trimethoprim–sulfamethoxazole combinations, proguanil, zidovudine, or cytostatic agents (e.g., methotrexate) may increase the risk of bone marrow suppression.

 ## DOSING

For treatment of toxoplasmosis

Starting dose is 50 to 75 mg of the drug daily for 1 to 3 weeks. Then half the dose previously given and continued for an additional 4 to 5 weeks.

For treatment of acute malaria

25 mg daily for 2 days with a sulfonamide will initiate transmission control and suppression of nonfalciparum malaria.

Should circumstances arise wherein pyrimethamine must be used alone in semi-immune persons, the adult dosage for acute malaria is 50 mg for 2 days.

For chemoprophylaxis of malaria

25 mg (1 tablet) once weekly

Antibiotics Manual: A Guide to Commonly Used Antimicrobials, Second Edition. David Schlossberg and Rafik Samuel.
© 2017 John Wiley & Sons Ltd. Published 2017 by John Wiley & Sons Ltd.

SPECIAL POPULATIONS

RENAL IMPAIRMENT: Use with caution.

HEPATIC DYSFUNCTION: Use with caution.

PEDIATRICS:

For toxoplasmosis

1 mg/kg/day divided into 2 equal daily doses; after 2 to 4 days this dose may be reduced to one half and continued for approximately 1 month.

For chemoprophylaxis of malaria

Pediatric patients over 10 years: 25 mg (1 tablet) once weekly.

Children 4 through 10 years: 12.5 mg (1/2 tablet) once weekly.

Infants and children under 4 years: 6.25 mg (1/4 tablet) once weekly.

 THE ART OF ANTIMICROBIAL THERAPY

Clinical Pearls

1. The action of pyrimethamine is enhanced when used with sulfa compounds.
2. Most Plasmodia around the world are resistant to pyrimethamine.
3. Folinic acid (leucovorin) should be administered in a dosage of 5 to 15 mg daily (orally, IV, or IM) to all patients receiving pyrimethamine.

DELTYBA (Delamanid)

BASIC CHARACTERISTICS

Class: Nitroimidazo-oxazole.

Mechanism of Action: Inhibits mycolic acid biosynthesis.

Mechanisms of Resistance: Limited information.

Metabolic Route: Primarily metabolized in plasma by albumin. Minimal metabolism in liver.

FDA-APPROVED INDICATIONS

Not available in the USA; approved by European Medicines Agency (EMA) for the treatment of MDR-TB.

SIDE EFFECTS/TOXICITY

Nausea, vomiting, dizziness, insomnia, abdominal pain, QTc prolongation.

Use with drugs that prolong the QT interval may cause additive QT prolongation. Monitor ECGs.

DRUG INTERACTIONS/FOOD INTERACTIONS

Delamanid exposure may be reduced during coadministration with inducers of CYP3A4 and increased during coadministration with inhibitors of CYP3A4.

Concomitant administration of strong CYP3A inducers should be avoided.

Should be taken with food.

DOSING

Adults: 100 mg twice daily for 24 weeks.

Children: Insufficient data. Safety and efficacy for children under 18 not established.

SPECIAL POPULATIONS

RENAL IMPAIRMENT: No adjustment needed for mild to moderate renal impairment; not recommended for severe renal impairment.

HEPATIC DYSFUNCTION: No adjustment necessary for mild impairment; not recommended for moderate to severe hepatic impairment. **Contraindicated** if serum albumin < 2.8 g/mL.

PEDIATRICS: Safety and effectiveness in patients under 18 not established.

Antibiotics Manual: A Guide to Commonly Used Antimicrobials, Second Edition. David Schlossberg and Rafik Samuel.
© 2017 John Wiley & Sons Ltd. Published 2017 by John Wiley & Sons Ltd.

THE ART OF ANTIMICROBIAL THERAPY

Clinical Pearls

1. Contraindicated with serum albumin < 2.8 g/mL because of increased risk of QTc prolongation.

2. Avoid if patient is taking other medications that are strong inducers of CYP3A, e.g., rifamycins.

3. EKG should be done before starting delamanid. If baseline QTc is prolonged, delamanid should not be given unless potential benefits outweigh the risks. All patients should have EKG monitored throughout treatment.

DESCOVY (Tenofovir Alafenamide + Emtricitabine)

 BASIC CHARACTERISTICS

Class: Nucleotide reverse transcriptase inhibitor + nucleoside reverse transcriptase inhibitor.

Mechanism of Action: Tenofovir and emtricitabine are converted by cellular enzymes to their active drugs tenofovir biphosphate (an analog of adenosine triphosphate) and emtricitabine triphosphate (an analog of cytosine triphosphate). These drugs compete with the naturally occurring nucleotides for incorporation in newly forming HIV DNA. Since they do not have a terminal hydroxyl group, they halt transcription and replication of the virus.

Mechanism of Resistance: Changes in the structure of HIV reverse transcriptase leads to preferred incorporation of adenosine triphosphate and cytosine triphosphate with decreased incorporation of tenofovir biphosphate and emtricitabine triphosphate, which allows transcription of DNA to continue. Resistance mutations include K65R, M184V, and "TAMS": 41 L, 67 N, 70R, 210 W, 215 F, and 219E.

Metabolic Route: Tenofovir and emtricitabine are excreted in the urine unchanged.

 FDA-APPROVED INDICATIONS

Treatment of HIV-1 in combination with other antiretrovirals.

 SIDE EFFECTS/TOXICITY

> **WARNING: Lactic acidosis and severe hepatomegaly** with steatosis, including fatal cases, have been reported with the use of nucleoside analogs.
>
> Descovy is not approved for the treatment of chronic hepatitis B virus (HBV) infection. Severe acute exacerbations of hepatitis B have been reported in patients who are coinfected with HIV-1 and HBV and have discontinued products containing emtricitabine (FTC) and/or tenofovir disoproxil fumarate (TDF), and may occur with discontinuation of Descovy. Hepatic function should be monitored closely in these patients. If appropriate, initiation of anti-hepatitis B therapy may be warranted.

Other adverse events: Immune reconstitution inflammatory syndrome, fat redistribution including central obesity and dorsocervical fat enlargement, peripheral wasting, facial wasting, breast enlargement, renal impairment, including acute renal failure and Fanconi syndrome, decreased bone mineral density, and nausea.

 DRUG INTERACTIONS/FOOD INTERACTIONS

Descovy can be taken with or without food.

Descovy should not be administered with tipranavir, rifampin, rifabutin, rifapentine, St John's wort, carbamazepine, oxcarbazepine, phenobarbital, or phenytoin.

Descovy should not be administered with any medication containing lamivudine because lamivudine and emtricitabine are both cytosine analogs and may be antagonistic.

Descovy contains both tenofovir and emtricitabine and should not be administered with Viread, Emtriva, Atripla, Complera, Odefsey, Stribild, or Genvoya.

Antibiotics Manual: A Guide to Commonly Used Antimicrobials, Second Edition. David Schlossberg and Rafik Samuel.
© 2017 John Wiley & Sons Ltd. Published 2017 by John Wiley & Sons Ltd.

DOSING

Descovy is a fixed dose tablet containing 25 mg of tenofovir and 200 mg of emtricitabine. The recommended adult dose is one tablet once daily.

 SPECIAL POPULATIONS

RENAL IMPAIRMENT: Descovy should not be administered in patients with a creatinine clearance under 30 mL/min.

HEPATIC DYSFUNCTION: No dose adjustment is necessary.

PEDIATRICS: Descovy has not been studied in children.

 THE ART OF ANTIMICROBIAL THERAPY

Clinical Pearls

1. Descovy should be used in combination with other antiretroviral agents.
2. Descovy contains both tenofovir and emtricitabine and should not be administered with Viread, Emtriva, Atripla, Complera, Odefsey, Stribild, or Genvoya.
3. Patients with HIV-1 should be tested for hepatitis B virus before initiating antiretroviral therapy with Descovy.
4. Descovy is not recommended for preexposure prophylaxis.
5. Descovy is not indicated for the treatment of hepatitis B.
6. Descovy is significantly smaller in size than Truvada.

DICLOXACILLIN

 BASIC CHARACTERISTICS

Class: Semisynthetic penicillin.

Mechanism of Action: Binds penicillin-binding protein, disrupting cell wall synthesis.

Mechanisms of Resistance:

1. The PBP can be altered, with reduced affinity.

2. Production of a beta-lactamase, resulting in hydrolysis of the beta-lactam ring.

3. Decreased ability of the antibiotic to reach the PBP when bacteria decrease porin production, resulting in reduced drug concentration within the cell.

Metabolic Route: Excreted as unchanged drug in the urine.

 FDA-APPROVED INDICATIONS

Dicloxacillin is indicated in the treatment of infections caused by susceptible penicillinase-producing staphylococci.

 SIDE EFFECTS/TOXICITY

A history of allergic reaction to any of the penicillins is a **contraindication.**

Side effects include *Clostridium difficile*-associated diarrhea (CDAD), interstitial nephritis including rash, fever, eosinophilia, hematuria, proteinuria and renal insufficiency, esophageal ulceration, thrombophlebitis, hypersensitivity reactions including rash, erythema multiforme, and Stevens–Johnson syndrome, hepatitis, nausea, vomiting, diarrhea, stomatitis, black or hairy tongue, hyperactivity and seizures, anemia, thrombocytopenia, neutropenia, and eosinophilia.

 DRUG INTERACTIONS/FOOD INTERACTIONS

Dicloxacillin is best absorbed when taken on an empty stomach and should be administered at least 1 hour before or 2 hours after meals. Chloramphenicol, macrolides, sulfonamides, and tetracyclines may interfere with the bactericidal effects of penicillins.

When dicloxacillin and warfarin are used concomitantly, the prothrombin time should be closely monitored. High urine concentrations of dicloxacillin may result in false-positive reactions when testing for the presence of glucose in urine using *Clinitest®*. It is recommended that glucose tests based on enzymatic glucose oxidase reactions (such as *Clinistix®*) be used.

DOSING

Dicloxacillin is supplied as 250 mg and 500 mg capsules.

Mild to moderate infections: 125 mg q 6 hours

Severe infections: 250 mg q 6 hours

Antibiotics Manual: A Guide to Commonly Used Antimicrobials, Second Edition. David Schlossberg and Rafik Samuel.
© 2017 John Wiley & Sons Ltd. Published 2017 by John Wiley & Sons Ltd.

SPECIAL POPULATIONS

RENAL IMPAIRMENT: No dose adjustment is necessary.

HEPATIC DYSFUNCTION: No dose adjustment is necessary.

COMBINED RENAL AND HEPATIC INSUFFICIENCY: Measurement of dicloxacillin serum levels should be performed and dosage adjusted accordingly.

PEDIATRICS: Dicloxacillin should be avoided in the neonate.
Mild to moderate infections: 12.5 mg/kg q 6 hours
Severe infections: 25 mg/kg q 6 hours

 THE ART OF ANTIMICROBIAL THERAPY

Clinical Pearls
1. Dicloxacillin does not need to be dose adjusted for renal dysfunction.
2. Dicloxacillin should be used with caution in patients with both renal and hepatic insufficiency.
3. Dicloxacillin should be taken with at least 4 fluid ounces (120 mL) of water and should not be taken in the supine position or immediately before going to bed.
4. Dicloxacillin should be taken on an empty stomach.

■ DIFICID (Fidaxomicin)

 BASIC CHARACTERISTICS

Class: Macrolide.

Mechanism of Action: Acts locally in the gastrointestinal tract. Bactericidal against *C. difficile in vitro*, inhibiting RNA synthesis by RNA polymerases.

Mechanisms of Resistance: Unknown.

Metabolic Route: Mainly excreted in feces.

 FDA-APPROVED INDICATIONS

Treatment of *Clostridium difficile*-associated diarrhea (CDAD).

 SIDE EFFECTS/TOXICITY

Toxicity includes **nausea**, **vomiting**, **abdominal pain**, **gastrointestinal hemorrhage**, **anemia**, **neutropenia**, hypersensitivity reactions, abdominal distension, abdominal tenderness, dyspepsia, dysphagia, flatulence, intestinal obstruction, megacolon, increased blood alkaline phosphatase, decreased blood bicarbonate, increased hepatic enzymes, decreased platelet count, hyperglycemia, and metabolic acidosis.

 DRUG INTERACTIONS/FOOD INTERACTIONS

Fidaxomicin tablets may be taken with or without food.

 DOSING

One 200 mg tablet orally twice daily for 10 days.

 SPECIAL POPULATIONS

RENAL IMPAIRMENT: No dose adjustment is recommended.

HEPATIC DYSFUNCTION: No dose adjustment is recommended.

PEDIATRICS: Safety and effectiveness in pediatric patients has not been studied in patients <18.

THE ART OF ANTIMICROBIAL THERAPY

Clinical Pearls

1. Fidaxomicin should not be used for systemic infections.
2. In clinical studies, fidaxomicin is associated with less recurrence and relapse than other agents for the treatment of *C. difficile* infection.
3. Fidaxomicin has less effect on the GI flora than other treatments for *C. difficile* infection.

Antibiotics Manual: A Guide to Commonly Used Antimicrobials, Second Edition. David Schlossberg and Rafik Samuel.
© 2017 John Wiley & Sons Ltd. Published 2017 by John Wiley & Sons Ltd.

BASIC CHARACTERISTICS

Class: Triazole.

Mechanism of Action: Inhibition of lanosterol 14-α-demethylase, which is involved in the synthesis of ergosterol, an essential component of fungal cell membranes.

Mechanisms of Resistance:

1. Point mutations in the gene (*ERG11*) encoding for the target enzyme lead to an altered target with decreased affinity for azoles.

2. Overexpression of *ERG11* results in the production of high concentrations of the target enzyme, creating the need for higher intracellular drug concentrations to inhibit all of the enzyme molecules in the cell.

3. Active efflux of fluconazole out of the cell through the activation of two types of multidrug efflux transporters.

Metabolic Route: Fluconazole can be administered orally or intravenously. It can be taken with or without food. It is metabolized by the liver; however, up to 22 % can be excreted unchanged in the urine.

 FDA-APPROVED INDICATIONS

Vaginal candidiasis, oropharyngeal and esophageal candidiasis, *Candida* urinary tract infections, peritonitis, candidemia, disseminated candidiasis, *Candida* pneumonia, cryptococcal meningitis, and prophylaxis of candidiasis in patients undergoing bone marrow transplantation who receive cytotoxic chemotherapy or radiation therapy.

Also Used for: *Coccidioides immitis* infections including meningitis.

 SIDE EFFECTS/TOXICITY

Fluconazole is contraindicated in patients who have shown hypersensitivity to fluconazole or to any of its excipients.

Hepatic toxicity, anaphylaxis and exfoliative skin disorder, prolongation of the QT interval and torsades de pointes, nausea, vomiting, abdominal pain, leukopenia, thrombocytopenia, hypercholesterolemia, hypertriglyceridemia, hypokalemia, and taste perversion.

 DRUG INTERACTIONS

Fluconazole can be taken with or without food.

Fluconazole is an inhibitor of the cytochrome p450-3A4; caution should be used when using fluconazole with other drugs that are metabolized by p450-3A4 as the serum levels of the coadministered drugs may be elevated.

Contraindicated with cisapride, astemizole, pimozide, voriconazole, or quinidine.

Monitor for toxicity if used with alfentanil, amitryptiline, benzodiazepines, calcium channel blockers, cyclophosphamide, cyclosporine, fentanyl, hydrochlorothiazide, losartan, oral hypoglycemics, oral contraceptives, nortryptiline, phenytoin, prednisone, rifabutin, saquinavir, sirolimus, tacrolimus, theophylin, or warfarin.

Fluconazole levels may be decreased if given with rifampin or rifabutin.

Antibiotics Manual: A Guide to Commonly Used Antimicrobials, Second Edition. David Schlossberg and Rafik Samuel.
© 2017 John Wiley & Sons Ltd. Published 2017 by John Wiley & Sons Ltd.

Terfenadine: The combined use of fluconazole at doses of 400 mg or greater with terfenadine is **contraindicated**. The coadministration of fluconazole at doses lower than 400 mg/day with terfenadine should be carefully monitored for QTc prolongation and dysrhythmias.

 DOSING

Fluconazole is supplied in 50 mg, 100 mg, 150 mg, and 200 mg tablets. It is also supplied as an oral suspension with 350 mg or 1400 mg per 350 mL.

Vaginal candidiasis: 150 mg as a single oral dose.

The following regimens utilize the same dose, either oral or intravenous:

Oropharyngeal candidiasis: 200 mg on the first day, followed by 100 mg once daily for 2 weeks.

Esophageal candidiasis: 200 mg on the first day, followed by 100 mg once daily. Doses up to 400 mg/day may be used for a minimum of three weeks and for at least two weeks following resolution of symptoms.

Systemic *Candida* infections: 800 mg on the first day followed by 400 mg daily. Duration of therapy has not been determined.

Urinary tract infections and peritonitis: 50–200 mg may be used.

Cryptococcal meningitis: 400 mg on the first day, followed by 200 mg once daily. A dosage of 400 mg once daily may be used based on medical judgment of the patient's response to therapy for 10–12 weeks after the cerebrospinal fluid becomes culture negative. The recommended dosage for suppression of relapse of cryptococcal meningitis in patients with AIDS is 200 mg once daily.

Prophylaxis in patients undergoing bone marrow transplantation: 400 mg, once daily. Patients who are anticipated to have severe granulocytopenia should start fluconazole prophylaxis several days before the anticipated onset of neutropenia, and continue for 7 days after the neutrophil count rises above 1000 cells per mm^3.

 SPECIAL POPULATIONS

RENAL IMPAIRMENT: There is no need to adjust single dose therapy for vaginal candidiasis because of impaired renal function. For multiple dose regimens:

Creatine clearance, mL/min	Daily dose
>50	Full dose
<50	Half the dose
Hemodialysis	Full dose after each dialysis; on nondialysis days, patients should receive the half dose
CRRT	400 mg–800 mg every 24 hours

HEPATIC DYSFUNCTION: Caution should be used when used in patients with hepatic dysfunction. Liver function tests should be monitored.

PEDIATRICS: Efficacy of fluconazole has not been established in infants less than 6 months of age.

3 mg/kg is equivalent for the adult 100 mg dose; 6 mg/kg for 200 mg and 12 mg/kg for 400 mg; etc.

THE ART OF ANTIMICROBIAL THERAPY

Clinical Pearls

1. Fluconazole is not active against *Candida krusei*.

2. Resistance in *Candida glabrata* is due to efflux of the azoles. If fluconazole is used, the highest dose is recommended.

3. Fluconazole does not have activity against molds, *Blastomyces* sp., or *Histoplasma* spp.

4. Fluconazole is an inhibitor of cytochrome P450 and can enhance the activity of many commonly used drugs, e.g., oral hypoglycemics and anticoagulants.

5. Fluconazole should be administered with caution to patients with potentially proarrhythmic conditions.

■ DORIBAX (Doripenem)

 ## BASIC CHARACTERISTICS

Class: Carbapenem.

Mechanism of Action: Binds penicillin-binding protein, disrupting cell wall synthesis.

Mechanisms of Resistance:

1. The PBP can be altered, with reduced affinity.
2. Production of a beta-lactamase, resulting in hydrolysis of the beta-lactam ring.
3. Decreased ability of the antibiotic to reach the PBP when bacteria decrease porins, resulting in a decrease of the drug concentration within the cell.
4. Increased expression of efflux pump components.

Metabolic Route: Doripenem is excreted in the urine.

 ## FDA-APROVED INDICATIONS

Doripenem is indicated for the treatment of serious infections caused by susceptible strains of microorganisms in the conditions listed below:

I. **Complicated intra-abdominal infections.**

II. **Complicated urinary tract infections, including pyelonephritis.**

✳ SIDE EFFECTS/TOXICITY

Doripenem is **contraindicated** in patients with known hypersensitivity to any component of this product or to other drugs in the same class or in patients who have demonstrated anaphylactic reactions to β-lactams. Before initiating therapy with doripenem, careful inquiry should be made concerning previous hypersensitivity reactions to carbapenems, penicillins, cephalosporins, other beta-lactams, and other allergens, because of the increased possibility of hypersensitivity.

Side effects include seizures, phlebitis, fever, anaphylaxis, rash including Stevens–Johnson syndrome, erythema multiforme and toxic epidermal necrolysis, angioedema, hypotension, encephalopathy, hearing loss, diarrhea, *Clostridium difficile*-associated diarrhea and pseudomembranous colitis, oral candidiasis, glossitis, anorexia, nausea, vomiting, stomach cramps, hepatitis, renal impairment, pyuria, hematuria, genital pruritis, dyspnea, polyarthralgia, prolonged prothrombin time, pancytopenia, positive Coombs' test, increased ALT (SGPT), AST (SGOT), alkaline phosphatase, bilirubin, and LDH, decreased serum sodium, increased potassium, and chloride.

 ## DRUG INTERACTIONS/FOOD INTERACTIONS

Doripenem may reduce serum valproic acid concentrations; levels should be monitored.

It is not recommended that probenecid be given with doripenem.

 ## DOSING

The recommended dosage of doripenem is 500 mg every 8 hours by intravenous infusion.

Antibiotics Manual: A Guide to Commonly Used Antimicrobials, Second Edition. David Schlossberg and Rafik Samuel.
© 2017 John Wiley & Sons Ltd. Published 2017 by John Wiley & Sons Ltd.

SPECIAL POPULATIONS

RENAL IMPAIRMENT:

Creatinine clearance	Dose
30–50 mL/min	250 mg q 8 hours
10-30 mL/min	250 mg q 12 hours
<10 mL/min	No information
After hemodialysis or peritoneal dialysis	No information
CRRT	No information

HEPATIC DYSFUNCTION: No dose adjustment is necessary.

PEDIATRICS: Safety and effectiveness in pediatric patients have not been established.

 THE ART OF ANTIMICROBIAL THERAPY

Clinical Pearls

1. Doripenem must be dose-adjusted for renal dysfunction.
2. Cross allergy with penicillins is <10%.
3. Doripenem is active against many organisms that carry extended spectrum betalactamases.
4. Among the carbapenems, doripenem has the most potent gram-negative activity and may be active in organisms resistant to other carbapenems.

◼ DORYX (Doxycycline Delayed Release), VIBRAMYCIN (Doxycycline)

 BASIC CHARACTERISTICS

Class: Tetracycline.

Mechanism of Action: They reversibly bind the 30s ribosomal subunit preventing the addition of new amino acids into the growing peptide chain.

Mechanisms of Resistance: Decreased entry into the cell or increased excretion of the drug. Rarely, the tetracyclines are inactivated.

Metabolic Route: They are concentrated by the liver in the bile and excreted in the urine and feces at high concentrations and in a biologically active form.

 FDA-APPROVED INDICATIONS

Doxycycline is indicated for the treatment of serious infections caused by susceptible strains of microorganisms in the conditions listed below:

> Respiratory and genitourinary tract infections due to susceptible organisms, Rocky Mountain spotted fever, typhus fever and the typhus group, Q fever, rickettsial pox and tick fevers caused by *Rickettsiae*, *Mycoplasma pneumonia*, lymphogranuloma venereum, psittacosis, trachoma, inclusion conjunctivitis, chlamydial genital and rectal infection, nongonococcal urethritis, relapsing fever, chancroid, plague, tularemia, cholera, *Campylobacter fetus* infections, brucellosis, bartonellosis, granuloma inguinale, gonorrhea, syphilis, yaws, listeriosis, anthrax, actinomycosis, Vincent's infection, intestinal amebiasis, *Clostridium* infections, intestinal amebiasis, prophylaxis of malaria, and severe acne.

Also Used for: Treatment of malaria, anaplasmosis, ehrlichiosis, borreliosis including Lyme disease, rapidly growing mycobacteria, community-acquired MRSA, and *M. marinum*.

 SIDE EFFECTS/TOXICITY

Doxycycline is **contraindicated** in persons who have shown hypersensitivity to any of the tetracyclines.

Tetracyclines should not be used during pregnancy or up to the age of 8 years unless absolutely necessary and no reasonable alternative exists.

Side effects include hypersensitivity reactions, including rash, anaphylaxis, urticaria, angioneurotic edema, serum sickness, photosensitivity, pericarditis, and exacerbation of systemic lupus erythematosus, nausea, vomiting, diarrhea, glossitis, esophagitis, hepatotoxicity, pseudomembranous colitis, bulging fontanels in infants and benign intracranial hypertension in adults, vertigo, pseudotumor cerebri, tinnitus and decreased hearing, dose-related rise in BUN, hemolytic anemia, thrombocytopenia, neutropenia, and eosinophilia.

 DRUG INTERACTIONS/FOOD INTERACTIONS

1. Doxycycline should be given with food or milk.
2. Concurrent use of tetracycline may render oral contraceptives less effective.
3. Patients who are on anticoagulant therapy may require downward adjustment of their anticoagulant dosage.

Antibiotics Manual: A Guide to Commonly Used Antimicrobials, Second Edition. David Schlossberg and Rafik Samuel.
© 2017 John Wiley & Sons Ltd. Published 2017 by John Wiley & Sons Ltd.

4. It is advisable to avoid giving tetracycline class drugs in conjunction with penicillin.

5. The concurrent use of tetracycline and methoxyflurane has been reported to result in fatal renal toxicity.

6. Absorption of tetracyclines is impaired by bismuth subsalicylate.

 DOSING

Doxycycline is supplied as 50 mg and 100 mg capsules, and a syrup containing 50 mg/5 mL. It is also administered intravenously; oral therapy should be instituted as soon as possible. If intravenous therapy is given over prolonged periods of time, thrombophlebitis may result

Usual dose of doxycycline: 200 mg on the first day of treatment (administered 100 mg every 12 hours) followed by a maintenance dose of 100 mg/day. The maintenance dose may be administered as a single dose or as 50 mg every 12 hours.

In the management of more severe infections, 100 mg every 12 hours is recommended.

Gonococcal infections, chlamydial genitourinary or rectal infections, nongonococcal urethritis: 100 mg bid × 7 days.

Syphilis: early – 100 mg bid × 2 weeks; syphilis of more than one year's duration – 100 mg bid × 4 weeks.

Gonococcal or chlamydial epididymo-orchitis: 100 mg bid × 10 days.

Malaria prophylaxis: 100 mg daily; children over 8 years – 2 mg/kg once daily up to the adult dose. Prophylaxis is begun 1–2 days before travel to the malarious area and continued during travel and for 4 weeks after leaving the malarious area.

Anthrax (treatment and prophylaxis): 100 mg bid × 60 days; children weighing less than 45 kg receive 2.2 mg/kg bid × 60 days. Children weighing 45 kg or more receive the adult dose.

Doxycycline delayed-release capsules are administered in 75 mg and 100 mg capsules. They are dosed similarly to regular doxycycline, but they may also be administered by carefully opening the capsules and sprinkling the capsule contents on a spoonful of apple sauce. However, any loss of pellets in the transfer would prevent using the dose. The apple sauce should be swallowed immediately without chewing and followed with a cool 8-ounce glass of water to ensure complete swallowing of the capsule contents.

 SPECIAL POPULATIONS

RENAL IMPAIRMENT: No dose adjustment is necessary.

HEPATIC DYSFUNCTION: No dose adjustment is necessary.

PEDIATRICS: **For children above eight years of age:** The recommended dosage schedule for children weighing 100 pounds or less is 2 mg/lb of body weight divided into two doses on the first day of treatment, followed by 1 mg/lb of body weight given as a single daily dose or divided into two doses, on subsequent days. For more severe infections up to 2 mg/lb of body weight may be used. For children over 100 lb the usual adult dose should be used.

 THE ART OF ANTIMICROBIAL THERAPY

Clinical Pearls

1. To reduce the risk of esophageal irritation and ulceration, doxycycline should be taken with adequate amounts of fluid and should not be taken immediately before going to bed.

2. Doxycycline can cause fetal harm when administered to a pregnant woman.

3. The use of drugs of the tetracycline class during tooth development (last half of pregnancy, infancy, and childhood to the age of 8 years) may cause permanent discoloration of the teeth (yellow–gray–brown).
4. The Oracea brand of doxycycline is indicated only for the treatment of inflammatory lesions (papules and pustules) of rosacea in adult patients. It has not been evaluated in the treatment or prevention of infections and should not be substituted for the doxycycline preparations discussed above.
5. The absorption of doxycycline is **not** markedly influenced by simultaneous ingestion of food or milk.

BASIC CHARACTERISTICS

Class: First generation cephalosporin.

Mechanism of Action: Binds penicillin-binding protein, disrupting cell wall synthesis.

Mechanisms of Resistance:

1. The PBP can be altered, with reduced affinity.

2. Production of a beta-lactamase resulting in hydrolysis of the beta-lactam ring.

3. Decreased ability of the antibiotic to reach the PBP when bacteria decrease porin production, resulting in a decrease of the drug concentration within the cell.

Metabolic Route: Cefadroxil is excreted unchanged in the urine.

 FDA-APPROVED INDICATIONS

Treatment of patients with infection caused by susceptible strains of the designated organisms in the following diseases:

Urinary tract infections

Skin and skin structure infections

Pharyngitis and/or tonsillitis

 SIDE EFFECTS/TOXICITY

> **WARNING:** To reduce the development of drug-resistant bacteria and maintain the effectiveness of cefadroxil for oral suspension and other antibacterial drugs, cefadroxil for oral suspension should be used only to treat or prevent infections that are proven or strongly suspected to be caused by bacteria.

Cefadroxil is **contraindicated** in patients with known allergy to the cephalosporins and should be used with caution if hypersensitivity exists to penicillin.

Toxicity includes fever, anaphylaxis, rash including Stevens–Johnson syndrome, erythema multiforme and toxic epidermal necrolysis, angioedema, flushing, serum-sickness-like reactions, encephalopathy, seizures, diarrhea, *Clostridium difficile*-associated diarrhea and pseudomembranous colitis, oral candidiasis, anorexia, nausea, vomiting, stomach cramps, flatulence, hepatitis, renal impairment, genital moniliasis, vaginitis, hemorrhage, prolonged prothrombin time, pancytopenia, hemolytic anemia, positive Coombs' test; cephalosporins may cause false-positive urine glucose determinations when using cupric sulfate solution (Benedict's solution, *Clinitest*®). Tests utilizing glucose oxidase (*Tes-Tape*®, *Clinistix*®) are not affected by cephalosporins.

 DRUG INTERACTIONS/FOOD INTERACTIONS

Cefadroxil may be given with or without food.

Probenecid may decrease renal tubular secretion of cephalosporins when used concurrently, resulting in increased and more prolonged cephalosporin blood levels.

Antibiotics Manual: A Guide to Commonly Used Antimicrobials, Second Edition. David Schlossberg and Rafik Samuel.
© 2017 John Wiley & Sons Ltd. Published 2017 by John Wiley & Sons Ltd.

DOSING

Cefadroxil is administered as 500 mg or 1 g tablets. It also can be administered as an oral suspension in the following concentrations: 125 mg/5 mL, 250 mg/5 mL, and 500 mg/5 mL.

Urinary tract infections: 1 or 2 g per day in single (q d) or divided doses (bid).

Skin and skin structure infections: 1 g per day in single (q d) or divided doses (bid).

Pharyngitis and tonsillitis: 1 g per day in single (q d) or divided doses (bid).

 SPECIAL POPULATIONS

RENAL IMPAIRMENT: An initial dose is 1 g of cefadroxil should be administered followed by 500 mg at the time intervals listed below.

Creatinine clearance	Timing
25–50 mL/min	Every 12 hours
10–25 mL/min	Every day
<10 mL/min	Every 36 hours
Hemodialysis	500 mg–1 gram after hemodialysis
CAPD	500 mg daily
CRRT	N/A

HEPATIC DYSFUNCTION: No dose adjustment is necessary.

PEDIATRICS: It is recommended to administer cefadroxil 30 mg/kg/day in divided doses every 12 hours.

 THE ART OF ANTIMICROBIAL THERAPY

Clinical Pearls

1. Cefadroxil needs to be adjusted for renal dysfunction.
2. Cross allergy with penicillins is <10 %.

BASIC CHARACTERISTICS

Class: Tetracycline.

Mechanism of Action: They reversibly bind the 30s ribosomal subunit preventing the addition of new amino acids into the growing peptide chain.

Mechanisms of Resistance: Decreased entry into the cell or increased excretion of the drug. Rarely, the tetracyclines are inactivated.

Metabolic Route: Minocycline is metabolized in the liver.

 FDA-APPROVED INDICATIONS

Minocycline is indicated for the treatment of serious infections caused by susceptible strains of microorganisms in the conditions listed below:

Respiratory tract and skin and skin structure infections infections due to susceptible organisms, Rocky Mountain spotted fever, typhus fever and the typhus group, Q fever, rickettsial pox and tick fevers caused by *Rickettsiae*; *Mycoplasma pneumonia*, lymphogranuloma venereum, psittacosis, trachoma, inclusion conjunctivitis, nongonococcal urethritis, relapsing fever, chancroid, plague, tularemia, cholera, infections caused by *Campylobacter fetus*, brucellosis, bartonellosis, granuloma inguinale, syphilis, yaws, listeriosis, anthrax, actinomycosis, Vincent's infection, intestinal amebiasis, *Clostridium* infections, acne, gonococcal infections, syphilis,

Mycobacterium marinum, and asymptomatic carriers of *Neisseria meningitidis*.

Also Used for: Community-acquired MRSA, nocardiosis, rapidly growing mycobacteria.

 SIDE EFFECTS/TOXICITY

Minocycline is **contraindicated** in persons who have shown hypersensitivity to any of the tetracyclines.

Tetracyclines should not be used during pregnancy or up to the age of 8 years unless absolutely necessary and no reasonable alternative exists.

Side effects include hypersensitivity reactions, including rash, anaphylaxis, urticaria, angioneurotic edema, serum sickness, photosensitivity, Lupus-like syndrome, nausea, vomiting, diarrhea, glossitis, esophagitis, hepatotoxicity, pseudomembranous colitis, renal failure, bulging fontanels in infants and benign intracranial hypertension in adults, vertigo, pseudotumor cerebri, tinnitus and decreased hearing, dose-related rise in BUN, hemolytic anemia, thrombocytopenia, neutropenia and eosinophilia, and drug rash with eosinophilia and systemic symptoms (DRESS).

 DRUG INTERACTIONS/FOOD INTERACTIONS

Minocycline hydrochloride tablets should be taken at least 1 hour before meals or 2 hours after meals.

1. Concurrent use of tetracycline may render oral contraceptives less effective.
2. Patients who are on anticoagulant therapy may require downward adjustment of their anticoagulant dosage.
3. It is advisable to avoid giving tetracycline class drugs in conjunction with penicillin.

Antibiotics Manual: A Guide to Commonly Used Antimicrobials, Second Edition. David Schlossberg and Rafik Samuel.
© 2017 John Wiley & Sons Ltd. Published 2017 by John Wiley & Sons Ltd.

4. Absorption of oral tetracyclines is impaired by antacids containing aluminum, calcium, or magnesium, and iron-containing preparations.

5. The concurrent use of tetracycline and methoxyflurane has been reported to result in fatal renal toxicity.

6. Administration of isotretinoin should be avoided shortly before, during, and shortly after minocycline therapy. Each drug alone has been associated with pseudotumor cerebri.

 ## DOSING

Minocycline is administered as 50 mg, 75 mg, and 100 mg tablets and capsules.

Usual dosage of minocycline is 200 mg initially followed by 100 mg every 12 hours.

Gonococcal urethritis: 100 mg q 12 × 5 days.

Other gonococcal infections: 200 mg initially, followed by 100 mg q 12 h for 4 days.

Syphilis: usual dosage, over 10–15 days.

Meningococcal carrier state: 100 mg q 12 hours × 5 days.

***M. marinum* infections:** 100 mg q 12 hours × 6–8 weeks.

Chlamydial genitourinary infection: 100 q 12 hours × 7 days.

 ## SPECIAL POPULATIONS

RENAL IMPAIRMENT: No dose adjustment is necessary.

HEPATIC DYSFUNCTION: Data insufficient.

PEDIATRICS: Above 8 years of age 4 mg/kg initially followed by 2 mg/kg every 12 hours.

THE ART OF ANTIMICROBIAL THERAPY

Clinical Pearls

1. To reduce the risk of esophageal irritation and ulceration, minocycline should be taken with adequate amounts of fluid and should not be take immediately before going to bed.

2. Minocycline can cause fetal harm when administered to a pregnant woman.

3. The use of drugs of the tetracycline class during tooth development (last half of pregnancy, infancy, and childhood to the age of 8 years) may cause permanent discoloration of the teeth (yellow–gray–brown).

4. Minocycline should not be administered with calcium or other cations.

5. Central nervous system side effects including lightheadedness, dizziness, or vertigo have been reported with minocycline therapy. Patients who experience these symptoms should be cautioned about driving vehicles or using hazardous machinery while on minocycline therapy. These symptoms may disappear during therapy and usually disappear rapidly when the drug is discontinued.

BASIC CHARACTERISTICS

Class: Nonnucleoside reverse transcriptase inhibitor.

Mechanism of Action: Rilpivirine inhibits reverse transcriptase activity by binding the enzyme.

Mechanism of Resistance: Changes in the structure of reverse transcriptase prevents rilpivirine from binding the enzyme and allowing transcription to continue. The most frequent resistance mutation is E138K.

Metabolic Route: Rilpivirine primarily undergoes oxidative metabolism mediated by the cytochrome P450 CYP 3A.

 FDA-APPROVED INDICATIONS

Treatment of HIV-1 in combinations with other antiretroviral agents.

 SIDE EFFECTS/TOXICITY

Rash and hypersensitivity

Depressive disorders

Hepatotoxicity

Fat redistribution

Immune reconstitution syndrome

Other side effects include diarrhea, abdominal discomfort, cholecystitis, cholelithiasis, decreased appetite, somnolence, sleep disorders, anxiety, glomerulonephritis, and nephrolithiasis.

 DRUG INTERACTIONS/FOOD INTERACTIONS

Rilpivirine should be administered with at least a 533 calorie meal.

Rilpivirine is primarily metabolized by cytochrome P450 (CYP)3A, and drugs that induce or inhibit CYP3A may affect the clearance of rilpivirine.

Rilpivirine should not be administered with delavirdine, efavirenz, etravirine, nevirapine, carbamazepine, oxcarbazepine, phenobarbital, phenytoin, rifampin, rifapentine, proton pump inhibitors, dexamethasone, or St John's wort.

If administered with antacids, rilpivirine should be given 4 hours before or 2 hours after.

If administered with H2 blockers, they should be given 12 hours apart.

If administered with rifabutin, the rilpivirine dose should be increased to 50 mg daily.

 DOSING

25 mg once daily.

 SPECIAL POPULATIONS

RENAL IMPAIRMENT: There is no adjustment needed.

Antibiotics Manual: A Guide to Commonly Used Antimicrobials, Second Edition. David Schlossberg and Rafik Samuel.
© 2017 John Wiley & Sons Ltd. Published 2017 by John Wiley & Sons Ltd.

HEPATIC DYSFUNCTION: Not studied in those with child Pugh class C hepatic dysfunction.

PEDIATRICS: for treatment: Recommended for those over 12 years of age.

 ## THE ART OF ANTIMICROBIAL THERAPY

Clinical Pearls

1. Edurant should not be used with other agents containing rilpivirine such as Complera or Odefsey.
2. Rilpivirine should not be used with other nonnucleoside reverse transcriptase inhibitors such as efavirenz, nevirapine, etravirine, or delavirdine.
3. Rilpivirine must be given with a meal of at least 533 calories.
4. Protein supplement drinks are not sufficient to ensure adequate levels of rilpivirine.
5. Do not initiate rilpivirine in patients who have a viral load of >100 000 copies.
6. Do not administer rilpivirine with a proton pump inhibitor.

Also available in Truvada, Descovy, Atripla, Stribild, Genvoya, Complera, and Odefsey.

 BASIC CHARACTERISTICS

Class: Nucleoside reverse transcriptase inhibitor (NRTI) with activity against HIV and hepatitis B.

Mechanism of Action: Converted by cellular enzymes to its active drug emtricitabine triphosphate, an analog of cytosine triphosphate. The emtricitabine triphosphate competes with the naturally occurring nucleotides for incorporation in newly forming HIV DNA. Since emtricitabine triphosphate does not have a terminal hydroxyl group, it halts transcription and replication of the virus.

Mechanism of Resistance: Changes in the structure of HIV reverse transcriptase leads to preferred incorporation of cytosine triphosphate and decreased incorporation of emtricitabine triphosphate, which allows transcription of DNA to continue. Resistance mutations include M184V.

Metabolic Route: Emtricitabine is mainly excreted unchanged in the urine.

 FDA-APPROVED INDICATIONS

Emtricitabine is approved to be used in combination with other antiretrovirals for the treatment of HIV infection.

Emtricitabine has activity against hepatitis B.

 SIDE EFFECTS/TOXICITY

> **WARNING: Lactic acidosis and severe hepatomegaly** with steatosis, including fatal cases, have been reported with the use of nucleoside analogs alone or in combination with other antiretrovirals.
>
> Emtricitabine is not approved for the treatment of chronic hepatitis B virus (HBV) infection and the safety and efficacy of emtricitabine have not been established in patients coinfected with HBV and HIV-1. Severe acute exacerbations of hepatitis B have been reported in patients who have discontinued emtricitabine. Hepatic function should be monitored closely with both clinical and laboratory follow-up for at least several months in patients who are coinfected with HIV-1 and HBV and discontinue emtricitabine. If appropriate, initiation of anti-hepatitis B therapy may be warranted.

Other side effects: Immune reconstitution inflammatory syndrome, fat redistribution including central obesity and dorsocervical fat enlargement, peripheral wasting, facial wasting, breast enlargement, headache, diarrhea, nausea, fatigue, dizziness, depression, insomnia, abnormal dreams, rash, abdominal pain, asthenia, increased cough, and rhinitis. Skin hyperpigmentation is common in pediatric patients.

 DRUG INTERACTIONS/FOOD INTERACTIONS

Emtricitabine can be taken with or without food and is unaffected by pH.

Emtricitabine should not be administered with any medication that contains lamivudine or emtricitabine, including Epivir, Combivir, Trizivir, Triumeq, Truvada, Descovy, Atripla, Complera, Odefsey, Stribild, or Genvoya.

Antibiotics Manual: A Guide to Commonly Used Antimicrobials, Second Edition. David Schlossberg and Rafik Samuel.
© 2017 John Wiley & Sons Ltd. Published 2017 by John Wiley & Sons Ltd.

DOSING

Emtricitabine is administered in a 200 mg tablet or in a clear orange liquid, which contains 10 mg/mL of emtricitabine. The recommended adult dose is 200 mg daily.

 SPECIAL POPULATIONS

RENAL IMPAIRMENT: Dose adjustment is necessary as follows:

For creatinine clearance:

30–49:	200 mg every 48 hours
15–29:	200 mg every 72 hours
<15 or hemodialysis:	200 mg every 96 hours

HEPATIC DYSFUNCTION: No dose adjustment is necessary.

PEDIATRICS: The approved dose is 6 mg/kg up to a maximum of 240 mg oral solution or a 200 mg capsule daily.

 THE ART OF ANTIMICROBIAL THERAPY

Clinical Pearls

1. Emtricitabine should be used in combination with other antiretroviral agents.
2. Emtricitabine is present in eight different medications: Emtriva, Truvada, Atripla, Descovy, Complera, Odefsey, Stribild, and Genvoya.
3. Patients with HIV-1 should be tested for hepatitis B virus before initiating antiretroviral therapy with emtricitabine.

BASIC CHARACTERISTICS

Class: Sofosbuvir is a nucleotide reverse transcriptase inhibitor for hepatitis C NS5B polymerase.

Velpatasvir is an NS5A inhibitor.

Mechanism of Action: Sofosbuvir undergoes intracellular metabolism to form the pharmacologically active uridine analog triphosphate, which can be incorporated into HCV RNA by the NS5B polymerase and acts as a chain terminator.

Velpatasvir inhibits viral replication by inhibiting the NS5A protein.

Mechanism of Resistance: The substitution S282T can decrease incorporation of the uridine analog triphosphate, allowing replication of the virus to continue.

Velpatasvir resistance develops with amino acid substitutions at NS5A positions 24, 28, 30, 31, 32, 58, 92, and 93.

Metabolic Route: Sofosbuvir is metabolized in the liver to its active form. It is predominantly excreted in the urine.

Velpatasvir is metabolized by the liver CYP 3A4, CYP2B6, and CYP 2C8 and excreted in the feces.

 FDA-APPROVED INDICATIONS

Epclusa is indicated for the treatment of adult patients with chronic hepatitis C virus (HCV) genotype 1, 2, 3, 4, 5, or 6:

1. Without cirrhosis or with compensated cirrhosis.
2. With decompensated cirrhosis for use in combination with ribavirin.

 SIDE EFFECTS/TOXICITY

Patients may be at increased risk for symptomatic bradycardia with coadministration of Epclusa and amiodarone.

Other side effects include: fatigue, headache, nausea, insomnia, asthenia, diarrhea, rash, anemia, and depression.

Lab abnormalities including elevated bilirubin, creatinine kinase, and lipase have been reported.

 DRUG INTERACTIONS/FOOD INTERACTIONS

Epclusa may be taken without regard to food.

When Epclusa is used in combination with ribavirin the **contraindications** applicable to ribavirin are applicable to combination therapies.

Do not coadminister Epclusa with Harvoni, sofosbuvir, amiodarone, proton pump inhibitors, topotecan, carbamazepine, phenytoin, phenobarbital, oxcarbazepine, rifampin, rifabutin, rifapentine, efavirenz, St John's wort, or tipranavir/ritonavir.

Separate Epclusa from antacids by 4 hours; H2 blockers by 12 hours.

Administer a maximum of rosuvastatin 10 mg when coadministered with Epclusa.

 DOSING

One tablet of Epclusa contains 400 mg of sofosbuvir and 100 mg of velpatasvir. The recommended dose is one tablet taken orally once daily with or without food.

Antibiotics Manual: A Guide to Commonly Used Antimicrobials, Second Edition. David Schlossberg and Rafik Samuel.
© 2017 John Wiley & Sons Ltd. Published 2017 by John Wiley & Sons Ltd.

Patient population	Medication	Duration
Patients without cirrhosis and patients with compensated cirrhosis	Epclusa	12 weeks
Patients with decompensated cirrhosis	Epclusa + ribavirin	12 weeks

 ## SPECIAL POPULATIONS

RENAL IMPAIRMENT: Do not use if creatinine clearance is < 30 mL/minute.

HEPATIC DYSFUNCTION: No dose adjustment necessary.

PEDIATRICS: Do not use in patients under 18 years of age.

 ## THE ART OF ANTIMICROBIAL THERAPY

Clinical Pearls

1. Epclusa is active against all hepatitis C genotypes.
2. The dose and duration of Epclusa does not change based on genotype, prior antiviral use, or liver impairment.
3. In patients with moderate or severe hepatic impairment, the addition of ribavirin is required.
4. Significant bradycardia has been reported if Epclusa is combined with amiodarone.
5. Do not administer Epclusa with Harvoni or sofosbuvir.
6. Review the most current hepatitis C treatment guidelines because they are changing rapidly: http://www.cdc.gov/hepatitis/HCV/index.htm.

Also available in Epzicom, Combivir, Trizivir, and Triumeq.

 BASIC CHARACTERISTICS

Class: Nucleoside reverse transcriptase inhibitor (NRTI) with activity against HIV and hepatitis B.

Mechanism of Action: Converted by cellular enzymes to its active drug lamivudine triphosphate, an analog of cytosine triphosphate. Lamivudine triphosphate competes with the naturally occurring nucleotide for incorporation in newly forming HIV DNA. Since lamivudine triphosphate does not have a terminal hydroxyl group, it halts transcription and replication of the virus.

Mechanism of Resistance: Changes in the structure of HIV reverse transcriptase leads to preferred incorporation of cytosine triphosphate and decreased incorporation of lamivudine triphosphate, which allows transcription of DNA to continue. Resistance mutations include M184V.

Metabolic Route:

The majority of lamivudine is eliminated unchanged in urine by active organic cationic secretion.

 FDA-APPROVED INDICATIONS

1. Treatment of HIV infection, in combination with other antiretrovirals.
2. Treatment of hepatitis B.

 SIDE EFFECTS/TOXICITY

> **WARNING: Lactic acidosis** and hepatomegaly with steatosis have been reported with nucleoside analogs, including lamivudine. If this syndrome occurs, the drug should be discontinued.
>
> **Severe acute exacerbations of hepatitis B** have been reported in patients who are coinfected with hepatitis B and HIV and have discontinued lamivudine. Hepatic function should be monitored closely with both clinical and laboratory follow-up for at least several months in patients who discontinue lamivudine and are coinfected with HIV and HBV. If appropriate, initiation of antihepatitis B therapy may be warranted.
>
> **Lamivudine tablets (HBV)** are not approved for the treatment of HIV-1 infection because the lamivudine dosage in lamivudine tablets (HBV) is subtherapeutic and monotherapy is inappropriate for the treatment of HIV-1 infection. HIV-1 resistance may emerge in chronic hepatitis B-infected patients with unrecognized or untreated HIV-1 infection. Counseling and testing should be offered to all patients before beginning treatment with lamivudine tablets (HBV) and periodically during treatment.

Other side effects: Immune reconstitution inflammatory syndrome, fat redistribution including central obesity and dorsocervical fat enlargement, peripheral wasting, facial wasting, breast enlargement, headache, nausea, malaise and fatigue, nasal signs and symptoms, diarrhea, and cough.

Antibiotics Manual: A Guide to Commonly Used Antimicrobials, Second Edition. David Schlossberg and Rafik Samuel.
© 2017 John Wiley & Sons Ltd. Published 2017 by John Wiley & Sons Ltd.

DRUG INTERACTIONS/FOOD INTERACTIONS

Lamivudine can be taken with or without food and is unaffected by pH.

Lamivudine should not be coadministered with emtricitabine because they are both cytosine analogs and may be antagonistic.

Lamivudine should not be coadminstered with any other medication containing either lamivudine or emtricitabine. These include: Combivir, Epzicom, Trizivir, Triumeq, Emtriva, Truvada, Descovy, Atripla, Complera, Odefsey, Stribild, or Genvoya.

 DOSING

Lamivudine is administered in 100 mg, 150 mg, and 300 mg tablets and a yellow strawberry–banana flavored liquid, which contains 10 mg/cc. The recommended adult dose is 300 mg once daily or 150 mg twice daily for HIV and 100 mg once daily for hepatitis B.

 SPECIAL POPULATIONS

RENAL IMPAIRMENT: Lamivudine dose must be reduced in patients with renal insufficiency. When creatinine clearance drops below 50, the recommended doses are as follows:

Creatinine clearance, mL/min	Dose
30–49	150 mg once daily
15–29	150 mg first dose, then 100 mg once daily
5–14	150 mg first dose, then 50 mg once daily
<5	50 mg first dose, then 25 mg once daily

HEPATIC DYSFUNCTION: No adjustment is necessary.

PEDIATRICS: The recommended dose is 4 mg/kg twice daily (up to a maximum of 150 mg twice a day), administered in combination with other antiretroviral agents.

 THE ART OF ANTIMICROBIAL THERAPY

Clinical Pearls

1. Lamivudine should be used in combination with other antiretroviral agents.
2. Lamivudine is present in five different medications: Epivir, Trizivir, Combivir, and Epzicom.
3. If lamivudine is used in hepatitis B infected patients, it is important to check Triumeq for HIV, since using lamivudine alone in HIV infected individuals leads to rapid resistance to lamivudine.
4. If you use lamivudine in HIV, it is important to check for hepatitis B, since using lamivudine alone in hepatitis B infected individuals leads to rapid resistance to lamivudine. For hepatitis B, lamivudine monotherapy leads to the YMDD mutation.

BASIC CHARACTERISTICS

Class: Nucleoside reverse transcriptase inhibitors (NRTI) with activity against HIV.

Mechanism of Action: Converted by cellular enzymes to its active drugs lamivudine triphosphate (a cytosine analog) and carbavir triphosphate (a guanasine triphosphate). These triphosphate analogs compete with the naturally occurring nucleotides for incorporation in newly forming HIV DNA. Since the triphosphate analogs do not have terminal hydroxyl groups, they halt transcription and replication of the virus.

Mechanism of Resistance: Lamivudine and abacavir lead to changes in the structure of HIV reverse transcriptase, leading to preferred incorporation of cytosine and guanasine triphosphate; this results in decreased incorporation of lamivudine and carbavir triphosphate, which allows transcription of DNA to continue. Resistance mutations that emerge in those on Epzicom include M184V, K65R, and L74V.

Metabolic Route: The majority of lamivudine is eliminated unchanged in urine by active organic cationic secretion.

Abacavir is metabolized by alcohol dehydrogenase and glucuronyl transferase into inactive metabolites that are eliminated primarily in the feces.

FDA-APPROVED INDICATIONS

Treatment of HIV infection, in combination with other antiretrovirals.

SIDE EFFECTS/TOXICITY

> **WARNINGS: Hypersensitivity Reactions**: Serious and sometimes fatal hypersensitivity reactions, with multiple organ involvement, have occurred with abacavir, a component of Epzicom. Patients who carry the HLA-B*5701 allele are at a higher risk of a hypersensitivity reaction to abacavir; although hypersensitivity reactions have occurred in patients who do not carry the HLA-B*5701 allele. Epzicom is contraindicated in patients with a prior hypersensitivity reaction to abacavir and in HLA-B*5701-positive patients. All patients should be screened for the HLA-B*5701 allele prior to initiating therapy with Epzicom or reinitiation of therapy with Epzicom, unless patients have a previously documented HLA-B*5701 allele assessment. Discontinue Epzicom immediately if a hypersensitivity reaction is suspected, regardless of HLA-B*5701 status and even when other diagnoses are possible. Following a hypersensitivity reaction to Epzicom, NEVER restart Epzicom or any other abacavir-containing product because more severe symptoms, including death, can occur within hours. Similar severe reactions have also occurred rarely following the reintroduction of abacavir-containing products in patients who have no history of abacavir hypersensitivity.
>
> **Lactic Acidosis and Severe Hepatomegaly with Steatosis**: Lactic acidosis and severe hepatomegaly with steatosis, including fatal cases, have been reported with the use of nucleoside analogs and other antiretrovirals. Discontinue Epzicom if clinical or laboratory findings suggestive of lactic acidosis or pronounced hepatotoxicity occur.
>
> **Exacerbations of Hepatitis B**: Severe acute exacerbations of hepatitis B have been reported in patients who are coinfected with hepatitis B virus (HBV) and human immunodeficiency virus (HIV-1) and have discontinued lamivudine, which is a component of Epzicom. Hepatic function should be monitored closely with both clinical and laboratory follow-up for at least several months in patients who discontinue Epzicom and are coinfected with HIV-1 and HBV. If appropriate, initiation of antihepatitis B therapy may be warranted.

Antibiotics Manual: A Guide to Commonly Used Antimicrobials, Second Edition. David Schlossberg and Rafik Samuel.
© 2017 John Wiley & Sons Ltd. Published 2017 by John Wiley & Sons Ltd.

Other side effects: Immune reconstitution inflammatory syndrome, fat redistribution including central obesity and dorsocervical fat enlargement, peripheral wasting, facial wasting, breast enlargement, GGT elevation, and pancreatitis.

 ## DRUG INTERACTIONS/FOOD INTERACTIONS

Epzicom can be taken with or without food and is unaffected by pH.

Epzicom should not be used with emtricitabine or any medications containing emtricitabine because both lamivudine and emtricitabine are cytosine analogs and may be antagonistic. These include Emtriva, Truvada, Atripla, Descovy, Complera, Odefsey, Stribild, and Genvoya.

Epzicom should not be given with other antiretrovirals containing lamivudine or abacavir. These include Epivir, Combivir, Ziagen, Epzicom, Triumeq, and Trizivir.

 ## DOSING

Epzicom is administered in a fixed dose combination of lamivudine 300 mg and abacavir 600 mg. The recommended adult dose is one tablet daily.

 ## SPECIAL POPULATIONS

RENAL IMPAIRMENT: Should not be used in patients with a creatinine clearance less than 50 mL/min.

HEPATIC DYSFUNCTION: In patients with hepatic insufficiency, this formulation should not be used.

PEDIATRICS: For pediatric patients weighing at least 25 kg is one tablet daily.

 ## THE ART OF ANTIMICROBIAL THERAPY

Clinical Pearls

1. Epzicom should be used in combination with other antiretroviral agents.
2. Epzicom contains lamivudine and abacavir and should not be used with medications containing these components, including Trizivir, Combivir, Epzicom, Ziagen, Triumeq, and Epivir.
3. An HLA-B5701 test should be done prior to starting and medication containing abacavir; if positive, abacavir should be avoided.
4. If a person has suspected hypersensitivity, abacavir and any medication containing abacavir should not be used.
5. Since lamivudine has activity against hepatitis B it is important to check for hepatitis B since using lamivudine or any medication containing lamivudine alone in hepatitis B infected individuals leads to rapid resistance to lamivudine.

BASIC CHARACTERISTICS

Class: Echinocandin.

Mechanism of Action: Inhibition of synthesis of 1,3-beta-D-glucan, an essential component of fungal cell walls.

Mechanism of Resistance: Data incomplete.

Metabolic Route: Slow chemical degradation to an open ring structure, which is then degraded to peptidic products and is eliminated in the feces. It is not metabolized by the cytochrome P450 enzymes.

 FDA-APPROVED INDICATIONS

Candidemia, intraabdominal abscess and peritonitis, and esophageal candidiasis.

Also Used for: *Aspergillus* infections, prevention of fungal infections in neutropenic patients, and other *Candida* infections such as endocarditis, osteomyelitis, or meningitis.

 SIDE EFFECTS/TOXICITY

Hepatotoxicity; possible histamine-related syndrome characterized by rash, urticaria, flushing, pruritus, and hypotension. Also seen are diarrhea, thrombocytopenia, arrhythmia, QT prolongation, seizures, hypercalcemia, hyperglycemia, hypokalemia, hyperkalemia, hypernatremia, and hypomagnesemia.

 DRUG INTERACTIONS

There are no significant drug interactions with anidulafungin.

 DOSING

Candidemia and other *Candida* infections: 200 mg IV loading dose and then 100 mg IV daily.

Esophageal candidiasis: 100 mg IV daily and then 50 mg a day.

 SPECIAL POPULATIONS

There is no dose adjustment needed for renal impairment or hepatic dysfunction.

PEDIATRICS: The safety and effectiveness of anidulafungin in patients ≤16 years old has not been established.

 THE ART OF ANTIMICROBIAL THERAPY

Clinical Pearls

1. Echinocandins have activity only against *Candida* species, *Pneumocystis jirovecii*, and *Aspergillus* species. They should not be used for any other fungal infections.
2. Anidulafungin is active against all pathogenic *Candida* species including those resistant to fluconazole.
3. Increasing resistance to echinocandins has been noted in *Candida glabrata* and *Candida parapsilosis*.

Antibiotics Manual: A Guide to Commonly Used Antimicrobials, Second Edition. David Schlossberg and Rafik Samuel.
© 2017 John Wiley & Sons Ltd. Published 2017 by John Wiley & Sons Ltd.

Also including: erythromycin ethylsuccinate tablets, suspension and delayed release formulation, erythromycin lactobionate for injection, erythromycin stearate (base), erythromycin estolate, erythromycin coated pellets and delayed release pellets.

 ## BASIC CHARACTERISTICS

Class: Macrolide.

Mechanism of Action: Erythromycin acts by binding to the 50S ribosomal subunit of susceptible microorganisms and, thus, interfering with microbial protein synthesis.

Mechanisms of Resistance:

1. Decreased permeability.
2. Active efflux.
3. Alteration of the 50S ribosomal unit.
4. Alteration of the 23S subunit of the 50S ribosomal unit.
5. Enzymatic inactivation of the macrolide.

Metabolic Route: Erythromycin is excreted in the bile.

 ## FDA-APPROVED INDICATIONS

All formulations of erythromycin have the following indications; any exceptions are noted:

Indicated in the treatment of infections caused by susceptible strains of the designated organisms in the diseases listed below:

Upper and lower respiratory tract infections

Mycoplasma infection

Listeriosis

Pertussis

Skin and skin structure infections

Diphtheria

Erythrasma due to *Corynebacterium minutissimum*

Intestinal amebiasis caused by *Entamoeba histolytica* (**oral erythromycins only**) *Chlamydia trachomatis* conjunctivitis of the newborn, pneumonia of infancy, and urogenital infections during pregnancy

Alternative to penicillin for **gonococcal pelvic inflammatory disease and syphilis**

Alternative to tetracyclines for uncomplicated urethral, endocervical, or rectal infections in adults due to *Chlamydia trachomatis*, nongonococcal urethritis caused by *Ureaplasma urealyticum*, **Legionnaires' disease**

Alternative to penicillin for prevention of rheumatic fever

 ## SIDE EFFECTS/TOXICITY

Contraindicated in patients with known hypersensitivity to this antibiotic.

Side effects include: allergic reactions, rash, nausea, vomiting, abdominal pain, diarrhea anorexia, elevations of liver enzymes, jaundice, pancreatitis, pseudomembranous colitis, rhabdomyolysis, exacerbation of symptoms of myasthenia gravis and new onset of symptoms of myasthenic syndrome, infantile hypertrophic pyloric stenosis (IHPS), QT prolongation and ventricular arrhythmias, convulsions, and reversible hearing loss.

 DRUG INTERACTIONS/FOOD INTERACTIONS

Erythromycin tablets and suspension can be administered with or without food.

Erythromycin is a substrate and inhibitor of the p450 enzyme system (CYP3A). Erythromycin is **contraindicated** in patients taking terfenadine, astemizole, pimozide, or cisapride,

Erythromycin should be used with **caution**, monitoring serum concentrations when possible, with the following medications: theophylline, oral anticoagulants, digoxin, verapamil, carbamazepine, sildenafil, midazolam, triazolam, HMG-CoA reductase inhibitors (e.g., lovastatin and simvastatin), ergotamine, cyclosporine, tacrolimus, alfentanil, disopyramide, rifabutin, quinidine, methylprednisolone, cilostazol, vinblastine, and bromocriptine.

Erythromycin interacts with other drugs not metabolized by the CYP3A system, including hexobarbital, phenytoin, and valproate.

 DOSING

There are multiple formulations of erythromycin.

Oral: Erythromycin ethylsuccinate: usual dose is 400 mg every 6 hours; delayed release formulations can be given in 6 h, 8 h, and 12 h intervals with a total of 1000 mg in the day; for severe infections, the dose can be increased to 4 grams in a 24 hour period.

For adult dosage calculation, use a ratio of 400 mg of erythromycin activity as the ethylsuccinate to 250 mg of erythromycin stearate (base) or estolate.

Intravenous (erythromycin lactobionate): 15 to 20 mg/kg/day, in divided doses every 6 hours. Higher doses, up to 4 g/day, may be given for severe infections.

 SPECIAL POPULATIONS

RENAL IMPAIRMENT: For creatinine clearance <10, administer half the usual daily dose.

HEPATIC DYSFUNCTION: Caution should be used.

PEDIATRICS: In mild to moderate infections the usual dosage of erythromycin ethylsuccinate for children is 30 to 50 mg/kg/day in equally divided doses every 6 hours. For more severe infections this dosage may be doubled. If twice-a-day dosage is desired, one-half of the total daily dose may be given every 12 hours. Doses may also be given three times daily by administering one-third of the total daily dose every 8 hours.

 THE ART OF ANTIMICROBIAL THERAPY

Clinical Pearls
1. Multiple formulations of erythromycin are available; caution should be used as the dosage regimens differ.
2. Macrolides prolong QT intervals and must be used with caution.

EVOTAZ (Atazanavir + Cobicistat)

 BASIC CHARACTERISTICS

Class: Protease inhibitor + CYP3A inhibitor.

Mechanism of Action: Atazanavir reversibly binds the active site of the enzyme protease. Inhibition of protease prevents cleavage of the *gag* and *gag-pol* polyprotein resulting in the production of immature, noninfectious virus.
Cobicistat is a mechanism-based CYP3A inhibitor.

Mechanism of Resistance: Development of mutations on the enzyme protease causes a conformational change that prevents atazanavir from binding the active site, allowing protease activity to continue. The most frequent resistance mutations include I50L.

Metabolic Route: Atazanavir and cobicistat are metabolized and excreted in the feces.

 FDA-APPROVED INDICATIONS

Treatment of HIV-1 in combinations with other antiretroviral agents.

SIDE EFFECTS/TOXICITY

Atazanavir has been associated with new onset diabetes mellitus, exacerbation of preexisting diabetes mellitus, hyperglycemia, increased bleeding, including spontaneous skin hematomas and hemarthrosis, in patients with hemophilia type A and B, redistribution/accumulation of body fat including central obesity, dorsocervical fat enlargement (buffalo hump), peripheral wasting, facial wasting, breast enlargement, "cushingoid appearance", immune reconstitution syndrome, rash, nephrolithiasis, prolongation of PR interval, QTc prolongation, torsades de pointes, abdominal pain, headache, anorexia, dyspepsia, epigastric pain, hepatitis, mouth ulceration, pancreatitis, vomiting, anemia, leucopenia, thrombocytopenia, increases in alkaline phosphatase, amylase, creatine phosphokinase, lactic dehydrogenase, SGOT, SGPT, indirect bilirubin and gamma glutamyl transpeptidase, hyperlipemia, hyperuricemia, hyperglycemia, hypoglycemia, and dehydration.

Cobicistat decreases estimated creatinine clearance due to inhibition of tubular secretion of creatinine without affecting actual renal glomerular function. Renal impairment, including cases of acute renal failure and Fanconi syndrome when combined with tenofovir DF. Other side effects reported include jaundice, rash, scleral icterus, nausea, diarrhea, and headache. In less than 2%: abdominal pain, vomiting, fatigue, rhabdomyolysis, depression, abnormal dreams, insomnia, nephropathy, and nephrolithiasis.

 DRUG INTERACTIONS/FOOD INTERACTIONS

Atazanavir/cobicistat should be taken with a meal.

Drugs that should not be coadministered with atazanavir/cobicistat include amiodarone, quinidine, rifampin, ergot derivatives, St John's wort, HMG-CoA reductase inhibitors simvastatin and lovastatin, pimozide, benzodiazepines, irinotecan, etravirine, nevirapine, indinavir, Kaletra, saquinavir, fosamprenavir, tipranavir, alfuzosin, dronedarone, carbamazapine, phenobarbatol, phenytoin, rivaroxaban, cisapride, avanafil, or sildenafil.

Atazanavir and cobicistat are inhibitors of the CYP3A enzyme and UGT1A1; coadministration of atazanavir/cobicistat and drugs primarily metabolized by CYP3A or UGT1A1 may result in increased plasma concentrations of the other drug that could increase or prolong its therapeutic and adverse effects.

Antibiotics Manual: A Guide to Commonly Used Antimicrobials, Second Edition. David Schlossberg and Rafik Samuel.
© 2017 John Wiley & Sons Ltd. Published 2017 by John Wiley & Sons Ltd.

Atazanavir is metabolized by CYP3A; coadministration of atazanavir and drugs that induce CYP3A may decrease atazanavir plasma concentrations and reduce its therapeutic effect. Coadministration of atazanavir and drugs that inhibit CYP3A may increase atazanavir plasma concentrations. Because of these metabolic affects, potential drug interactions that may require dosage change or clinical/laboratory monitoring are listed below:

Medication	Adjustment or action
Itraconzole	Monitor for toxicity
Voriconazole	Monitor for toxicity
Rifabutin	Rifabutin 150 mg/d or 300 mg 3 times/week
Contraceptives	Use alternative method of contraception
Atorvastatin	Use lowest possible dose of atorvastatin and monitor
Phenobarbital, phenytoin, or carbamazepine	Monitor anticonvulsant level; consider alternative
Sildenafil	25 mg every 48 hours
Tadalafil	5 mg, no more than 10 mg in 72 hours
Vardenafil	2.5 mg in 24 hours
Diltiazem	ECG monitoring recommended
H2 receptors	Dose should not exceed 40 mg bid equivalent of famotidine
PPI	Dose should not exceed 20 mg equivalent of omeprazole and should be given 12 hours before
Antacids	Administer 2 hours apart
Didanosine	Administer separately from atazanavir
Maraviroc	Maraviroc dose is 150 mg bid
Colchicine	Not recommended in renal or hepatic impairment
Bosentan	Bosentan dose is 62.5 mg daily or qod
Cyclosporine, tacrolimus	Monitor levels of the immunosuppressants

 ## DOSING

Atazanavir/cobicistat is a fixed dose combination of atazanavir 300 mg and cobicistat 150 mg. The recommended dose is 1 pill daily with food.

 ## SPECIAL POPULATIONS

RENAL IMPAIRMENT: Not recommended in HIV-treatment-experienced adults with endstage renal disease managed with hemodialysis.

HEPATIC DYSFUNCTION: Not recommended for use in patients with hepatic impairment.

PEDIATRICS: Not recommended in patients under 18 years of age.

THE ART OF ANTIMICROBIAL THERAPY

Clinical Pearls

1. Atazanavir/cobicistat should always be used in combination with other antiretrovirals.
2. Atazanavir/cobicsitat should be taken with food to increase absorption.
3. Whenever initiating atazanavir/cobicistat, make sure to review all medications the patient is receiving to minimize drug interactions.
4. Atazanavir causes an increase in indirect bilirubin by inhibiting glucuronidation.
5. Atazanavir causes nephrolithiasis; patients should be advised to drink adequate water.
6. Rash is not infrequent on atazanavir even though it does not contain a sulfa moiety.
7. Do not use with agents that contain cobicistat or atazanavir: Reyataz, Tybost, Stribild, Genvoya, or Prezcobix.

BASIC CHARACTERISTICS

Class: Fluoroquinolone.

Mechanism of Action: Inhibition of bacterial topoisomerase IV and DNA gyrase.

Mechanisms of Resistance: Mutations in DNA gyrase and/or topoisomerase IV.

Metabolic Route: Approximately two-thirds of the gemifloxacin is excreted in the feces with the remainder excreted in the urine.

 ## FDA-APPROVED INDICATIONS

Gemifloxacin is indicated for the treatment of serious infections caused by susceptible strains of microorganisms in the diseases listed below:

Acute bacterial exacerbation of chronic bronchitis

Community-acquired pneumonia of mild to moderate severity

 ## SIDE EFFECTS/TOXICITY

> **WARNING:** Serious adverse reactions including tendinitis, tendon rupture, peripheral neuropathy, central nervous system effects and exacerbation of myasthenia gravis. Fluoroquinolones, including gemifloxacin, have been associated with disabling and potentially irreversible serious adverse reactions that have occurred together, including tendinitis and tendon rupture, peripheral neuropathy, and central nervous system effects. Discontinue gemifloxacin immediately and avoid the use of fluoroquinolones, including gemifloxacin in patients who experience any of these serious adverse reactions. Fluoroquinolones, including gemifloxacin, may exacerbate muscle weakness in patients with myasthenia gravis. Avoid gemifloxacin in patients with a known history of myasthenia gravis. Because fluoroquinolones, including gemifloxacin, have been associated with serious adverse reactions, reserve for use in patients who have no alternative treatment options for acute bacterial exacerbation of chronic bronchitis.

Gemifloxacin is **contraindicated** in persons with a history of hypersensitivity associated with the use of gemifloxacin or any quinolone.

Other adverse effects include anaphylactic reactions with cardiovascular collapse, angioedema, allergic skin reactions including toxic epidermal necrolysis and Stevens-Johnson syndrome, photosensitivity, tendinitis and tendon rupture, renal toxicity, hepatotoxicity (sometimes fatal), central nervous system effects including headache, dizziness, seizures, anxiety, confusion, depression, and insomnia (use with caution in patients at risk of seizures), peripheral neuropathy, nausea, diarrhea, constipation, *Clostridium difficile*-associated colitis, prolongation of the QT interval and torsade de pointes (avoid use in patients with known prolongation of QT, hypokalemia, and with other drugs that prolong the QT interval), and pancytopenia.

Antibiotics Manual: A Guide to Commonly Used Antimicrobials, Second Edition. David Schlossberg and Rafik Samuel.
© 2017 John Wiley & Sons Ltd. Published 2017 by John Wiley & Sons Ltd.

DRUG INTERACTIONS/FOOD INTERACTIONS

Gemifloxacin can be taken with or without food.

1. Antacids containing calcium, magnesium, or aluminum; sucralfate; divalent or trivalent cations such as iron; or multivitamins containing zinc should not be taken within the three-hour period before or within the two-hour period after taking gemifloxacin.
2. The concomitant administration of a nonsteroidal anti-inflammatory drug with a quinolone may increase the risk of seizures.
3. The concomitant use of probenecid with quinolones decreases renal tubular secretion.

 DOSING

Gemifloxacin is administered as a 320 mg tablet once daily.

 SPECIAL POPULATIONS

RENAL IMPAIRMENT: If creatinine clearance is <40 mL/min, the dose should be 160 mg daily.

HEPATIC DYSFUNCTION: No dose adjustment is necessary.

PEDIATRICS: Safety and efficacy in pediatric patients less than 18 years of age have not yet been established.

 THE ART OF ANTIMICROBIAL THERAPY

Clinical Pearls

1. Gemifloxacin should be given at least 3 hours after or 2 hours before cations.
2. All fluoroquinolones can lead to tendon rupture, especially in patients over 60 years of age.
3. All fluoroquinolones can prolong QT intervals, so caution should be used when given with medications that affect QT intervals.
4. All fluoroquinolones can cause phototoxicity.
5. All fluoroquinolones can lower the seizure threshold.
6. Fluoroquinolones should be avoided if possible in children, pregnant women, and nursing mothers, due to possible disturbance in cartilage development.
7. Fluoroquinolones have activity against Mycobacteria; therefore gemifloxacin monotherapy should be avoided if mycobacterial infection is possible.
8. Gemifloxacin is not recommended for urinary tract infections.
9. In 2016, an FDA Safety Communication advised that the serious side effects associated with fluoroquinolones generally outweigh the benefits for patients with sinusitis, bronchitis, and uncomplicated urinary tract infections who have other treatment options.

BASIC CHARACTERISTICS

Class: Nucleoside analog.

Mechanism of Action: Famciclovir is the prodrug of penciclovir. Penciclovir is a guanine analog. After hydrolysis, it is phosphorylated by thymadine kinase to the active triphosphate form. Penciclovir triphosphate stops replication of herpes viral DNA. This is accomplished in three ways: (1) competitive inhibition of viral DNA polymerase, (2) incorporation into and termination of the growing viral DNA chain, and (3) inactivation of the viral DNA polymerase. The greater antiviral activity of acyclovir against HSV compared to VZV is due to its more efficient phosphorylation by the viral thymadine kinase.

Mechanism of Resistance: Resistance of HSV and VZV to penciclovir can result from qualitative or quantitative changes in the viral TK or DNA polymerase.

Metabolic Route: After oral administration, famciclovir is deacetylated and hydrolyzed to penciclovir. Penciclovir is excreted in the urine.

 FDA-APPROVED INDICATIONS

Famciclovir is indicated for the treatment of recurrent herpes labialis, recurrent genital herpes, herpes zoster, suppression of recurrent genital herpes in immunocompetent patients, and the treatment of recurrent herpes simplex infections in HIV-infected patients.

 SIDE EFFECTS/TOXICITY

Acute renal failure, headache, parasthesia, migraine, confusion, hallucinations, nausea, vomiting, diarrhea, flatulence, abdominal pain, fatigue, pruritus, rash, and dysmenorrhea.

 DRUG INTERACTIONS/FOOD INTERACTIONS

Famciclovir can be administered orally with or without food.

Concurrent use with probenecid or other drugs significantly eliminated by active renal tubular secretion may result in increased plasma concentrations of penciclovir.

 DOSING

Famciclovir is supplied in 125 mg, 250 mg, and 500 mg tablets.

Herpes labialis	1500 mg single dose
Treatment of recurrent genital herpes	1000 mg twice daily for 1 day
Herpes Zoster	500 mg every 8 hours for 7 days
Suppression of recurrent genital herpes	250 mg twice daily
Recurrent orolabial or genital herpes simplex in HIV-infected individuals	500 mg twice daily for 7 days

Antibiotics Manual: A Guide to Commonly Used Antimicrobials, Second Edition. David Schlossberg and Rafik Samuel.
© 2017 John Wiley & Sons Ltd. Published 2017 by John Wiley & Sons Ltd.

SPECIAL POPULATIONS

RENAL IMPAIRMENT:

Indication	Creatinine clearance, mL/min			
	40–59	20–39	<20	HD*
Herpes labialis	750 mg (×1)	500 mg (×1)	250 mg (×1)	250 p HD
Recurrent genital herpes	500 mg q 12 h (×2)	500 mg (×1)	250 mg (×1)	250 p HD
Herpes Zoster	500 mg q 12 h	500 mg q 24 h	250 mg q 24 h	250 p HD
Suppression genital herpes	250 mg q 12 h	125 mg q 12 h	125 mg q 24 h	125 p HD
Treatment of recurrent orolabial and genital herpes in HIV	500 mg q 12 h	500 mg q 24 h	250 mg q 24 h	250 p HD

* Hemodialysis.

HEPATIC DYSFUNCTION: No dose adjustment is needed.

PEDIATRIC: Famciclovir has not been studied in patients under the age of 18. Use acyclovir.

 THE ART OF ANTIMICROBIAL THERAPY

Clinical Pearls

1. Famciclovir is effective against HSV and VZV. It has no activity against the other herpes viruses.

2. Famciclovir is not recommended for children; acyclovir is recommended in this age group.

BASIC CHARACTERISTICS

Class: Nitroimidazole.

Mechanism of Action: After entry into the bacteria, it is reduced into multiple products that are toxic to intracellular targets.

Mechanism of Resistance: Decreased pyruvate:ferredoxin oxidoreductase activity, which reduces uptake of the drug.

Metabolic Route: The major route of elimination of metronidazole and its metabolites is via the urine (60–80 % of the dose), with fecal excretion accounting for 6–15 % of the dose.

 FDA-APPROVED INDICATIONS

Intravenous metronidazole: Treatment of susceptible anaerobic infections, including:

Intra-abdominal infections

Skin and skin structure infections

Gynecologic infections

Bacterial septicemia

Bone and joint infections

Central nervous system (CNS) infections

Lower respiratory tract infections

Endocarditis

Surgical prophylaxis

Oral metronidazole:

Symptomatic trichomoniasis

Asymptomatic trichomoniasis

Treatment of asymptomatic consorts with trichomoniasis

Amebiasis

Anaerobic bacterial infections (often treated orally after initial IV therapy)

   Intra-abdominal infections

   Skin and skin structure infections

   Gynecologic infections

   Bacterial septicemia

   Bone and joint infections

   Central nervous system infections

   Lower respiratory tract infections

   Endocarditis

Also Used for:

Clostridium difficile-associated diarrhea

Giardiasis

Antibiotics Manual: A Guide to Commonly Used Antimicrobials, Second Edition. David Schlossberg and Rafik Samuel.
© 2017 John Wiley & Sons Ltd. Published 2017 by John Wiley & Sons Ltd.

Balantidiasis, Blastocystis, Dientamoeba fragilis

In combination with amoxicillin, clarithromycin, and a proton pump inhibitor for *H. pylori* infections

Bacterial vaginosis

Bacterial overgrowth syndromes

 ## SIDE EFFECTS/TOXICITY

> **WARNING:** Metronidazole has been shown to be carcinogenic in mice and rats. Unnecessary use of the drug should be avoided.

Contraindicated in patients with a prior history of hypersensitivity to metronidazole or other nitroimidazole derivatives.

Side effects include seizures, peripheral neuropathy, fever, thrombophlebitis, pruritus, rash, urticaria, flushing, nasal congestion, anorexia, furry tongue, glossitis, metallic taste, nausea, vomiting, abdominal discomfort, pancreatitis, diarrhea, headache, dizziness, syncope, vertigo, ataxia, confusion, incoordination, dysuria, cystitis, polyuria, incontinence, darkened urine, neutropenia, thrombocytopenia, flattening of the T-wave, interference with laboratory determinations of AST, ALT, LDH, triglycerides, and glucose.

 ## DRUG INTERACTIONS/FOOD INTERACTIONS

Metronidazole may potentiate the anticoagulant effect of warfarin and other oral coumarin anticoagulants.

Phenytoin or phenobarbital and other drugs that induce hepatic microsomal enzymes may accelerate the elimination of metronidazole.

Drugs that decrease hepatic microsomal enzyme activity, e.g., cimetidine, may prolong the half-life and decrease plasma clearance of metronidazole.

Alcoholic beverages should not be consumed during metronidazole therapy because abdominal cramps, nausea, vomiting, headaches, and flushing may occur.

Metronidazole should not be given to patients who have taken disulfiram within the last two weeks; psychotic reactions have been reported.

 ## DOSING

Metronidazole is administered as 250 mg and 500 mg capsules. It is also administered intravenously.

IV

Treatment of anaerobic infections

The recommended dose is 15 mg/kg loading dose followed by 7.5 mg/kg every 6 hours, with a maximum of 4 g during a 24-hour period.

Prophylaxis

15 mg/kg followed by 7.5 mg/kg at 6 and 12 hours after the initial dose. The first dose should be administered 30–60 minutes prior to incision.

Oral

Trichomoniasis

One-day treatment: two grams as a single dose or in two divided doses of one gram each given in the same day.

Seven-day course of treatment: 250 mg three times daily for seven consecutive days.

Amebiasis

For mild to moderate intestinal disease: 500–750 mg PO tid × 7–10 d.

For severe intestinal and extraintestinal disease: 750 mg PO (or IV) tid × 7–10 d.

Giardiasis: 250 mg PO tid × 5–7 d.

 ## SPECIAL POPULATIONS

RENAL IMPAIRMENT:

Creatinine clearance, mL/min	Dose
>10	Usual dose and intervals
<10	Usual dose every 8 hours (max.)
Hemodialysis	Administer after dialysis only
CAPD	Usual dose every 8 hours (max.)
CRRT	Usual dose and intervals

HEPATIC DYSFUNCTION: Patients with severe hepatic disease metabolize metronidazole slowly, with resultant accumulation of metronidazole and its metabolites in the plasma. Accordingly, for such patients, doses below those usually recommended should be administered cautiously. Close monitoring of plasma metronidazole levels and toxicity is recommended.

PEDIATRICS:

Amebiasis:

Mild to moderate intestinal disease; 35–50 mg/kg/d PO in 3 doses × 7–10 d.

Severe intestinal and extraintestinal disease: 35–50 mg/kg/d PO or IV in 3 doses × 7–10 d.

Giardiasis: 15 mg/kg/d PO in 3 doses × 5–7 d.

 ## THE ART OF ANTIMICROBIAL THERAPY

Clinical Pearls

1. Ethanol should be avoided when taking metronidazole.
2. Metronidazole should not be used in the first trimester of pregnancy.
3. Metronidazole has poor activity against anaerobic nonspore-forming gram-positive bacilli, e.g., bifidobacterium, eubacterium, actinomyces, propionibacterium, and lactobacillus.
4. In a mixed aerobic and anaerobic infection, antimicrobials appropriate for the treatment of the aerobic infection and gram-positive anaerobes (see above) should be used in addition to metronidazole.

■ FLOXIN (Ofloxacin)

 BASIC CHARACTERISTICS

Class: Fluoroquinolone.

Mechanism of Action: Inhibition of bacterial topoisomerase IV and DNA gyrase.

Mechanisms of Resistance: Mutations in DNA gyrase and/or topoisomerase IV; or through altered efflux.

Metabolic Route: Ofloxacin is predominantly excreted in the urine.

 FDA-APPROVED INDICATIONS

Ofloxacin is indicated for the treatment of serious infections caused by susceptible strains of microorganisms in the diseases listed below:

Acute bacterial exacerbations of chronic bronchitis

Community-acquired pneumonia

Uncomplicated skin and skin structure infections

Acute, uncomplicated urethral and cervical gonorrhea

Nongonococcal urethritis and cervicitis

Mixed infections of the urethra and cervix

Acute pelvic inflammatory disease

Uncomplicated cystitis

Complicated urinary tract infections

Prostatitis

 SIDE EFFECTS/TOXICITY

> **WARNING:** Fluoroquinolones, including ofloxacin, are associated with an increased risk of tendinitis and tendon rupture in all ages. This risk is further increased in older patients usually over 60 years of age, in patients taking corticosteroid drugs and in patients with kidney, heart, or lung transplants. Fluoroquinolones, including ofloxacin, may exacerbate muscle weakness in persons with myasthenia gravis. Avoid ofloxacin in patients with a known history of myasthenia gravis. Ofloxacin is **contraindicated** in persons with a history of hypersensitivity associated with the use of ofloxacin or any quinolone.

Other adverse effects include anaphylactic reactions and allergic skin reactions including toxic epidermal necrolysis and Stevens–Johnson syndrome, photosensitivity, renal toxicity, hepatotoxicity (sometimes fatal), central nervous system effects including headache, dizziness, seizures, anxiety, confusion, depression, and insomnia (use with caution in patients at risk of seizures), peripheral neuropathy, nausea, diarrhea, constipation, *Clostridium difficile*-associated colitis, prolongation of the QT interval, and torsade de pointes (avoid use in patients with known prolongation of QT, hypokalemia, and with other drugs that prolong the QT interval), and pancytopenia.

Antibiotics Manual: A Guide to Commonly Used Antimicrobials, Second Edition. David Schlossberg and Rafik Samuel.
© 2017 John Wiley & Sons Ltd. Published 2017 by John Wiley & Sons Ltd.

DRUG INTERACTIONS/FOOD INTERACTIONS

1. Antacids containing calcium, magnesium, or aluminum; sucralfate; divalent or trivalent cations such as iron; or multivitamins containing zinc should not be taken within the two-hour period before or after taking ofloxacin.
2. Cimetidine results in significant increases in half-life of some quinolones, possibly including ofloxacin.
3. Ofloxacin may enhance the effect of theophylline, cyclosporine, and warfarin, via inhibition of P450 enzyme activity.
4. The concomitant administration of a nonsteroidal anti-inflammatory drug with a quinolone may increase the risk of CNS stimulation and convulsive seizures.
5. The concomitant use of probenecid with quinolones decreases renal tubular secretion.
6. Disturbances of blood glucose, including hyperglycemia and hypoglycemia, in patients treated concurrently with quinolones and antidiabetic agents.
7. Ofloxacin may produce false-positive urine screening results for opiates.

 DOSING

Ofloxacin is supplied as 200 mg, 300 mg, and 400 mg tablets.

The usual dose of ofloxacin is 200 mg to 400 mg orally every 12 h.

Infection	Dose	Frequency	Duration
Acute exacerbation of bronchitis	400 mg	q 12 h	10 days
Community-acquired pneumonia	400 mg	q 12 h	10 days
Uncomplicated skin infections	400 mg	q 12 h	10 days
Acute urethral and cervical gonorrhea	400 mg	Single dose	1 day
Nongonococcal cervicitis/urethritis	300 mg	q 12 h	7 days
Infection of the urethra and cervix	300 mg	q 12 h	7 days
Acute pelvic inflammatory disease	400 mg	q 12 h	10–14 days
Cystitis	200 mg	q 12 h	3 days
Uncomplicated UTI	200 mg	q 12 h	7 days
Complicated UTIs	200 mg	q 12 h	10 days
Prostatitis	300 mg	q 12 h	6 weeks

 SPECIAL POPULATIONS

RENAL IMPAIRMENT:

Creatinine clearance	Maintenance dose	Frequency
20–50 mL/min	The usual recommended unit dose	q 24 h
<20 mL/min	Half the usual recommended unit dose	q 24 h
Hemodialysis	Half the usual recommended unit dose	q 12
CAPD	Half the usual recommended unit dose	q 24 h
CRRT	300 mg	q 24 h

HEPATIC DYSFUNCTION: A maximum dose of 400 mg of ofloxacin per day should not be exceeded.

PEDIATRICS: Safety and efficacy in pediatric patients less than 18 years of age have not yet been established.

THE ART OF ANTIMICROBIAL THERAPY

Clinical Pearls

1. Ofloxacin should be given at least 2 hours separately from cations.
2. All fluoroquinolones can lead to tendon rupture, especially patients over 65 years of age.
3. All fluoroquinolones can prolong QT intervals, and caution should be used when given with medications that affect QT intervals
4. All fluoroquinolones can cause phototoxicity.
5. All fluoroquinolones can lower the seizure threshold.
6. Fluoroquinolones should be avoided if possible in children, pregnant women, and nursing mothers, due to possible disturbance in cartilage development.
7. Treatment of gonorrhea with fluoroquinolones should be undertaken with caution because of rising resistance.
8. In 2016, an FDA Safety Communication advised that the serious side effects associated with fluoroquinolones generally outweigh the benefits for patients with sinusitis, bronchitis, and uncomplicated urinary tract infections who have other treatment options.

BASIC CHARACTERISTICS

Class: Third generation cephalosporin.

Mechanism of Action: Binds penicillin-binding protein, disrupting cell wall synthesis.

Mechanisms of Resistance:

1. The PBP can be altered, with reduced affinity.
2. Production of a beta-lactamase, resulting in hydrolysis of the beta-lactam ring.
3. Decreased ability of the antibiotic to reach the PBP when bacteria decrease porin production, resulting in a decrease of the drug concentration within the cell.

Metabolic Route: Excreted unchanged in the urine.

 FDA-APPROVED INDICATIONS

Treatment of patients with infections caused by susceptible strains of organisms in the following diseases:

Lower respiratory tract infections

Skin and skin structure infections

Urinary tract infections

Bacterial septicemia

Bone and joint infections

Gynecologic infections

Intra-abdominal infections

Central nervous system infections

 SIDE EFFECTS/TOXICITY

Ceftazidime is **contraindicated** in patients who have shown immediate hypersensitivity to ceftazidime or the cephalosporin group of antibiotics.

Ceftazidime should be used with caution if other forms of hypersensitivity exist to penicillin.

Toxicity includes inflammation at the site of injection, fever, anaphylaxis, rash including Stevens–Johnson syndrome, erythema multiforme and toxic epidermal necrolysis, angioedema, flushing, serum-sickness-like reactions, encephalopathy, seizures, myoclonus, diarrhea, *Clostridium difficile*-associated diarrhea and pseudomembranous colitis, oral candidiasis, anorexia, nausea, vomiting, stomach cramps, flatulence, hepatitis, renal impairment, genital moniliasis, vaginitis, hemorrhage, prolonged prothrombin time, pancytopenia, hemolytic anemia, positive Coombs' test.

 DRUG INTERACTIONS/FOOD INTERACTIONS

Nephrotoxicity has been reported following concomitant administration of cephalosporins with aminoglycoside antibiotics or potent diuretics such as furosemide. Cephalosporins may cause false-positive urine glucose determinations when using cupric sulfate solution (Benedict's solution, *Clinitest®*). Tests utilizing glucose oxidase (*Tes-Tape®*, *Clinistix®*) are not affected by cephalosporins.

Antibiotics Manual: A Guide to Commonly Used Antimicrobials, Second Edition. David Schlossberg and Rafik Samuel.
© 2017 John Wiley & Sons Ltd. Published 2017 by John Wiley & Sons Ltd.

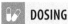 **DOSING**

Infection	Dose
Urinary tract infections	250 mg q 12 hours IV or IM
Bone and joint infections	2 g q 12 hours IV
Complicated urinary tract infections	500 mg q 8–12 hours IV or IM
Pneumonia	500 mg–1 gram q 8 hours IV or IM
Skin and skin structure infections	500 mg–1 gram q 8 hours IV or IM
Gyn and abdominal infections	2 g q 8 hours IV
Meningitis	2 g q 8 hours IV
Severe life-threatening infections	2 g q 8 hours IV
Severe pseudomonas lung infections	30–50 mg/kg up to 6 grams/day IV

 SPECIAL POPULATIONS

RENAL IMPAIRMENT:

Creatinine clearance	Dose
31–50 mL/min	1 gram q 12 hours
16–30 mL/min	1 gram q 24 hours
6–15 mL/min	500 mg q 24 hours
<5 mL/min	500 mg q 48 hours
Hemodialysis	1 gram after dialysis
CAPD	500 mg daily
CRRT	1 gram q 12–24 hours

HEPATIC DYSFUNCTION: No dose adjustment is necessary.

PEDIATRICS:

Neonates under 1 month of age: 30 mg/kg q 12 hours.

Children 1 month–12 years: 30–50 mg/kg q 8 hours up to 6 grams/day.

 THE ART OF ANTIMICROBIAL THERAPY

Clinical Pearls

1. Ceftazidime is dose adjusted for renal dysfunction.
2. Cross allergy with penicillins is <10% and can be used in life-threatening infections with caution if the allergy is not severe.
3. Inducible type I beta-lactamase resistance has been noted with some organisms (e.g., *Enterobacter* spp., *Pseudomonas* spp., and *Serratia* spp.) and can develop during therapy.

BASIC CHARACTERISTICS

Class: Organic pyrophosphate.

Mechanism of Action: Foscarnet sodium is an organic analog of inorganic pyrophosphate that inhibits replication of cytomegalovirus (CMV) and herpes simplex virus types 1 and 2.

HSV strains resistant to acyclovir or CMV strains resistant to ganciclovir may be sensitive to foscarnet sodium.

Mechanism of Resistance: Mutation in the viral DNA polymerase gene.

Metabolic Route: Most of administered dose is excreted unchanged in the urine.

 FDA-APPROVED INDICATIONS

Treatment of CMV retinitis in patients with acquired immunodeficiency syndrome (AIDS).

Foscarnet is also indicated for the treatment of acyclovir-resistant mucocutaneous HSV infections in immunocompromised patients.

Also Used for: Treatment of varicella zoster virus infections and cytomegalovirus infections in transplant recipients.

 SIDE EFFECTS/TOXICITY

> **WARNING:** Renal impairment is the major toxicity of foscarnet. Frequent monitoring of serum creatinine with dose adjustment for changes in renal function and adequate hydration with administration of foscarnet is imperative.
>
> Seizures related to alterations in plasma minerals and electrolytes have been associated with foscarnet treatment. Therefore, patients must be carefully monitored for such changes and their potential sequelae. Mineral and electrolyte supplementation may be required.
>
> Foscarnet is indicated for use only in immunocompromised patients with CMV retinitis and mucocutaneous acyclovir-resistant HSV infections.

Other toxic effects include rash, genital irritation from urinary drug levels, possibly ameliorated by adequate hydration, bone marrow toxicity, rigors, paresthesia, nausea, vomiting, diarrhea, abdominal pain, depression, dementia, cough, vision abnormalities, ECG abnormalities and electrolyte disturbances (hypocalcemia, hypophosphatemia, hyperphosphatemia, hypomagnesemia, and hypokalemia) related to chelation of divalent metal ions by foscarnet, and seizures. The rate of foscarnet sodium infusion may affect the decrease in ionized calcium.

 DRUG INTERACTIONS/FOOD INTERACTIONS

Since foscarnet decreases serum concentrations of ionized calcium, concurrent treatment with other drugs known to influence serum calcium concentrations should be used with particular caution, including pentamidine.

Because of foscarnet's tendency to cause renal impairment, the use of foscarnet sodium should be avoided in combination with potentially nephrotoxic drugs such as aminoglycosides, amphotericin B, and intravenous pentamidine unless the potential benefits outweigh the risks to the patient.

Antibiotics Manual: A Guide to Commonly Used Antimicrobials, Second Edition. David Schlossberg and Rafik Samuel.
© 2017 John Wiley & Sons Ltd. Published 2017 by John Wiley & Sons Ltd.

Abnormal renal function has been observed in clinical practice during the use of foscarnet sodium and ritonavir, or foscarnet sodium, ritonavir, and saquinavir.

 ## DOSING (BY CONTROLLED INFUSION)

For **CMV retinitis** patients, either 90 mg/kg every 12 hours or 60 mg/kg every 8 hours over 2 to 3 weeks. Following induction treatment the recommended maintenance dose is 90 mg/kg/day to 120 mg/kg/day.

For **acyclovir-resistant HSV** patients, 40 mg/kg either every 8 or 12 hours for 2 to 3 weeks or until healed.

 ## SPECIAL POPULATIONS

RENAL IMPAIRMENT:

Creatinine clearance, mL/min/kg	Dose for HSV	Induction dose for CMV	Maintenance dose for CMV
>1.4	40 mg/kg q 12 hours	90 mg/kg q 12 hours	90 mg/kg q day
1.0–1.4	30 mg/kg q 12 hours	70 mg/kg q 12 hours	70 mg/kg q day
0.8–1	20 mg/kg q 12 hours	50 mg/kg q 12 hours	50 mg/kg q day
0.6–0.8	35 mg/kg q day	80 mg/kg q day	80 mg/kg q 48 hours
0.5–0.6	25 mg/kg q day	60 mg/kg q day	60 mg/kg q 48 hours
0.4–0.5	20 mg/kg q day	50 mg/kg q day	50 mg/kg q 48 hours
<0.4	Not recommended	Not recommended	Not recommended

It is not recommended to administer in CRRT.

HEPATIC DYSFUNCTION: Caution should be used when administered to those with hepatic dysfunction.

PEDIATRICS: Foscarnet is not recommended for use in pediatric patients.

 ## THE ART OF ANTIMICROBIAL THERAPY

Clinical Pearls

1. The combination of foscarnet and ganciclovir has been shown to have enhanced activity for the treatment of CMV encephalitis.
2. Even though not FDA approved, foscarnet is used to treat other CMV infections in HIV patients and those who have received transplants.
3. Renal impairment is most likely to become clinically evident during the second week of induction therapy.
4. Hydration is recommended with each dose of foscarnet to decrease renal toxicity.
5. The chelation of calcium is related to the rate of infusion; slowing down the infusion can decrease this complication.
6. Infusion should be carefully controlled **per the manufacturer's instructions**.

BASIC CHARACTERISTICS

Class: Polyene.

Mechanism of Action: Amphotericin B inserts into the cytoplasmic membrane through ergosterol, leading to increased permeability of the fungal membrane and loss of intracellular ions.

Amphotericin B also affects oxidation and may cause fungal death in this manner.

Mechanism of Resistance: Resistance is rare, but is due to changes in the cell membrane that prevent amphotericin from inserting into the membrane.

Metabolic Route: Amphotericin B is excreted very slowly by the kidneys. After discontinuation of treatment, amphotericin is detectable in urine for at least seven weeks.

 FDA-APPROVED INDICATIONS

Potentially life-threatening fungal infections: aspergillosis, cryptococcosis, blastomycosis, systemic candidiasis, coccidioidomycosis, histoplasmosis, zygomycosis, and infections due to related susceptible species of *Conidiobolus* and *Basidiobolus*, and sporotrichosis.

Also Used for: Amphotericin B has been used to treat American mucocutaneous leishmaniasis and *Naegleria fowleri*, but it is not the drug of choice as primary therapy.

 SIDE EFFECTS/TOXICITY

> **WARNING:** This drug should be used *primarily* for treatment of patients with progressive and potentially life-threatening fungal infections: it should not be used to treat noninvasive forms of fungal disease such as oral thrush, vaginal candidiasis, and esophageal candidiasis in patients with normal neutrophil counts.
>
> Amphotericin B should not be given in doses greater than 1.5 mg/kg.
>
> **EXERCISE CAUTION** to prevent inadvertent overdosage, which may result in potentially fatal cardiac or cardiopulmonary arrest. Verify the product name and dosage if the dose exceeds 1.5 mg/kg.

Contraindicated in patients who have shown hypersensitivity to amphotericin B or any other component in the formulation.

Acute reactions including fever, shaking chills, hypotension, anorexia, nausea, vomiting, headache, and tachypnea are common 1 to 3 hours after starting an intravenous infusion. Rapid intravenous infusion has been associated with hypotension, hypokalemia, arrhythmias, and shock and should therefore be avoided.

Amphotericin B should be used with care in patients with reduced renal function; frequent monitoring of renal function is recommended.

Since acute pulmonary reactions have been reported in patients given amphotericin B during or shortly after leukocyte transfusions, it is advisable to temporarily separate these infusions as far as possible and to monitor pulmonary function.

Leukoencephalopathy has been reported following use of amphotericin B.

Antibiotics Manual: A Guide to Commonly Used Antimicrobials, Second Edition. David Schlossberg and Rafik Samuel.
© 2017 John Wiley & Sons Ltd. Published 2017 by John Wiley & Sons Ltd.

DRUG INTERACTIONS

Antineoplastic agents may enhance the potential for renal toxicity, bronchospasm, and hypotension and should be given concomitantly only with great caution.

Corticosteroids and corticotropin (ACTH): closely monitor serum electrolytes and cardiac function.

Digitalis glycosides: amphotericin B-induced hypokalemia may potentiate digitalis toxicity.

Flucytosine: concomitant use may increase the toxicity of flucytosine.

Imidazoles (e.g., **fluconazole**): imidazoles may induce fungal resistance to amphotericin B. Combination therapy should be administered with caution.

Other nephrotoxic medications: may enhance the potential for drug-induced renal toxicity and should be used concomitantly only with great caution.

Skeletal muscle relaxants: amphotericin B-induced hypokalemia may enhance the curariform effect of skeletal muscle relaxants.

Leukocyte transfusions: acute pulmonary toxicity has been reported in patients receiving intravenous amphotericin B and leukocyte transfusions.

 DOSING

A single intravenous test dose (1 mg in 20 mL of 5 % dextrose solution) administered over 20 to 30 minutes may be preferred. The patient's temperature, pulse, respiration, and blood pressure should be recorded every 30 minutes for 2 to 4 hours.

Therapy is usually initiated with a daily dose of 0.25 mg/kg of body weight and can be increased by 5 to 10 mg per day to final daily dosage of 0.5 to 0.7 mg/kg. Total daily dosage may range up to 1.0 mg/kg per day or up to 1.5 mg/kg when given on alternate days.

 SPECIAL POPULATIONS

RENAL IMPAIRMENT: Technically not contraindicated; however, monitor renal function closely or use lipid formulation. No dosage adjustment recommended.

HEPATIC DYSFUNCTION: Liver tests should be monitored routinely.

PEDIATRICS: Safety and effectiveness in pediatric patients have not been established. Amphotericin B, when administered to pediatric patients, should be limited to the smallest dose compatible with an effective therapeutic regimen.

 THE ART OF ANTIMICROBIAL THERAPY

Clinical Pearls
1. There are various forms of amphotericin with many important differences: amphotericin B deoxycholate, amphotericin B lipid dispersion, amphotericin B lipid complex, or liposomal amphotericin B. This chapter pertains only to amphotericin B deoxycholate.
2. Premedication with acetaminophen, diphenhydramine, meperidine, and even hydrocortisone can decrease infusion-related toxicity.
3. Hydration and sodium repletion prior to amphotericin B administration may reduce the risk of developing nephrotoxicity.

4. Under no circumstances should a total daily dose of 1.5 mg/kg be exceeded.

5. In patients with poor underlying renal function or those with worsening renal function, a lipid formulation of amphotericin is preferred.

6. Some experts believe that mold infections should be treated with the lipid forms of amphotericin B to allow more drug delivery.

7. For candida infections, the echinocandins and azoles may be preferred options for selected patients.

8. *Candida lusitaniae*, *Pseudallescheria boydii*, and *Fusarium* sp. are often resistant to amphotericin B. Voriconazole is frequently used for these infections.

9. It is advisable to monitor on a regular basis liver function, serum electrolytes (particularly magnesium and potassium), blood counts, and hemoglobin concentrations.

FURADANTIN, MACROBID, MACRODANTIN (Nitrofurantoin)

 ## BASIC CHARACTERISTICS

Class: Imidazolidinedione.

Mechanism of Action: Nitrofurantoin is reduced by bacterial flavoproteins to reactive intermediates that inactivate or alter bacterial ribosomal proteins and other macromolecules.

Mechanisms of Resistance: Development of resistance to nitrofurantoin has not been a significant problem.

Metabolic Route: Nitrofurantoin is excreted in the urine.

 ## FDA-APPROVED INDICATIONS

Macrobid is indicated for the treatment of acute uncomplicated urinary tract infections (acute cystitis) caused by susceptible strains of *Escherichia coli* or *Staphylococcus saprophyticus* (not pyelonephritis or perinephric abscesses).

Furadantin is indicated for the treatment of urinary tract infections when due to susceptible strains of *Escherichia coli*, enterococci, *Staphylococcus aureus*, and certain susceptible strains of *Klebsiella* and *Enterobacter* species (not pyelonephritis or perinephric abscesses).

Macrodantin is indicated for the treatment of urinary tract infections when due to susceptible strains of *Escherichia coli*, *Enterococci*, *Staphylococcus aureus*, and certain susceptible strains of *Klebsiella* and *Enterobacter* species (not pyelonephritis or perinephric abscesses).

 ## SIDE EFFECTS/TOXICITY

Contraindications: hypersensitivity to nitrofurantoin, history of hepatotoxicity from nitrofurantoin, anuria, oliguria, creatinine clearance <60 mL/min, pregnancy at term, neonates < 1 month of age.

Adverse events: hypersensitivity with fever and rash, exfoliative dermatitis and erythema multiforme, acute, subacute, or chronic pulmonary reactions with consolidation, pleural effusion, diffuse interstitial pneumonitis or pulmonary fibrosis, nausea, vomiting, hepatitis, jaundice, pancreatitis, *Clostridium difficile*-associated diarrhea, changes in EKG, peripheral neuropathy, optic neuritis, vertigo, nystagmus, headache, benign intracranial hypertension (pseudotumor cerebri), confusion, depression, psychosis, sialadenitis, lupus-like syndrome, leukopenia, thrombocytopenia, megaloblastic anemia, hemolytic anemia in G6PDH-deficient patients, cyanosis secondary to methemoglobinemia.

DRUG INTERACTIONS/FOOD INTERACTIONS

Nitrofurantoin should be given with food to improve absorption.

Antacids containing magnesium trisilicate should not be administered with nitrofurantoin. Probenecid and sulfinpyrazone can inhibit secretion of nitrofurantoin.

A false-positive reaction for glucose in the urine may occur with Benedict's and Fehling's solutions but not with the glucose enzymatic test.

Antibiotics Manual: A Guide to Commonly Used Antimicrobials, Second Edition. David Schlossberg and Rafik Samuel.
© 2017 John Wiley & Sons Ltd. Published 2017 by John Wiley & Sons Ltd.

DOSING

Furadantin is available in a 25 mg/5 mL liquid suspension and the usual dose is 50–100 mg four times a day × 7 days.

Macrobid is available as 100 mg capsules and the usual dose is 100 mg every 12 hours × 7 days.

Macrodantin is available in 25 mg, 50 mg, and 100 mg capsules and the usual dose is 50–100 four times a day × 7 days.

 SPECIAL POPULATIONS

RENAL IMPAIRMENT: Do not administer if creatinine clearance is < 60 mL/min.

HEPATIC DYSFUNCTION: Monitor liver function tests.

PEDIATRICS: Safety and effectiveness of nitrofurantoin in neonates below the age of one month have not been established.

The usual dose of **Furadantin** and **Macrodantin** is 5–7 mg/kg of body weight per 24 hours, given in four divided doses × 7 days.

Macrobid is indicated in patients over 12 years of age and the dose is similar to adults: 100 mg twice daily × 7 days.

 THE ART OF ANTIMICROBIAL THERAPY

Clinical Pearls

1. Nitrofurantoin is most consistently active against *E. coli*; it is not active against most strains of *Proteus* or *Serratia* species and has no activity against *Pseudomonas* species.

2. Antagonism has been demonstrated *in vitro* between nitrofurantoin and quinolone antimicrobial agents.

3. Nitrofurantoin is not indicated for the treatment of pyelonephritis or any systemic infections.

4. Nitrofurantoin can cause pulmonary fibrosis, especially if given for long durations of time.

5. Nitrofurantoin should be administered with food.

6. The different formulations of nitrofurantoin have different dosage recommendations and are absorbed differently; therefore they are not interchangeable.

▪ FUZEON (Enfuvirtide)

 BASIC CHARACTERISTICS

Class: Fusion inhibitor.

Mechanism of Action: Enfuvirtide interferes with the entry of HIV-1 into cells by inhibiting fusion of viral and cellular membranes.

Mechanism of Resistance: Resistant isolates showed mutations that resulted in amino acid substitutions at the enfuvirtide binding HR1 domain positions 36 to 38 of the HIV-1 envelope glycoprotein gp41.

Metabolic Route: Enfuvirtide undergoes catabolism to its constituent amino acids, with subsequent recycling of the amino acids in the body pool.

 FDA-APPROVED INDICATIONS

Treatment of HIV-1 in combinations with other antiretroviral agents in treatment-experienced patients with evidence of HIV-1 replication despite ongoing antiretroviral therapy.

 SIDE EFFECTS/TOXICITY

Hypersensitivity reactions including rash and fever, nausea, vomiting, chills, rigors, hypotension, and/or elevated serum liver transaminases; injection site reactions that include pain and discomfort, induration, erythema, nodules and cysts, pruritus, and ecchymosis; immune reconstitution syndrome, bacterial pneumonia; primary immune complex reaction, respiratory distress, glomerulonephritis, and Guillain–Barre syndrome. There is a theoretical risk that enfuvirtide use may lead to the production of antienfuvirtide antibodies, which cross-react with HIV gp41. This could result in a false positive HIV test with an ELISA assay.

 DRUG INTERACTIONS/FOOD INTERACTIONS

There are no drug interactions.

 DOSING

The recommended dose of enfuvirtide is 90 mg (1 mL) twice daily injected subcutaneously into the upper arm, anterior thigh, or abdomen. Each injection should be given at a site different from the preceding injection site.

 SPECIAL POPULATIONS

RENAL IMPAIRMENT: There is no adjustment needed.

HEPATIC DYSFUNCTION: There is no adjustment needed.

PEDIATRICS: Should not be used in children under 6 years. In those 6 years through 16 years of age, the recommended dosage of enfuvirtide is 2 mg/kg twice daily up to a maximum dose of 90 mg twice daily injected subcutaneously.

Antibiotics Manual: A Guide to Commonly Used Antimicrobials, Second Edition. David Schlossberg and Rafik Samuel.
© 2017 John Wiley & Sons Ltd. Published 2017 by John Wiley & Sons Ltd.

THE ART OF ANTIMICROBIAL THERAPY

Clinical Pearls

1. Enfuvirtide should always be used in combination with other antiretrovirals.
2. Enfuvirtide must be administered within 24 hours of reconstitution.
3. Injection site reactions may be decreased if the enfuvirtide is at room temperature or warmer.
4. Enfuvirtide should only be administered subcutaneously in the anterior thigh, abdomen, or back of arms to ensure good absorption.

■ GARAMYCIN (Gentamicin)

 BASIC CHARACTERISTICS

Class: Aminoglycoside.

Mechanisms of Action:

1. Rearranges lipopolysaccharide in the outer membrane of the bacterial cell wall, resulting in disruption of the cell wall.
2. Binds the 30S subunit of the bacterial ribosome, which terminates protein synthesis.

Mechanism of Resistance

1. Gram-negative bacteria inactivate aminoglycosides by acetylation.
2. Some bacteria alter the 30S ribosomal subunit, which prevents gentamicin's interference with protein synthesis.
3. Low-level resistance may result from inhibition of gentamicin uptake by the bacteria.

Metabolic Route: The drug is excreted unchanged in the urine.

 FDA-APPROVED INDICATIONS

Treatment of susceptible gram-negative bacteria causing bacteremia, pneumonia, osteomyelitis, arthritis, meningitis, skin and soft tissue infection, intra-abdominal infections, in burns and postoperative infections, and urinary tract infections.

Also Used for: Combination therapy with beta-lactams for the treatment of gram-positive endovascular infections.

 SIDE EFFECTS/TOXICITY

> **WARNING**
>
> **Ototoxicity**: vestibular toxicity and auditory ototoxicity, especially in patients with renal damage, those treated with higher doses, and those with prolonged treatment. Avoid use with potent diuretics such as ethacrynic acid because of additive ototoxicity.
>
> **Nephrotoxicity**: especially in patients with impaired renal function and those treated with higher doses or prolonged treatment. Avoid concurrent use with other nephrotoxic agents and potent diuretics, which can cause dehydration.
>
> **Neurotoxicity, including** numbness, skin tingling, muscle twitching and convulsions.

Other adverse effects include fever, rash, anaphylactoid reactions, encephalopathy, pseudotumor cerebri, peripheral neuropathy, neuromuscular blockade, nausea, vomiting, abnormal liver function tests, myasthenia gravis-like syndrome, leucopenia, thrombocytopenia, decreased serum calcium, magnesium, sodium, and potassium.

 DRUG INTERACTIONS

Gentamicin should not be administered with other medications that are nephrotoxic or ototoxic.

Antibiotics Manual: A Guide to Commonly Used Antimicrobials, Second Edition. David Schlossberg and Rafik Samuel.
© 2017 John Wiley & Sons Ltd. Published 2017 by John Wiley & Sons Ltd.

DOSING

3–5 mg/kg/day IM or IV divided q 8 h; desired serum levels are peak 6–12 µg/mL and trough <2 µg/mL. Can also be given once daily as 5–7 mg/kg/24 h; desired serum levels are peak 16–24 µg/mL, trough < 1 µg/mL. Infuse over 60 minutes to avoid neuromuscular blockade.

Intrathecal dose: 4–8 mg/day.

Synergistic dose: 1 mg/kg q 8 h.

 SPECIAL POPULATIONS

RENAL IMPAIRMENT: Adjust dose either by increased interval (serum creatinine multiplied by 8) or by lowering the dose by dividing the dose by the serum creatinine. With either approach, adjustments should be made by following serum assays for q 8 h dosing, above.

Hemodialysis: 3 mg/kg loading dose followed by 1–1.7 mg/kg after hemodialysis.

Peritoneal dialysis: 1 mg/2 L dialysate removed.

CRRT: 3 mg/kg loading dose followed by 2 mg/kg q 24–48 hours or 1 mg/kg q 24–36 hours for gram-positive synergy.

HEPATIC DYSFUNCTION: No dose adjustment necessary.

PEDIATRICS: 3–7.5 mg/kg/d; divide IV q 8 h (newborn: 0–7 d: 2.5 mg/kg q 12 h; 1–4 weeks: 7.5 mg/kg/d q 8 h).

 THE ART OF ANTIMICROBIAL THERAPY

Clinical Pearls

1. Gentamicin is more likely to be active against gram-positive cocci when compared to the other aminoglycosides when used in synergy.
2. Aminoglycosides require oxygen to be active and thus are less effective in anaerobic environments such as an abscess or infected bone.
3. Aminoglycosides have decreased activity in low pH environments such as respiratory secretions or abscesses.
4. When dosing aminoglycosides, use the ideal body weight not the true body weight.
5. Gentamicin has a postantibiotic effect, which allows it to be used once daily.
6. Gentamicin is a good option for treatment of *Tularemia* and *Yersinia pestis* infections.

■ GENVOYA (Tenofovir Alafenamide + Emtricitabine + Elvitegravir + Cobicistat)

 BASIC CHARACTERISTICS

Class: Nucleotide reverse transcriptase inhibitor + nucleotide reverse transcriptase inhibitor + integrase inhibitor + CYP3A inhibitor.

Mechanism of Action: Tenofovir and emtricitabine are converted by cellular enzymes to their active drugs tenofovir biphosphate (an analog of adenosine triphosphate) and emtricitabine triphosphate (an analog of cytosine triphosphate). These drugs compete with the naturally occurring nucleotides for incorporation in newly forming HIV DNA. Since they do not have a terminal hydroxyl group, they halt transcription and replication of the virus.

Elvitegravir is an HIV-1 integrase strand transfer inhibitor (INSTI). Inhibition of integrase prevents the integration of HIV-1 DNA into host genomic DNA, blocking propagation of the viral infection.

Cobicistat is a CYP3A inhibitor indicated to increase systemic exposure of elvitegravir.

Mechanism of Resistance: Changes in the structure of HIV reverse transcriptase leads to preferred incorporation of adenosine triphosphate and cytosine triphosphate with decreased incorporation of tenofovir biphosphate and emtricitabine triphosphate, which allows transcription of DNA to continue. Resistance mutations include K65R, M184V, and "TAMS": 41 L, 67 N, 70R, 210 W, 215 F, and 219E.

Changes in the structure of HIV integrase prevents elvitegravir from binding to the active site of the enzyme and allowing integrase activity to continue. Resistance mutations that emerge in patients taking elvitegravir include T66A/I, E92G/Q, S147G, and Q148R.

Metabolic Route: Tenofovir and emtricitabine are excreted in the urine unchanged.

Elvitegravir undergoes primarily oxidative metabolism via CYP3A and is secondarily glucuronidated via UGT1A1/3 enzymes in the liver and excreted.

Metabolized by CYP3A and to a minor extent by CYP2D6 enzymes in the liver and excreted.

 FDA-APPROVED INDICATIONS

Genvoya is indicated as a complete regimen for the treatment of HIV-1 infection in adults and pediatric patients 12 years of age and older who have no antiretroviral treatment history or to replace the current antiretroviral regimen in those who are virologically suppressed on a stable antiretroviral regimen for at least 6 months with no history of treatment failure and no known substitutions associated with resistance to the individual components of Genvoya.

 SIDE EFFECTS/TOXICITY

> **WARNING: Lactic acidosis and severe hepatomegaly** with steatosis, including fatal cases, have been reported with the use of nucleoside analogs in combination with other antiretrovirals.
>
> Genvoya is not approved for the treatment of chronic hepatitis B virus (HBV) infection and the safety and efficacy of Genvoya have not been established in patients coinfected with human immunodeficiency virus-1 (HIV-1) and HBV. Severe acute exacerbations of hepatitis B have been reported in patients who are coinfected with HIV-1 and HBV and have discontinued products containing emtricitabine and/or tenofovir disoproxil fumarate (TDF), and may occur with Genvoya. Hepatic function should be monitored closely with both clinical and laboratory follow-up for at least several months in patients who are coinfected with HIV-1 and HBV and discontinue Genvoya. If appropriate, initiation of anti-hepatitis B therapy may be warranted.

Antibiotics Manual: A Guide to Commonly Used Antimicrobials, Second Edition. David Schlossberg and Rafik Samuel.
© 2017 John Wiley & Sons Ltd. Published 2017 by John Wiley & Sons Ltd.

Other adverse events: Immune reconstitution inflammatory syndrome, fat redistribution including central obesity and dorso-cervical fat enlargement, peripheral wasting, facial wasting, breast enlargement, renal impairment, including acute renal failure and Fanconi syndrome, and decreased bone mineral density, diarrhea, nausea, fatigue, headache, and decreased estimated creatinine clearance due to inhibition of tubular secretion of creatinine without affecting actual renal glomerular function.

 ## DRUG INTERACTIONS/FOOD INTERACTIONS

Genvoya should be administered with food.

Elvitegravir and cobicistat are metabolized by CYP3A. Drugs that induce or inhibit CYP3A activity are expected to affect the clearance of elvitegravir and cobicistat.

Do not coadminister Genvoya with alfuzosin, phenobarbital, phenytoin, carbamazepine, oxcarbazepine, rifampin, rifabutin, rifapentine, dihydroergotamine, ergotamine, dexamethasone, salmeterol, methylergonovine, St John's wort, cisapride, lovastatin, simvastatin, pimozide, avanafil, sildenafil, triazolam, or midazolam.

Medication	Adjustment or action
Antacid	Administer 2 hours apart
Ketoconazole or itraconzole	Maximum dose of the azoles should be 200 mg
Voriconazole	Only if benefit outweighs risk
Colchicine	Not recommended in renal or hepatic impairment
Quetiapine	Decrease quetiapine dose to one-sixteenth of original dose
Diazepam	Close monitoring
Bosentan	Bosentan 62.5 mg daily or qod
Atorvastatin	Atorvastatin should be given at lowest dose
Cyclosporine, tacrolimus	Monitor levels of the immunosuppressants
Sildenafil	25 mg every 48 hours
Tadalafil	No more than 10 mg in 72 hours
Vardenafil	No more than 2.5 mg in 24 hours

 ## DOSING

Genvoya is a fixed formulation of tenofovir alafenamide 10 mg + emtricitabine 200 mg + elvitegravir 150 mg + cobicistat 150 mg. The recommended adult dose is one tablet once daily.

 ## SPECIAL POPULATIONS

RENAL IMPAIRMENT: The safety of Genvoya has not been established in patients with estimated creatinine clearance that declines below 30 mL per minute.

HEPATIC DYSFUNCTION: Not recommended for use in patients with severe hepatic impairment.

PEDIATRICS: Safety and effectiveness of Genvoya in pediatric patients less than 12 years of age have not been established.

THE ART OF ANTIMICROBIAL THERAPY

Clinical Pearls

1. Genvoya should not be used with any medications that include its components, including: Viread, Emtriva, Truvada, Descovy, Atripla, Stribild, Complera, Odefsey, Vitekta, or Tybost.

2. Genvoya is an integrase inhibitor and should not be used with Triumeq, Isentress, or Tivicay.

3. Genvoya contains emtricitabine and should not be used with any medication containing lamivudine, including: Epivir, Triumeq, Epzicom, Trizivir, or Combivir.

4. Genvoya should be given with food.

5. Genvoya is not indicated to treat hepatitis B.

BASIC CHARACTERIZATION

Class: Hexasulfated naphthylamide.

Mechanism of Action: Binding to several enzymes in the Trypanosomes; however, the mechanism is not fully understood.

Mechanisms of Resistance: Data incomplete.

Metabolic Route: Excreted in the urine unchanged.

Used for: Treatment of *Trypanosoma brucei gambiense* (West African trypanosomiasis) *and Trypanosoma brucei rhodesiense* (East African trypanosomiasis).

 SIDE EFFECTS/TOXICITY

Shock after first dose (rare), fever, renal failure, skin reactions including fatal toxic epidermal necrolysis, polyneuropathy, optic atrophy, corneal deposits, photophobia, coagulopathy, adrenal insufficiency, liver function test anomalies, proteinuria, thrombocytopenia, and neutropenia.

 DRUG INTERACTIONS/FOOD INTERACTIONS

Data incomplete.

 DOSING

100 mg (test dose) IV, then 1 g IV on days 1, 3, 5, 14, and 21.

 SPECIAL POPULATIONS

RENAL IMPAIRMENT: Dose should be reduced or alternative agent should be used.

HEPATIC DYSFUNCTION: No dose adjustment is necessary.

PEDIATRICS: 2 mg/kg (test dose) IV, then 20 mg/kg IV on days 1, 3, 5, 14, and 21.

 THE ART OF ANTIMICROBIAL THERAPY

Clinical Pearls

1. Suramin is available from the CDC Drug Service, 404-639-3670. Evenings, weekends and holidays: 770-488-7100; FAX 404-639-3717.
2. Suramin is considered the drug of choice for *Trypanosoma brucei rhodesiense*.
3. Patients with concomitant onchocerciasis may show aggravation of ocular lesions and hypersensitivity, and such patients should be pretreated with ivermectin, if possible, before receiving suramin.
4. Because of poor CSF penetration, suramin monotherapy should be avoided in patients with CNS trypanosomiasis.

Antibiotics Manual: A Guide to Commonly Used Antimicrobials, Second Edition. David Schlossberg and Rafik Samuel.
© 2017 John Wiley & Sons Ltd. Published 2017 by John Wiley & Sons Ltd.

■ GLUCANTIME (Meglumine Antimonite)

 BASIC CHARACTERISTICS

Class: Organometallic pentavalent antimonial.

Mechanism of Action: Inhibits DNA topoisomerase, glycolytic enzymes, and fatty acid oxidation.

Metabolic Route: Eliminated rapidly, mainly via the urine.

Used for: Active against all *Leishmania* spp. Used for visceral, cutaneous, and mucosal infection.

 SIDE EFFECTS/TOXICITY

Elevated serum amylase, hepatitis, arthralgias, myalgias, anorexia, thrombophlebitis, headache, abdominal pain, nausea, vomiting, pancreatitis, metallic taste, pruritus, arrhythmias, prolongation of QTc interval, thrombocytopenia, and leukopenia.

 DRUG INTERACTIONS/FOOD INTERACTIONS

No interactions are known, but drugs that may impair renal function or prolong the QT interval should be used with caution.

 DOSING

The recommended daily dose is 20 mg/kg/day; however, bid or tid doses of 10 mg/kg have been used. It is given by slow intravenous infusion; IM administration is painful and PO absorption is inadequate.

Cutaneous leishmaniasis is treated for 20 days.

Visceral leishmaniasis is treated for 28–30 days.

Mucocutaneous leishmaniasis is treated for 28 days.

 SPECIAL POPULATIONS

RENAL IMPAIRMENT: An alternative drug such as liposomal amphotericin B should be used in patients with renal failure.

HEPATIC DYSFUNCTION: No dose adjustment is necessary.

PEDIATRICS: The dose is 20 mg/kg with an upper daily dose limit of 850 mg/day.

 THE ART OF ANTIMICROBIAL THERAPY

Clinical Pearls

1. Antimonials are more toxic in HIV infected patients.
2. Children tolerate antimonials better than adults.
3. Alcohol should be avoided during therapy.
4. EKG should be monitored and treatment interrupted for significant QTc prolongation.
5. Not available commercially in the US. It may be obtained through compounding pharmacies via the National Association of Compounding Pharmacies (800-687-7850) or the Professional Compounding Centers of America (800-331-2498, www.pccarx.com).

Antibiotics Manual: A Guide to Commonly Used Antimicrobials, Second Edition. David Schlossberg and Rafik Samuel.
© 2017 John Wiley & Sons Ltd. Published 2017 by John Wiley & Sons Ltd.

BASIC CHARACTERISTICS

Class: Antifungal.

Mechanism of Action: Griseofulvin has activity against *Microsporum*, *Epidermophyton*, and *Trichophyton*. Griseofulvin is deposited in the keratin precursor cells and has a greater affinity for diseased tissue. The drug is tightly bound to the new keratin, which becomes highly resistant to fungal invasion.

Mechanism of Resistance: Data incomplete.

Metabolic Route: Metabolized in the liver and excreted in GI tract and urine.

 FDA-APPROVED INDICATIONS

Tinea capitis, tinea corporis, tinea pedis, tinea unguium, tinea cruris, and tinea barbae, when caused by one or more of the following genera of fungi: *Trichophyton rubrum*, *Trichophyton tonsurans*, *Trichophyton mentagrophytes*, *Trichophyton interdigitalis*, *Trichophyton verrucosum*, *Trichophyton megnini*, *Trichophyton gallinae*, *Trichophyton crateriform*, *Trichophyton sulphureum*, *Trichophyton schoenleini*, *Microsporum audouinii*, *Microsporum canis*, *Microsporum gypseum*, and *Epidermophyton floccosum*.

 SIDE EFFECTS/TOXICITY

Contraindicated in pregnancy, porphyria, hepatocellular failure, and in patients with a history of hypersensitivity to griseofulvin.

Cross-sensitivity with penicillin exists.

Adverse events include photosensitivity, paresthesias, oral thrush, nausea, vomiting, epigastric distress, diarrhea, headache, fatigue, dizziness, insomnia, confusion and impairment of performance of routine activities, lupus-like syndrome, proteinuria, and leucopenia. Administration of the drug should be discontinued if granulocytopenia occurs. Periodic monitoring of renal, hepatic, and hematopoietic function is recommended.

 DRUG INTERACTIONS

Patients on warfarin therapy may require dosage adjustment of the anticoagulant during and after griseofulvin therapy.

Concomitant use of barbiturates usually depresses griseofulvin activity and may necessitate raising the dosage.

Griseofulvin has been reported to reduce the efficacy of oral contraceptives and to increase the incidence of breakthrough bleeding. The effects of ethanol ingestion may be potentiated.

Antibiotics Manual: A Guide to Commonly Used Antimicrobials, Second Edition. David Schlossberg and Rafik Samuel.
© 2017 John Wiley & Sons Ltd. Published 2017 by John Wiley & Sons Ltd.

DOSING

Disease	PO dose Ultramicrosize crystals	Microsize	Duration
Tinea capitis	375	500 mg	4 to 6 weeks
Tinea corporis	375	500 mg	2 to 4 weeks
Tinea pedis	750 divided	1 g	4 to 8 weeks
Tinea unguium of fingernails	750 divided	1 g	>4 months
Tinea unguium of toenails	750 divided	1 g	>6 months

 SPECIAL POPULATIONS

RENAL IMPAIRMENT: Monitoring of renal function is recommended.

HEPATIC DYSFUNCTION: Should not be administered to those with severe hepatic dysfunction; hepatic function should be monitored.

PEDIATRICS:

Ultramicrosize:

Children weighing 30 to 60 pounds: 125 mg to 187.5 mg daily.

Children weighing over 60 pounds: 187.5 mg to 375 mg daily.

Microsize:

Children 30–50 pounds: 125–250 mg daily.

Children over 50 pounds: 250–500 mg daily.

 THE ART OF ANTIMICROBIAL THERAPY

Clinical Pearls

1. Griseofulvin should be used only for tinea infections.
2. Griseofulvin is better absorbed with a high fat diet.
3. Periodic monitoring of renal, hepatic, and hemopoietic function is recommended.

BASIC CHARACTERISTICS

Class: Ledipasvir is an inhibitor of the HCV NS5A protein.

Sofosbuvir is a nucleotide reverse transcriptase inhibitor for HCV NS5B polymerase.

Mechanism of Action: Ledipasvir is an inhibitor of the HCV NS5A protein, which is required for viral replication.

Sofosbuvir undergoes intracellular metabolism to form the pharmacologically active uridine analog triphosphate, which can be incorporated into HCV RNA by the NS5B polymerase and acts as a chain terminator.

Mechanism of Resistance: Reduced susceptibility to ledipasvir was associated with the primary NS5A amino acid substitution Y93H in both genotypes 1a and 1b.

The substitution S282T can lead to decreased incorporation of the uridine analog triphosphate of sofosbuvir, allowing replication of the virus to continue.

Metabolic Route: Ledipasvir is excreted in the feces.

Sofosbuvir is metabolized in the liver to its active form. It is predominantly excreted in the urine.

 FDA-APPROVED INDICATIONS

Harvoni is indicated with or without ribavirin for the treatment of patients with chronic hepatitis C virus (HCV) genotype 1, 4, 5, or 6 infection.

 SIDE EFFECTS/TOXICITY

Patients may be at increased risk for symptomatic bradycardia with coadministration of Harvoni and amiodarone.

Other side effects include: fatigue, headache, nausea, diarrhea, insomnia, asthenia, myalgias, rash, and dizziness.

Lab abnormalities including elevated bilirubin, lipase, and creatinine kinase have been reported.

 DRUG INTERACTIONS/FOOD INTERACTIONS

Harvoni may be taken without regard to food.

If Harvoni is administered with ribavirin, the contraindications to ribavirin also apply to this combination regimen.

Do not coadminister Harvoni with sofosbuvir, amiodarone, carbamazepine, phenytoin, phenobarbital, oxcarbazepine, rifampin, rifabutin, rifapentine, Stribild, simeprevir, tipranavir/ritonavir, St John's wort, or rasuvastatin.

It is recommended to separate Harvoni and antacids by 4 hours.

It is recommended to separate Harvoni and H2 blockers by 12 hours.

 DOSING

Each tablet contains 90 mg ledipasvir and 400 mg sofosbuvir, administered once daily with or without food.

Antibiotics Manual: A Guide to Commonly Used Antimicrobials, Second Edition. David Schlossberg and Rafik Samuel.
© 2017 John Wiley & Sons Ltd. Published 2017 by John Wiley & Sons Ltd.

Patient population	Medication	Duration
Genotype 1, treatment naïve without cirrhosis or with compensated cirrhosis	Harvoni	12 weeks
Genotype 1, treatment experienced without cirrhosis	Harvoni	12 weeks
Genotype 1, treatment experienced with cirrhosis	Harvoni	24 weeks
Genotype 1, with decompensated cirrhosis	Harvoni + ribavirin	12 weeks
Genotype 1 or 4 after liver transplant	Harvoni + ribavirin	12 weeks
Genotype 4, 5, or 6 without cirrhosis or with compensated cirrhosis	Harvoni	12 weeks

 SPECIAL POPULATIONS

RENAL IMPAIRMENT: Do not use if creatinine clearance is < 30 mL/minute.

HEPATIC DYSFUNCTION: No dose adjustment necessary.

PEDIATRICS: Do not use in patients under 18 years of age.

 THE ART OF ANTIMICROBIAL THERAPY

Clinical Pearls

1. Harvoni is active against HCV genotypes 1, 4, 5, and 6 only.
2. Harvoni for 8 weeks can be considered in treatment-naïve genotype 1 patients without cirrhosis who have pretreatment HCV RNA less than 6 million IU/mL.
3. Harvoni + ribavirin for 12 weeks can be considered in treatment-experienced genotype 1 patients with cirrhosis who are eligible for ribavirin.
4. Significant bradycardia has been reported if Harvoni is combined with amiodarone.
5. Do not administer Harvoni with Sovaldi.
6. Separate Harvoni and antacids by 4 hours.
7. Separate Harvoni and H2 blockers by 12 hours.
8. Harvoni can be used in HIV coinfected patients.
9. Review the most current hepatitis C treatment guidelines because they are changing rapidly: http://www.cdc.gov/hepatitis/HCV/index.htm.

BASIC CHARACTERISTICS

Class: Nucleotide reverse transcriptase inhibitor for hepatitis B.

Mechanism of Action: Adefovir is an acyclic nucleotide analog of adenosine monophosphate, which is phosphorylated to the active metabolite adefovir diphosphate by cellular kinases. Adefovir diphosphate inhibits HBV DNA polymerase by competing with the natural substrate deoxyadenosine triphosphate and by causing DNA chain termination after its incorporation into viral DNA.

Mechanism of Resistance: Amino acid substitutions rtN236T and rtA181T/V have been observed in association with adefovir resistance, leading to decreased incorporation of adefovir diphosphate.

Metabolic Route: Adefovir dipivoxil is rapidly converted to adefovir. Adefovir is renally excreted by a combination of glomerular filtration and active tubular secretion.

 FDA-APPROVED INDICATIONS

Adefovir is indicated for the treatment of chronic hepatitis B with evidence of active viral replication and either evidence of persistent elevations in serum aminotransferases (ALT or AST) or histologically active disease.

 SIDE EFFECTS/TOXICITY

> **WARNING: Severe acute exacerbations of hepatitis** have been reported in patients who have discontinued antihepatitis B therapy including adefovir dipivoxil tablets. Hepatic function should be monitored closely with both clinical and laboratory follow-up for at least several months in patients who discontinue anthepatitis B therapy. If appropriate, resumption of antihepatitis B therapy may be warranted.
>
> In patients at risk of or having underlying renal dysfunction, chronic administration of adefovir dipivoxil tablets may result in nephrotoxicity. These patients should be monitored closely for renal function and may require dose adjustment.
>
> HIV resistance may emerge in chronic hepatitis B patients with unrecognized or untreated human immunodeficiency virus (HIV) infection treated with antihepatitis B therapies, such as adefovir dipivoxil tablets, that may have activity against HIV.
>
> Lactic acidosis and severe hepatomegaly with steatosis, including fatal cases, have been reported with the use of nucleoside analogs alone or in combination with other antiretrovirals.

Possible **additional adverse effects** include hypophosphatemia, myopathy, osteomalacia, proximal renal tubulopathy, and Fanconi syndrome.

 DRUG INTERACTIONS/FOOD INTERACTIONS

Adefovir may be taken without regard to food.

Patients should be monitored closely for adverse events when adefovir is coadministered with drugs that are excreted renally or with other drugs known to affect renal function.

Adefovir should not be used with any compound that includes tenofovir. These include Viread, Vemlidy, Truvada, Complera, Odefsey, Descovy, Stribild, Atripla, and Genvoya.

Antibiotics Manual: A Guide to Commonly Used Antimicrobials, Second Edition. David Schlossberg and Rafik Samuel.
© 2017 John Wiley & Sons Ltd. Published 2017 by John Wiley & Sons Ltd.

DOSING

Adefovir is available in a 10 mg of adefovir dipivoxil. The recommended dose is 10 mg once daily.

 SPECIAL POPULATIONS

RENAL IMPAIRMENT:

Creatinine clearance, mL/min	Dose
>50	10 mg daily
30–49	10 mg q 48 hours
10–29	10 mg q 72 hours
HD	10 mg q week postdialysis

HEPATIC DYSFUNCTION: Caution should be used when administered to those with hepatic impairment.

PEDIATRICS: Adefovir is contraindicated in children <12 years of age.

 THE ART OF ANTIMICROBIAL THERAPY

Clinical Pearls

1. In order to reduce the risk of resistance in patients with lamivudine-resistant HBV, adefovir dipivoxil should be used in combination with lamivudine and not as adefovir dipivoxil monotherapy.
2. All patients should be tested for HIV before initiating adefovir.
3. Renal function must be monitored closely in those receiving adefovir.
4. Hepatic function should be monitored for months after discontinuing adefovir.

BASIC CHARACTERISTICS

Class: Piperazine derivative.

Mechanism of Action (incompletely understood):

1. Killing of microfilariae involving free radicals, from platelet-mediated release of antigen from microfilariae.
2. Alteration of prostaglandin metabolism, leading to immobilization of microfilariae.
3. Inhibition of microtubule polymerization.

Metabolic Route: Excreted in the urine, 50 % in unchanged form.

Used for: *Wuchereria bancrofti*, *Brugia malayi*, Brugia timori, and loa loa.

 SIDE EFFECTS/TOXICITY

Anorexia, nausea, vomiting, headache, somnolence.

The Mazzotti reaction (fever, tachypnea, tachycardia, and hypotension) is seen predominantly in individuals with onchocerciasis; milder forms of the Mazzotti reaction may also be seen in patients with bancroftian filariasis and loa loa.

May also see local inflammatory reaction at site of dying worms or microfilariae, e.g., pain, abscess formation, adenitis, and lymphangitis.

In loaiasis, encephalitis may develop if level of parasitemia is high.

 DRUG INTERACTIONS/FOOD INTERACTIONS

Efficacy may be reduced by corticosteroids.

Synergism is seen with albendazole or ivermectin.

 DOSING

DEC is administered in 50 mg tablets.

Disease	Dose and duration
Bancroftian filariasis	6 mg/kg/day, divided into 3 doses for 12 days
	6 mg/kg/day for 12 days + albendazole or ivermectin
Loaiasis	8–10 mg/kg/day divided into 3 doses for 21 days
Prophylaxis of loa loa	300 mg weekly

 SPECIAL POPULATIONS

RENAL IMPAIRMENT: Should decrease the dose if used in renal insufficiency.

HEPATIC DYSFUNCTION: Data incomplete.

PEDIATRICS: Same dose as adults.

Antibiotics Manual: A Guide to Commonly Used Antimicrobials, Second Edition. David Schlossberg and Rafik Samuel.
© 2017 John Wiley & Sons Ltd. Published 2017 by John Wiley & Sons Ltd.

THE ART OF ANTIMICROBIAL THERAPY

Clinical Pearls

1. Diethylcarbamazine can be obtained from the Centers for Disease Control Parasitic Diseases Drug Service (770-488-7775).

2. DEC is not used for onchocerciasis because of the Mazzotti reaction and the risk of increased ocular side effects including blindness. Before treating a patient with DEC for lymphatic filariasis or loa loa, coinfection with Onchocerca should be excluded.

3. Corticosteroids may ameliorate the Mazzotti reaction but may also reduce the efficacy of DEC.

4. In individuals with high-level loa loa infection, pretreatment apheresis may decrease the likelihood of encephalitis.

5. If DEC is given as a single large daily dose it should be administered at night to minimize symptoms.

BASIC CHARACTERISTICS

Mechanism of Action: Unknown.

Mechanisms of Resistance: May be due to a decrease in miltefosine accumulation within a *Leishmania* parasite, which is thought to be due to either an increase in drug efflux or a decrease in the drug.

Metabolic Route: Data incomplete.

 FDA-APPROVED INDICATIONS

Visceral leishmaniasis due to *Leishmania donovani*.

Cutaneous leishmaniasis due to *Leishmania braziliensis*, *Leishmania guyanensis*, and *Leishmania panamensis*.

Mucosal leishmaniasis due to *Leishmania braziliensis*.

Also Used for: Available from CDC for treatment of amebic encephalitis.

 SIDE EFFECTS/TOXICITY

> **WARNING:** May cause fetal harm. Fetal death and teratogenicity occurred in animals administered miltefosine at doses lower than the recommended human dose. Do not administer to pregnant women. Obtain a serum or urine pregnancy test in females of reproductive potential prior to prescribing. Advise females of reproductive potential to use effective contraception during therapy and for 5 months after therapy.

Contraindications: Pregnancy, Sjögren–Larsson Syndrome, hypersensitivity to miltefosine or any of its excipients.

Toxicity: **Vomiting**, **diarrhea**, **nausea**, **abdominal pain**, thrombocytopenia, Stevens–Johnson syndrome, anemia, lymphadenopathy, abdominal distension, constipation, dysphagia, flatulence, fatigue, malaise, abscess, cellulitis, ecthyma, paresthesia, testicular pain, testicular swelling, urticaria, rash, pyoderma, thrombocytopenia, agranulocytosis, melena, generalized edema, peripheral edema, jaundice, elevation of transaminases, elevated creatinine, seizure, scrotal pain, decreased ejaculate volume, absent ejaculation, and epistaxis.

 DRUG INTERACTIONS/FOOD INTERACTIONS

Administer with food to ameliorate gastrointestinal adverse reactions.

 DOSING

30 to 44 kg: one 50 mg capsule twice daily for 28 consecutive days.

45 kg or greater: one 50 mg capsule three times daily for 28 consecutive days.

Antibiotics Manual: A Guide to Commonly Used Antimicrobials, Second Edition. David Schlossberg and Rafik Samuel.
© 2017 John Wiley & Sons Ltd. Published 2017 by John Wiley & Sons Ltd.

SPECIAL POPULATIONS

RENAL IMPAIRMENT: Has not been studied in patients with renal impairment.

HEPATIC DYSFUNCTION: Has not been studied in patients with hepatic renal impairment.

PEDIATRICS: Safety and effectiveness in pediatric patients < 12 years have not been established.

 THE ART OF ANTIMICROBIAL THERAPY

Clinical Pearls

1. *Leishmania* species evaluated in clinical trials were based on epidemiologic data. The efficacy of miltefosine in the treatment of other *Leishmania* species has not been evaluated.
2. Monitor renal function weekly in patients receiving miltefosine during therapy and for 4 weeks after end of therapy
3. Females and males of reproductive potential: advise females to use effective contraception during therapy and for 5 months after therapy.

BASIC CHARACTERISTICS

Class: Alpha interferon.

Mechanism of Action: After binding to the cell-surface receptor, production of several interferon-stimulated gene products lead to antiviral, antiproliferative, and immunomodulatory effects, regulation of cell surface major histocompatibility antigen (HLA class I and class II) expression, and regulation of cytokine expression.

Mechanism of Resistance: Unknown.

Metabolic Route: Interferon is metabolized into amino acids.

 FDA-APPROVED INDICATIONS

Both Infergen and Intron A are indicated for treatment of chronic hepatitis C in patients 18 years and older.

Intron A is also indicated for the treatment of hepatitis B.

Intron A is also indicated for hairy cell leukemia, malignant melanoma, follicular lymphoma, condylomata acuminata, and AIDS-related Kaposi sarcoma.

Other uses: Hepatitis B.

 SIDE EFFECTS/TOXICITY

> **WARNING:** Alpha interferons cause or aggravate fatal or life-threatening neuropsychiatric, autoimmune, ischemic, and infectious disorders. Patients should be monitored closely with periodic clinical and laboratory evaluations. Patients with persistently severe or worsening signs or symptoms of these conditions should be withdrawn from therapy. In many but not all cases these disorders resolve after stopping alpha interferon therapy.

Interferon is **contraindicated** in patients with known hypersensitivity to alpha interferons or to any component of the product, decompensated hepatic disease, or autoimmune hepatitis.

Other adverse events:

General: fever, hypersensitivity.

Neuropsychiatric disorders: depression, suicide, psychosis, aggressive behavior, nervousness, anxiety, emotional lability, abnormal thinking, agitation, apathy, and relapse of drug addiction.

Infections

Bone marrow suppression

Cardiovascular disorders, including hypertension, tachycardia, palpitation, tachyarrhythmias, supraventricular arrhythmias, chest pain, and myocardial infarction.

Hypersensitivity

Endocrine disorders: hyperthyroidism, hypothyroidism, hyperglycemia, diabetes mellitus, elevated serum triglycerides.

Antibiotics Manual: A Guide to Commonly Used Antimicrobials, Second Edition. David Schlossberg and Rafik Samuel.
© 2017 John Wiley & Sons Ltd. Published 2017 by John Wiley & Sons Ltd.

Autoimmune disorders: autoimmune thrombocytopenia, idiopathic thrombocytopenic purpura, psoriasis, SLE, thyroiditis, and rheumatoid arthritis.

Pulmonary: pneumonia and interstitial pneumonitis.

Gastrointestinal disorders: hemorrhagic/ischemic, ulcerative colitis, pancreatitis, and hepatic decompensation.

Ophthalmologic disorders: decrease or loss of vision, macular edema, retinal artery or vein thrombosis, retinal hemorrhages, cotton wool spots, optic neuritis, and papilledema.

Cerebrovascular disorders: ischemic and hemorrhagic cerebrovascular events.

 ## DRUG INTERACTIONS/FOOD INTERACTIONS

None.

 ## DOSING

Chronic hepatitis C

Infergen (interferon alfacon-1): nine mcg three times weekly administered subcutaneously as a single injection for 24 weeks. At least 48 hours should elapse between doses.

Patients who did not respond or relapsed following its discontinuation may be subsequently treated with 15 mcg times a week (tiw) administered SC as a single injection for up to 48 weeks.

Dose reduction to 7.5 mcg may be necessary following an intolerable adverse event.

Intron A: 3 MIU three times a week (tiw) administered subcutaneously or intramuscularly for 18–24 months in patients who tolerate therapy and normalize ALT at 16 weeks of treatment. If severe adverse reactions develop during Intron A treatment, the dose should be modified (50 % reduction) or therapy should be temporarily discontinued until the adverse reactions abate.

Chronic hepatitis B

Intron A: 30 to 35 million IU per week, administered subcutaneously or intramuscularly, either as 5 million IU daily (q d) or as 10 million IU three times a week (tiw) for 16 weeks.

 ## SPECIAL POPULATIONS

RENAL IMPAIRMENT: Interferon should be used with caution in patients with renal insufficiency.

HEPATIC DYSFUNCTION: Interferon should not be administered to those with decompensated liver disease. LFTs should be monitored closely.

PEDIATRICS: **Infergen** is not recommended for those under 18 years of age.

Intron A can be used to treat chronic hepatitis B in children. The recommended dose is 3 MIU/m^2 three times for the first week, followed by 6 MIU/m^2 three times a week for a total of 16–24 weeks.

 ## THE ART OF ANTIMICROBIAL THERAPY

Clinical Pearls

1. Interferon alpha is not indicated for multiple sclerosis (MS); interferon **beta** is used for MS.
2. Before initiating interferon alpha, evaluate for psychiatric issues including depression.

3. Complete blood counts should be monitored during therapy. Alpha interferon therapy should be discontinued in patients who develop severe decreases in neutrophil ($<0.5 \times 109/L$) or platelet counts ($<50 \times 109/L$).

4. Hepatic function should be closely monitored, and interferon treatment should be immediately discontinued for signs of hepatic decompensation, such as jaundice, ascites, coagulopathy, or decreased serum albumin.

5. Many options with better tolerability exist to treat chronic hepatitis B and chronic hepatitis C. Please review the most updated guidelines for current recommendations.

■ INTELENCE (Etravirine)

 BASIC CHARACTERISTICS

Class: Nonnucleoside reverse transcriptase inhibitor.

Mechanism of Action: Etravirine inhibits reverse transcriptase activity by binding the enzyme.

Mechanism of Resistance: Changes in the structure of reverse transcriptase leads to the inability of etravirine to bind the enzyme and allow transcription to continue. The most frequent resistance mutations that lead to resistance to other NNRTIs do not affect etravirine.

Metabolic Route: Etravirine is metabolized by the cytochrome P450 system and excreted in both urine and feces.

 FDA-APPROVED INDICATIONS

Treatment of HIV-1 in combination with other antiretroviral agents.

 SIDE EFFECTS/TOXICITY

Hypersensitivity with fever, general malaise, fatigue, muscle or joint aches, blisters, oral lesions, conjunctivitis, facial edema, hepatitis, eosinophilia, Stevens–Johnson syndrome, and erythema multiforme; elevated liver enzymes, elevated cholesterol, fat redistribution, and immune reconstitution syndrome.

 DRUG INTERACTIONS/FOOD INTERACTIONS

Etravirine must be administered with food.

Etravirine should not be administered concurrently with astemizole, bepridil, cisapride, midazolam, pimozide, triazolam, ergot derivatives, St John's wort, rifampin, phenobarbitol, phenytoin, carbamazepine, clopidogrel, efavirenz, delavirdine, rilpivirine, fosamprenavir, atazanavir, indinavir, nevirapine, full-dose ritonavir, or tipranavir.

Etravirine causes hepatic enzyme induction of CYP3A4; coadministration of etravirine with drugs primarily metabolized by 2C9, 2C19, and 3A4 isozymes may result in altered plasma concentrations of the coadministered drug. Drugs that induce CYP3A4 activity would be expected to increase the clearance of etravirine, resulting in lowered plasma concentrations. Because of these metabolic activities, the following drug interactions warrant consideration of dosage adjustment and monitoring of clinical effects and serum levels of affected drugs:

Medication	Adjustment or action
Maraviroc	Maraviroc 600 mg twice daily
Maraviroc/darunavir/ritonavir	Maraviroc 150 mg twice daily
Itraconazole, ketoconazole, and voriconazole	Monitor azole levels
Clarithromycin	Consider alternative agent
Rifabutin	Normal dose unless etravirine is combined with ritonavir; then consider an alternative to etravirine
Methadone	Monitor for methadone withdrawal
Warfarin	Monitor INR closely

Antibiotics Manual: A Guide to Commonly Used Antimicrobials, Second Edition. David Schlossberg and Rafik Samuel.
© 2017 John Wiley & Sons Ltd. Published 2017 by John Wiley & Sons Ltd.

Medication	Adjustment or action
Dexamethasone	Use with caution
Diazepam	Decrease diazepam as needed
Cyclosporine, sirolimus tacrolimus	Monitor immunosuppressant levels
Atorvastatin, fluvastatin, simvastatin, lovastatin	Dose adjustment of the HMG-CoA may be necessary
Antiarrhythmics	Use with caution

 DOSING

Etravirine is formulated as 25 mg, 100 mg, and 200 mg tablets. The recommended oral dose of etravirine is 200 mg twice daily. Etravirine tablets may be dispersed in a glass of water.

 SPECIAL POPULATIONS

RENAL IMPAIRMENT: There is no adjustment needed.

HEPATIC DYSFUNCTION: Do not administer in patients with severe hepatic dysfunction.

PEDIATRICS: for treatment: For children over the age of 6 years:

Weight in kg	Dose
Greater than or equal to 16 kg to less than 20 kg	100 mg twice daily
Greater than or equal to 20 kg to less than 25 kg	125 mg twice daily
Greater than or equal to 25 kg to less than 30 kg	150 mg twice daily
Greater than or equal to 30 kg	200 mg twice daily

 THE ART OF ANTIMICROBIAL THERAPY

Clinical Pearls

1. Etravirine should always be used in combination with other antiretrovirals.
2. Etravirine should be dosed with food.
3. Etravirine can be dissolved in water to create a slurry.
4. Whenever initiating etravirine, make sure to review all medications the patient is receiving, to limit drug interactions.
5. Etravirine has a higher barrier to resistance when compared to the other NNRTI.
6. The only PIs that can be coadministered with etravirine are darunavir, lopinavir, or saquinavir.
7. Etravirine is not recommended for naïve antiretroviral therapy.
8. Etravirine should not be used alone with 2 NRTI; it is recommended to be used in the salvage setting with at least one other class in addition to the NRTI.

■ INTRON A (Interferon Alpha) Infergen (Interferon Alfacon-1) Injection
Intron A (Interferon Alfa-2a) Injection

 ## BASIC CHARACTERISTICS

Class: Alpha interferon.

Mechanism of Action: After binding to the cell-surface receptor, production of several interferon-stimulated gene products lead to antiviral, antiproliferative, and immunomodulatory effects, regulation of cell surface major histocompatibility antigen (HLA class I and class II) expression, and regulation of cytokine expression.

Mechanism of Resistance: Unknown.

Metabolic Route: Interferon is metabolized into amino acids.

 ## FDA-APPROVED INDICATIONS

Both Infergen and Intron A are indicated for treatment of chronic hepatitis C in patients 18 years and older.

Intron A is also indicated for the treatment of hepatitis B.

Intron A is also indicated for hairy cell leukemia, malignant melanoma, follicular lymphoma, condylomata acuminata, and AIDS-related Kaposi sarcoma.

Other uses: Hepatitis B.

 ## SIDE EFFECTS/TOXICITY

> **WARNING:** Alpha interferons cause or aggravate fatal or life-threatening neuropsychiatric, autoimmune, ischemic, and infectious disorders. Patients should be monitored closely with periodic clinical and laboratory evaluations. Patients with persistently severe or worsening signs or symptoms of these conditions should be withdrawn from therapy. In many but not all cases these disorders resolve after stopping alpha interferon therapy.

Interferon is **contraindicated** in patients with known hypersensitivity to alpha interferons or to any component of the product, decompensated hepatic disease, or autoimmune hepatitis.

Other adverse events:

General: fever, hypersensitivity.

Neuropsychiatric disorders: depression, suicide, psychosis, aggressive behavior, nervousness, anxiety, emotional lability, abnormal thinking, agitation, apathy, and relapse of drug addiction.

Infections

Bone marrow suppression

Cardiovascular disorders, including hypertension, tachycardia, palpitation, tachyarrhythmias, supraventricular arrhythmias, chest pain, and myocardial infarction.

Hypersensitivity

Endocrine disorders: hyperthyroidism, hypothyroidism, hyperglycemia, diabetes mellitus, elevated serum triglycerides.

Antibiotics Manual: A Guide to Commonly Used Antimicrobials, Second Edition. David Schlossberg and Rafik Samuel.
© 2017 John Wiley & Sons Ltd. Published 2017 by John Wiley & Sons Ltd.

Autoimmune disorders: autoimmune thrombocytopenia, idiopathic thrombocytopenic purpura, psoriasis, SLE, thyroiditis, and rheumatoid arthritis.

Pulmonary: pneumonia and interstitial pneumonitis.

Gastrointestinal disorders: hemorrhagic/ischemic, ulcerative colitis, pancreatitis, and hepatic decompensation.

Ophthalmologic disorders: decrease or loss of vision, macular edema, retinal artery or vein thrombosis, retinal hemorrhages, cotton wool spots, optic neuritis, and papilledema.

Cerebrovascular disorders: ischemic and hemorrhagic cerebrovascular events.

 ## DRUG INTERACTIONS/FOOD INTERACTIONS

None.

 ## DOSING

Chronic hepatitis C

Infergen (interferon alfacon-1): nine mcg three times weekly administered subcutaneously as a single injection for 24 weeks. At least 48 hours should elapse between doses.

Patients who did not respond or relapsed following its discontinuation may be subsequently treated with 15 mcg times a week (tiw) administered SC as a single injection for up to 48 weeks.

Dose reduction to 7.5 mcg may be necessary following an intolerable adverse event.

Intron A: 3 MIU three times a week (tiw) administered subcutaneously or intramuscularly for 18–24 months in patients who tolerate therapy and normalize ALT at 16 weeks of treatment. If severe adverse reactions develop during Intron A treatment, the dose should be modified (50 % reduction) or therapy should be temporarily discontinued until the adverse reactions abate.

Chronic hepatitis B

Intron A: 30 to 35 million IU per week, administered subcutaneously or intramuscularly, either as 5 million IU daily (q d) or as 10 million IU three times a week (tiw) for 16 weeks.

 ## SPECIAL POPULATIONS

RENAL IMPAIRMENT: Interferon should be used with caution in patients with renal insufficiency.

HEPATIC DYSFUNCTION: Interferon should not be administered to those with decompensated liver disease. LFTs should be monitored closely.

PEDIATRICS: **Infergen** is not recommended for those under 18 years of age.

Intron A can be used to treat chronic hepatitis B in children. The recommended dose is 3 MIU/m^2 three times for the first week, followed by 6 MIU/m^2 three times a week for a total of 16–24 weeks.

 ## THE ART OF ANTIMICROBIAL THERAPY

Clinical Pearls

1. Interferon alpha is not indicated for multiple sclerosis (MS); interferon **beta** is used for MS.
2. Before initiating interferon alpha, evaluate for psychiatric issues including depression.

3. Complete blood counts should be monitored during therapy. Alpha interferon therapy should be discontinued in patients who develop severe decreases in neutrophil ($<0.5 \times 109/L$) or platelet counts ($<50 \times 109/L$).

4. Hepatic function should be closely monitored and interferon treatment should be immediately discontinued for signs of hepatic decompensation, such as jaundice, ascites, coagulopathy, or decreased serum albumin.

5. Many options with better tolerability exist to treat chronic hepatitis B and chronic hepatitis C. Please review the most updated guidelines for current recommendations.

BASIC CHARACTERISTICS

Class: Carbapenem.

Mechanism of Action: Binds penicillin-binding protein, disrupting cell wall synthesis.

Mechanisms of Resistance:

1. The PBP can be altered, with reduced affinity.
2. Production of a beta-lactamase, resulting in hydrolysis of the beta-lactam ring.
3. Decreased ability of the antibiotic to reach the PBP when bacteria decrease porin production, resulting in a decrease of the drug concentration within the cell.
4. Increased expression of efflux pump components.

Metabolic Route: Ertapenem is excreted in the urine.

 FDA-APPROVED INDICATIONS

Treatment of serious infections caused by susceptible strains of microorganisms in the conditions listed below:

1. Complicated intra-abdominal infections.
2. Complicated skin and skin structure infections, including diabetic foot infections without osteomyelitis.
3. Community acquired pneumonia.
4. Complicated rrinary tract infections including pyelonephritis including cases with concurrent bacteremia.
5. Acute pelvic infections including postpartum endomyometritis, septic abortion, and postsurgical gynecologic infections.
6. Prophylaxis of surgical site infection following elective colorectal surgery.

 SIDE EFFECTS/TOXICITY

Ertapenem is **contraindicated** in patients with known hypersensitivity to any component of this product or to other drugs in the same class or in patients who have demonstrated anaphylactic reactions to beta-lactams. Before initiating therapy with ertapenem, careful inquiry should be made concerning previous hypersensitivity reactions to penicillins, cephalosporins, other beta-lactams, and other allergens, because of the increased possibility of hypersensitivity.

Side effects include phlebitis, fever, anaphylaxis, rash including Stevens–Johnson syndrome, erythema multiforme and toxic epidermal necrolysis, angioedema, hypotension, encephalopathy, seizures, hearing loss, diarrhea, *Clostridium difficile*-associated diarrhea and pseudomembranous colitis, oral candidiasis, glossitis, anorexia, nausea, vomiting, stomach cramps, hepatitis, renal impairment, pyuria, hematuria, genital pruritis, dyspnea, polyarthralgia, prolonged prothrombin time, pancytopenia, positive Coombs' test, increased ALT (SGPT), AST (SGOT), alkaline phosphatase, bilirubin, and LDH, decreased serum sodium, increased potassium and chloride.

 DRUG INTERACTIONS/FOOD INTERACTIONS

Ertapenem may reduce serum valproic acid concentrations; levels should be monitored.

It is not recommended that probenecid be given with ertapenem.

Antibiotics Manual: A Guide to Commonly Used Antimicrobials, Second Edition. David Schlossberg and Rafik Samuel.
© 2017 John Wiley & Sons Ltd. Published 2017 by John Wiley & Sons Ltd.

DOSING

The dose of ertapenem in patients 13 years of age and older is 1 g given once a day by intravenous infusion or intramuscular injection.

Type of infection	Dose (patients > 13 years)	Duration
Complicated skin and skin structure	1 gram daily	7–14 days
Community acquired pneumonia	1 gram daily	10–14 days
Complicated UTI	1 gram daily	10–14 days
Acute pelvic infections	1 gram daily	3–10 days
Prophylaxis	1 gram	given 60 minutes before incision

 SPECIAL POPULATIONS

RENAL IMPAIRMENT:

Creatinine clearance	Dose
<30 mL/min	500 mg daily
After hemodialysis	If dose <6 hours before hemodialysis, give supplemental dose of 150 mg
CRRT or peritoneal dialysis	Unknown

HEPATIC DYSFUNCTION: No dose adjustment is necessary.

PEDIATRICS:

Type of infection	Dose (patients < 13 years)	Duration
Complicated skin and skin structure	15 mg/kg q 12 hours	7–14 days
Community acquired pneumonia	15 mg/kg q 12 hours	10–14 days
Complicated UTI	15 mg/kg q 12 hours	10–14 days
Acute pelvic infections	15 mg/kg q 12 hours	3–10 days

 THE ART OF ANTIMICROBIAL THERAPY

Clinical Pearls

1. Eretapenem must be dose-adjusted for renal dysfunction.
2. Cross allergy with penicillins is <10%.
3. Unlike other carbapenems, ertapenem is not active against *Pseudomonas* spp. and other highly resistant gram-negative rods.
4. Ertapenem is active against ESBL-producing gram-negative enteric rods.
5. Seizure risk predominantly in patients with CNS disease or renal dysfunction.

BASIC CHARACTERISTICS

Class: Integrase inhibitor.

Mechanism of Action: Raltegravir inhibits the catalytic activity of HIV-1 integrase, which terminates integration of HIV DNA into the host genome.

Mechanism of Resistance: Development of mutations on the enzyme integrase leads to the inability of raltegravir to bind the active site of the enzyme and allow integrase activity to continue. Mutations that lead to resistance to raltegravir include Q148H/K/R or N155H.

Metabolic Route: Raltegravir is glucuronidated by the enzyme UGT1A1 in the liver and then excreted.

 FDA-APPROVED INDICATIONS

Treatment of HIV-1 in combination with other antiretroviral agents.

 SIDE EFFECTS/TOXICITY

Immune reconstitution syndrome

Severe skin and hypersensitivity reaction

Raltegravir chewable tablets contain phenylalanine

Other side effects include fever, headaches, dizziness, diarrhea, nausea, myopathy and rhabdomyolysis, abdominal pain, gastritis, hepatitis, genital herpes, herpes zoster, and renal failure.

 DRUG INTERACTIONS/FOOD INTERACTIONS

Raltegravir can be taken with or without food.

Raltegravir is not a substrate, inhibitor, or inducer of the CYP3A4. Raltegravir is metabolized by UGT1A1.

When administering with rifampin, increase the raltegravir dose to 800 mg twice daily.

Raltegravir should not be coadministered with magnesium or aluminum containing antacids.

 DOSING

Formulations include 400 mg film coated tablets.

25 mg and 100 mg chewable tablets.

Granular powder for oral suspension, which should be mixed 100 mg in 5 mL to give 20 mg per mL.

The recommended adult dose is 400 mg orally, twice daily.

 SPECIAL POPULATIONS

RENAL IMPAIRMENT: There is no adjustment needed.

HEPATIC DYSFUNCTION: There is no adjustment needed.

Antibiotics Manual: A Guide to Commonly Used Antimicrobials, Second Edition. David Schlossberg and Rafik Samuel.
© 2017 John Wiley & Sons Ltd. Published 2017 by John Wiley & Sons Ltd.

PEDIATRICS: For children over 25 kg. The dose is 400 mg twice daily of the regular tablet. If unable to swallow the tablet, chewable tablets can be used as follows:

Weight	Dose
20 to <28 kg	150 mg twice daily
28 to <40 kg	200 mg twice daily
40 kg or more	300 mg twice daily

For children less than 20 kg:

Body weight	Volume (dose) of suspension
3 to <4 kg	1 mL (20 mg) twice daily
4 to <6 kg	1.5 mL (30 mg) twice daily
6 to <8 kg	2 mL (40 mg) twice daily
8 to <11 kg	3 mL (60 mg) twice daily
11 to <14 kg	4 mL (80 mg) twice daily
14 to <20 kg	6 mL (100 mg) twice daily

THE ART OF ANTIMICROBIAL THERAPY

Clinical Pearls

1. Raltegravir should always be used in combination with other antiretrovirals.
2. Raltegravir should be given twice daily.
3. Raltegravir is not a substrate, inducer or inhibitor of the CYP 3A4 enzymes.

BASIC CHARACTERISTICS

Class: Isonicotinic acid hydrazide.

Mechanisms of Action:

1. Inhibits the synthesis of mycolic acid, a constituent of the cell wall.
2. Inhibits catalase-peroxidase.

Mechanisms of Resistance:

1. Point mutations in the catalase-peroxidase gene.
2. Mutations of the regulatory genes involved in mycolic acid synthesis.

Metabolic Route: Metabolized by acetylation and dehydrazination. The rate of acetylation is genetically determined.

 FDA-APPROVED INDICATIONS

Treatment of active tuberculosis in combination with other antimycobacterials.

Latent tuberculosis (LTBI).

 SIDE EFFECTS/TOXICITY

> **WARNING:** Severe and sometimes fatal **hepatitis** has been associated with isoniazid. The risk of hepatitis is greatest in older and peripartum patients, Asian males, and possibly black and Hispanic women, and risk is increased with acetaminophen, elevated baseline transaminases, chronic HBV and HBC infection, and possibly HIV infection.

Other adverse events: Peripheral neuropathy, hypersensitivity, fever, skin eruptions, vasculitis, a systemic lupus erythematosus-like syndrome, nausea, vomiting, epigastric distress, seizures, encephalopathy, metabolic acidosis, optic neuritis, arthralgias, agranulocytosis, hemolytic or sideroblastic anemia, thrombocytopenia, and gynecomastia.

 DRUG INTERACTIONS/FOOD INTERACTIONS

When taken with food, the absorption of isoniazid is reduced but still adequate for most patients and is much better tolerated. Foods rich in histamine (e.g., cheese, wine, tuna) or tyramine (e.g., cured meats, soybeans, aged cheese) may produce flushing and headache. Antacids may impair absorption and should be separated from INH ingestion by 2 hours.

Isoniazid inhibits the metabolism of many drugs, potentially increasing their serum levels; patients on anticoagulants, anticonvulsants, benzodiazepines, haloperidol, theophylline and cycloserine should be monitored for toxic effects; levels of carbamazepine, phenytoin, and valproate should be measured.

Acetaminophen and alcohol should be avoided, as they may increase hepatotoxicity, as should disulfiram, enflurane, stavudine, and vincristine.

Antibiotics Manual: A Guide to Commonly Used Antimicrobials, Second Edition. David Schlossberg and Rafik Samuel.
© 2017 John Wiley & Sons Ltd. Published 2017 by John Wiley & Sons Ltd.

DOSING (dose should never be divided, but should be given as a single dose)

Isoniazid is available as an elixir and for oral, intravenous, and intramuscular administration; the dose is 5 mg/kg/day up to 300 mg daily. It may also be given twice or thrice weekly, 15 mg/kg up to 900 mg per dose.

 SPECIAL POPULATIONS

RENAL IMPAIRMENT: No dose adjustment is necessary.

HEPATIC DYSFUNCTION: No dose adjustment, but use with caution.

PEDIATRICS: 10–15 mg/kg/day with a maximum of 300 mg daily. Twice or thrice weekly dose is 20–30 mg/kg/dose, with a maximum of 900 mg per dose.

 THE ART OF ANTIMICROBIAL THERAPY

Clinical Pearls

1. Isoniazid should not be used alone in the treatment of active tuberculosis.
2. Liver function tests, symptoms of gastrointolerance, and CBC should be monitored at least monthly in all patients receiving isoniazid.
3. Pyroxidine (25 mg/day) should be given to prevent B6 deficiency in those at risk for peripheral neuropathy, i.e., nutritional deficiency, diabetes, HIV infection, renal failure, alcoholism, pregnancy, and breastfeeding mothers.
4. When used to treat latent tuberculosis in pregnant patients, INH therapy should be deferred 2–3 months after delivery because of increased hepatotoxicity. Exceptions, whose treatment should not be deferred, are women with recently acquired infection and those who are HIV-positive.
5. INH dosage should never be split but should be given as a single dose.
6. Serum levels should be assayed in HIV-positive patients, diabetics, patients with gastrointestinal disease and those responding poorly to therapy.

BASIC CHARACTERISTICS

Class: Protease inhibitor.

Mechanism of Action: Lopinavir reversibly binds the active site of the enzyme protease. Inhibition of protease prevents cleavage of the *gag* and *gag-pol* polyprotein, resulting in the production of an immature, non-infectious virus.

Mechanism of Resistance: Development of mutations on the enzyme protease causes a conformational change that prevents lopinavir from binding the active site allowing protease activity to continue. Many protease mutations are required for the virus to become resistant to lopinavir.

Metabolic Route: Lopinavir is metabolized by the liver and excreted in the feces.

 FDA-APPROVED INDICATIONS

Treatment of HIV-1 in combinations with other antiretroviral agents.

 SIDE EFFECTS/TOXICITY

New-onset diabetes mellitus, exacerbation of preexisting diabetes mellitus, hyperglycemia, increased bleeding, including spontaneous skin hematomas and hemarthrosis, in patients with hemophilia types A and B, redistribution/accumulation of body fat including central obesity, dorsocervical fat enlargement (buffalo hump), peripheral wasting, facial wasting, breast enlargement, "cushingoid appearance", immune reconstitution syndrome, diarrhea, QTc prolongation, torsades de pointes, abdominal pain, headache, anorexia, dyspepsia, epigastric pain, hepatitis, mouth ulceration, vomiting, anemia, leucopenia, thrombocytopenia, increases in alkaline phosphatase, amylase, creatine phosphokinase, lactic dehydrogenase, SGOT, SGPT, gamma-glutamyl transpeptidase, hyperlipemia, hyperuricemia, hyperglycemia, hypoglycemia, and dehydration.

 DRUG INTERACTIONS/FOOD INTERACTIONS

Lopinavir/ritonavir tablets may be taken with or without food. The tablets should be swallowed whole and not chewed, broken, or crushed. Lopinavir/ritonavir oral solution must be taken with food.

Drugs that should not be coadministered with lopinavir/ritonavir include alfuzosin, amiodarone, quinidine, rifampin, ergot derivatives, St John's wort, simvastatin, lovastatin, lurasidone, pimozide, triazolam, midazolam, voriconazole, ritonavir, phenobarbitol, phenytoin, carbamazepine, tipranavir, fosamprenavir, darunavir, salmeterol, fluticasone, budesonide, simepravir, and sildenafil for pulmonary hypertension.

Lopinavir is an inhibitor of the CYP3A enzyme; coadministration of lopinavir and drugs primarily metabolized by CYP3A may result in increased plasma concentrations of the other drug that could increase or prolong its therapeutic and adverse effects.

Lopinavir is metabolized by CYP3A; coadministration of lopinavir and drugs that induce CYP3A may decrease lopinavir plasma concentrations and reduce its therapeutic effect. Coadministration of lopinavir and drugs that inhibit CYP3A may increase

Antibiotics Manual: A Guide to Commonly Used Antimicrobials, Second Edition. David Schlossberg and Rafik Samuel.
© 2017 John Wiley & Sons Ltd. Published 2017 by John Wiley & Sons Ltd.

lopinavir plasma concentrations. Because of these metabolic affects, potential drug interactions that may require dosage change or clinical/laboratory monitoring are listed below:

Medication	Adjustment or action
Itraconazole	Do not exceed 200 mg/day; monitor for toxicity
Ketoconazole	Do not exceed 200 mg/day
Clarithromycin	Reduce clarithromycin dose in moderate to severe renal impairment
Rifabutin	Decrease rifabutin to 150/qod or 3 × week
Contraceptives	Use alternative or additional method
Atorvastatin	Use lowest possible dose with close monitoring
Methadone	Monitor, may require higher methadone dose
Sildenafil	25 mg every 48 hours (maximum)
Tadalafil	10 mg in 72 hours (maximum)
Vardenafil	2.5 mg in 72 hours (maximum)
Tenofovir	Monitor for tenofovir toxicity
Efavirenz, nevirapine	Increase lopinavir/ritonavir to 600/150 mg in treatment experienced patients receiving efavirenz or nevirapine. No dose adjustment in treatment naïve patients
Maraviroc	Maraviroc dose should be 150 mg bid
Cyclosporine, tacrolimus, rapamycin	Monitor concentration of immunosuppressant
Colchicine	Do not coadminister in renal or hepatic impairment
Quetiapine	Administer one-sixth of the quetiapine dose
Bosentan	Bosentan dose 62.5 mg daily

 DOSING

Lopinavir/ritonavir is supplied in 200 mg lopinavir/50 mg ritonavir tablets, 100 mg lopinavir/25 mg ritonavir tablets and a light yellow to orange colored liquid containing 80 mg lopinavir/20 mg ritonavir per mL. For therapy naïve patients, the recommended dose is lopinavir 400/100 mg (2 tablets or 5 mL) twice daily or 800/200 mg (4 tablets or 10 mL) once daily.

For therapy experienced patients the recommended dose is 400/100 mg (2 tablets or 5.0 mL) twice daily.

 SPECIAL POPULATIONS

RENAL IMPAIRMENT: There is no adjustment needed.

HEPATIC DYSFUNCTION: Administer with caution.

PEDIATRICS: Lopinavir/ritonavir should not be administered once daily in patients < 18 years of age.

14 days to 6 months: the recommended dosage is 16/4 mg/kg or 300/75 mg/m^{2*} twice daily.

6 months to 18 years: the recommended dosage of lopinavir/ritonavir is 230/57.5 mg/m^{2*} given twice daily, not to exceed the recommended adult dose, or lopinavir/ritonavir for patients <15 kg is 12/3 mg/kg given twice daily and the dosage for patients ≥15 kg to 40 kg is 10/2.5 mg/kg given twice daily.

THE ART OF ANTIMICROBIAL THERAPY

Clinical Pearls

1. Lopinavir/ritonavir should always be used in combination with other antiretrovirals.
2. Even though lopinavir/ritonavir can be administered with or without food, it is likely that gastrointestinal side effects are decreased when taken with food.
3. Kaletra contains ritonavir, and all side effects of ritonavir should be considered when administering it.
4. When assessing for resistance to lopinavir/ritonavir, a phenotype assay may be helpful.
5. Whenever initiating lopinavir/ritonavir, make sure to review all medications the patient is receiving to limit drug interactions.

* See Helpful Formulas, Equations, and Definitions for body surface determination.

KANTREX (Kanamycin)

 BASIC CHARACTERISTICS

Class: Aminoglycoside.

Mechanisms of Action: Binds the 30S subunit of the bacterial ribosome, which terminates protein synthesis.

Mechanism of Resistance:

1. Gram-negative bacteria inactivate aminoglycosides by acetylation.
2. Some bacteria alter the 30S ribosomal subunit, which prevents kanamycin's interference with protein synthesis.
3. Low-level resistance may result from inhibition of kanamycin uptake by the bacteria.

Metabolic Route: The drug is excreted unchanged in the urine.

 FDA-APPROVED INDICATIONS

Treatment of serious infections caused by susceptible bacteria.

Other uses: Kanamycin is also used for the treatment of *M. tuberculosis*.

 SIDE EFFECTS/TOXICITY

> **WARNING: Ototoxicity**: vestibular toxicity and auditory ototoxicity, especially in patients with renal damage, those treated with higher doses, and those with prolonged treatment. Avoid use with potent diuretics such as ethacrynic acid because of additive ototoxicity.
>
> **Nephrotoxicity**: especially in patients with impaired renal function and those treated with higher doses or prolonged treatment. Avoid concurrent use with other nephrotoxic agents and potent diuretics, which can cause dehydration.
>
> **Neuromuscular** blockade: especially in those receiving anesthetics, neuromuscular blocking agents or massive transfusions; neuromuscular blockade has been reported after intraperitoneal instillation and oral use.

Other neurotoxic reactions include numbness, skin tingling, muscle twitching, and seizures. Also reported are rash, fever, headache, nausea, vomiting, and diarrhea. The "malabsorption syndrome" characterized by an increase in fecal fat, decrease in serum carotene, and fall in xylose absorption, reportedly has occurred with prolonged therapy.

 DRUG INTERACTIONS

Kanamycin should not be administered with other medications that are nephrotoxic or ototoxic.

DOSING

Kanamycin may be given intramuscularly or intravenously.

Intramuscular or intravascular route: 7.5 mg/kg q 12 hours.

For tuberculosis: 15 mg/kg/day (maximum 1 gm), reduced to 15 mg/kg/dose 2–3 times/week after an initial period of daily administration. For patients >59 years of age, dose is 10 mg/kg (maximum 750 mg).

Aerosol treatment: 250 mg 2 to 4 times a day.

Antibiotics Manual: A Guide to Commonly Used Antimicrobials, Second Edition. David Schlossberg and Rafik Samuel.
© 2017 John Wiley & Sons Ltd. Published 2017 by John Wiley & Sons Ltd.

SPECIAL POPULATIONS

RENAL IMPAIRMENT: Creatinine clearance < 30 mL/min or in dialysis patients: 12–15 mg/kg 2–3 times a week.

PEDIATRICS: 7.5 mg/kg q 12 hours.

 THE ART OF ANTIMICROBIAL THERAPY

Clinical Pearls

1. When dosing aminoglycosides, use the ideal body weight not the true body weight.
2. Peak concentrations should be between 35 and 45 mcg/mL.
3. Kanamycin should be used in combination with other medications when treating tuberculosis.
4. Monitor renal function and hearing and auditory function.
5. *Mycobacterium tuberculosis* cross-resistance is seen with amikacin and possibly with capreomycin.

■ KEFLEX (Cephalexin)

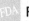 ## BASIC CHARACTERISTICS

Class: First generation cephalosporin.

Mechanism of Action: Binds penicillin-binding protein, disrupting cell wall synthesis.

Mechanisms of Resistance:

1. The PBP can be altered, with reduced affinity.
2. Production of a beta-lactamase, resulting in hydrolysis of the beta-lactam ring.
3. Decreased ability of the antibiotic to reach the PBP when bacteria decrease porin production, resulting in a decrease of the drug concentration within the cell.

Metabolic Route: Excreted unchanged in the urine.

FDA-APPROVED INDICATIONS

Treatment of the following infections when caused by susceptible strains of organisms:

Respiratory tract infections

Otitis media

Skin and skin structure infections

Bone infections

Genitourinary tract infections

 ## SIDE EFFECTS/TOXICITY

> **WARNING:** To reduce the development of drug-resistant bacteria and maintain the effectiveness of cephalexin capsules and cephalexin for oral suspension and other antibacterial drugs, cephalexin capsules and cephalexin for oral suspension should be used only to treat or prevent infections that are proven or strongly suspected to be caused by bacteria.

Cephalexin is **contraindicated** in patients with known allergy to the cephalosporin group of antibiotics.

Cephalexin should be used with caution if hypersensitivity exists to penicillin.

Toxicity includes fever, anaphylaxis, rash including Stevens–Johnson syndrome, erythema multiforme and toxic epidermal necrolysis, angioedema, flushing, hypotension, serum-sickness-like reactions, encephalopathy, seizures, diarrhea, *Clostridium difficile*-associated diarrhea and pseudomembranous colitis, oral candidiasis, anorexia, nausea, vomiting, stomach cramps, flatulence, hepatitis, renal impairment, genital moniliasis, vaginitis, hemorrhage, arthritis, prolonged prothrombin time, pancytopenia, hemolytic anemia, positive Coombs' test.

 ## DRUG INTERACTIONS/FOOD INTERACTIONS

Cephalexin can be administered with or without food.

Probenecid may decrease renal tubular secretion of cephalosporins when used concurrently, resulting in increased and more prolonged cephalosporin blood levels. Cephalosporins may cause false-positive urine glucose determinations when using cupric sulfate solution (Benedict's solution, *Clinitest®*). Tests utilizing glucose oxidase (*Tes-Tape®*, *Clinistix®*) are not affected by cephalosporins.

Antibiotics Manual: A Guide to Commonly Used Antimicrobials, Second Edition. David Schlossberg and Rafik Samuel.
© 2017 John Wiley & Sons Ltd. Published 2017 by John Wiley & Sons Ltd.

DOSING

Cephalexin is administered in 250 mg and 500 mg tablets. It can also be administered in a suspension of 125 mg/5 mL or 250 mg/5 mL.

The usual adult dose is 250 mg every 6 hours.

Streptococcal pharyngitis, skin and skin structure infections, and uncomplicated cystitis: a dosage of 500 mg may be administered every 12 hours.

Severe infections: daily doses of cephalexin up to 4 g may be administered.

SPECIAL POPULATIONS

RENAL IMPAIRMENT:

Creatinine clearance	Dose
>50 mL/min	q 6 hours
10–50 mL/min	q 8–12 hours
<10 mL/min	q 24–48 hours
Supplemental dose after hemodialysis	250 mg–1 gm
CRRT	N/A

HEPATIC DYSFUNCTION: No dose adjustment is necessary.

PEDIATRICS: The usual recommended daily dosage for pediatric patients is 25 to 50 mg/kg in divided doses.
Streptococcal pharyngitis: total daily dose may be divided and administered every 12 hours.

Severe infections: the dosage may be doubled.

Otitis media: 75 to 100 mg/kg/day in 4 divided doses is required.

THE ART OF ANTIMICROBIAL THERAPY

Clinical Pearls

1. Cephalexin is adjusted for renal dysfunction.
2. Cross allergy with penicillins is <10%.
3. If more than 4 grams of cephalexin are required, parenteral cephalosporins should be used.

■ KETOCONAZOLE

 BASIC CHARACTERISTICS

Class: Imidazole.

Mechanism of Action: Inhibition of lanosterol 14-α-demethylase, which is involved in the synthesis of ergosterol, an essential component of fungal cell membranes.

Mechanisms of Resistance:

1. Point mutations in the gene (*ERG11*) encoding for the target enzyme lead to an altered target with decreased affinity for azoles.
2. Overexpression of *ERG11* results in the production of high concentrations of the target enzyme, creating the need for a higher intracellular drug concentrations to inhibit all of the enzyme molecules in the cell.
3. Active efflux of itraconazole out of the cell through the activation of two types of multidrug efflux transporters.

Metabolic Route: Ketoconazole is metabolized in the liver and excreted in the bile.

 FDA-APPROVED INDICATIONS

Ketoconazole tablets should be used only when other effective antifungal therapy is not available or tolerated and the potential benefits are considered to outweigh the potential risks: blastomycosis, coccidioidomycosis, histoplasmosis, chromomycosis, and *para*-coccidioidomycosis.

 SIDE EFFECTS/TOXICITY

> **WARNING:** Ketoconazole tablets should be used only when other effective antifungal therapy is not available or tolerated and the potential benefits are considered to outweigh the potential risks.
>
> **Hepatotoxicity**: Serious hepatotoxicity, including cases with a fatal outcome or requiring liver transplantation has occurred with the use of oral ketoconazole. Some patients had no obvious risk factors for liver disease. Patients receiving this drug should be informed by the physician of the risk and should be closely monitored.
>
> **QT prolongation and drug interactions leading to QT Prolongation**: Coadministration of the following drugs with keto-conazole is contraindicated: dofetilide, quinidine, pimozide, and cisapride. Ketoconazole can cause elevated plasma con-centrations of these drugs and may prolong QT intervals, sometimes resulting in life-threatening ventricular dysrhythmias such as torsades de pointes.

Other adverse events include hypersensitivity, fever and chills, pruritus, suppression of adrenal corticosteroid and testosterone secretion, nausea, vomiting, diarrhea, abdominal pain, headache, photophobia, gynecomastia, impotence, dizziness, somnolence, suicidal tendencies, severe depression, bulging fontanelles, thrombocytopenia, leukopenia, and hemolytic anemia.

Antibiotics Manual: A Guide to Commonly Used Antimicrobials, Second Edition. David Schlossberg and Rafik Samuel.
© 2017 John Wiley & Sons Ltd. Published 2017 by John Wiley & Sons Ltd.

214

DRUG INTERACTIONS/ADMINISTRATION

Ketoconazole can be taken with or without food; however, in studies, Ketoconazole was administered with meals. Ketoconazole requires a low pH for absorption. If concomitant antacids, anticholinergics, and H2-blockers are needed, they should be given at least two hours after administration of Ketoconazole.

Ketoconazole is an inhibitor of the cytochrome P450 3A4 enzyme system. Coadministration of Ketoconazole tablets and drugs primarily metabolized by the cytochrome P450 3A4 enzyme system may result in increased plasma concentrations of the latter drugs, possibly requiring dosage adjustments. The following list includes significant drug interactions with Ketoconazole.

Do not administer Ketoconazole with the following: astemizole, cisapride, dofetilide, quinidine, pimozide methadone, disopyramide, dronedarone, ergot alkaloids such as dihydroergotamine, ergometrine, ergotamine, methylergometrine, irinotecan, lurasidone, oral midazolam, alprazolam, triazolam, felodipine, nisoldipine, ranolazine, tolvaptan, eplerenone, lovastatin, simvastatin, tamsulosin, rifabutin, rifampin, rivaroxaban, carbamazapine, dasatanib, lapatanib, nilotinib, everolimus, sirolimus, salmeterol, terfenadine, and colchicine.

Cyclosporine, tacrolimus: levels of cyclosporine, tacrolimus may be elevated.

Digoxin: levels of digoxin may be elevated.

Ethanol: may see a disulfiram-like reaction.

Isoniazid: may lower ketoconazole concentrations.

Methylprednisolone: levels of methylprednisolone may be elevated.

Oral hypoglycemics: may increase levels of oral hypoglycemic.

Warfarin: elevated levels of warfarin.

Phenytoin: monitor for altered levels of both phenytoin and ketoconazole.

Rifampin: may lower ketoconazole levels.

 DOSING

Adults

Ketoconazole is available in 200 mg tablets.

Ketoconazole should be started at 200 mg daily; in very serious infections or if clinical responsiveness is insufficient within the expected time, the dose may be increased to 400 mg once daily.

 SPECIAL POPULATIONS

RENAL IMPAIRMENT: No dose adjustment.

HEPATIC DYSFUNCTION: Do not use in acute or chronic liver disease.

PEDIATRICS: Ketoconazole should not be used in pediatric patients unless the potential benefit outweighs the risks. In pediatric patients over 2 years of age, a single daily dose of 3.3 to 6.6 mg/kg has been used. Ketoconazole tablets have not been studied in pediatric patients under 2 years of age.

THE ART OF ANTIMICROBIAL THERAPY

Clinical Pearls

1. Ketoconazole should only be used if the benefits outweigh the risk of using it.

2. Ketoconazole requires a low pH for absorption. If concomitant antacids, anticholinergics, and H2-blockers are needed, they should be given at least two hours after administration of Ketoconazole tablets. In achlorhydric patients, dissolve each tablet in 4 mL of aqueous solution of 0.2 N HCl. For ingesting the resulting mixture, they should use a drinking straw so as to avoid contact with the teeth. This administration should be followed with a cup of tap water.

3. Ketoconazole should not be used for fungal meningitis because it penetrates poorly into the cerebro-spinal fluid.

4. Ketoconazole is an inhibitor of cytochrome P450 and can enhance the activity of many commonly used drugs, e.g., oral hypoglycemics and anticoagulants.

BASIC CHARACTERISTICS

Class: Allylamine derivative.

Mechanism of Action: Inhibition of squalene epoxidase, blocking the biosynthesis of ergosterol, an essential component of fungal cell membranes.

Active against *Trichophyton mentagrophytes*, *Trichophyton rubrum*, *Candida albicans*, *Epidermophyton floccosum*, and *Scopulariopsis brevicaulis*.

Mechanism of Resistance: Not defined.

Metabolic Route: Eliminated in the urine.

 FDA-APPROVED INDICATIONS

Tablet: treatment of onychomycosis of the toenail or fingernail due to dermatophytes (tinea unguium).

Oral granules: treatment of tinea capitis in patients 4 years of age and older.

 SIDE EFFECTS/TOXICITY

Contraindicated in individuals with hypersensitivity to terbinafine or to any other ingredients of the formulation.

Liver failure in individuals with and without preexisting liver disease. Serious skin reactions (e.g., Stevens–Johnson syndrome and toxic epidermal necrolysis, and psoriasisiform eruptions). Precipitation and exacerbation of cutaneous and systemic lupus erythematosus. Changes in the ocular lens and retina, reversible lymphopenia and neutropenia, malaise, fatigue, depression, vomiting, arthralgia, myalgia, taste and smell disturbance, and hair loss.

 DRUG INTERACTIONS

Terbinafine is an inhibitor of the CYP450 2D6 isozyme. Drugs predominantly metabolized by the CYP450 2D6 isozyme include tricyclic antidepressants, selective serotonin reuptake inhibitors, beta-blockers, antiarrhythmics class 1C (e.g., flecainide and propafenone), and monoamine oxidase inhibitors type B. Coadministration of these drugs with terbinafine hydrochloride should be done with careful monitoring and may require a reduction in dose of the 2D6-metabolized drug.

Terbinafine clearance is increased 100 % by rifampin and decreased 33 % by cimetidine.

 DOSING

Tablets (250 mg):

Fingernail onychomycosis: 250 mg once daily for 6 weeks.

Toenail onychomycosis: 250 mg once daily for 12 weeks.

Oral granules: once a day for 6 weeks based upon body weight (see table below). Sprinkle the contents of each packet on a spoonful of pudding or other soft, non-acidic food such as mashed potatoes and swallow the entire spoonful (without chewing); do not use apple sauce or fruit-based foods. Take with food. If two packets (250 mg) are required with each dose, either the content of both packets may be sprinkled on one spoonful or the contents of both packets may be sprinkled on two spoonfuls of nonacidic food as directed above.

Antibiotics Manual: A Guide to Commonly Used Antimicrobials, Second Edition. David Schlossberg and Rafik Samuel.
© 2017 John Wiley & Sons Ltd. Published 2017 by John Wiley & Sons Ltd.

Dosage of oral granules by body weight

Body weight	Dosage
<25 kg	125 mg/day
25–35 kg	187.5 mg/day
>35 kg	250 mg/day

 ## SPECIAL POPULATIONS

RENAL IMPAIRMENT: Not recommended in patients with creatinine clearance ≤50 mL/min.

HEPATIC DYSFUNCTION: Not recommended for patients with chronic or active liver disease.

PEDIATRICS: Safety and dosing has not been studied in children.

THE ART OF ANTIMICROBIAL THERAPY

Clinical Pearls

1. Prior to initiating treatment, a KOH preparation, fungal culture, or nail biopsy should be obtained to confirm the diagnosis of onychomycosis.
2. Hepatic and hematologic function should be monitored throughout therapy.

BASIC CHARACTERISTICS

Class: Nitrofuran derivative.

Mechanism of Action: Formation of nitro anion radicals resulting in decreased protein and nucleic acid synthesis, breakage of DNA, and inhibition of growth of the organism

Metabolic route: Data incomplete.

Used for: *Trypanosoma cruzii* infections; also used for CNS *T. brucei gambiense*, in combination with eflornithine.

 SIDE EFFECTS/TOXICITY

Nausea, vomiting, abdominal pain, anorexia, insomnia, twitching, paresthesias, disorientation, seizures, and rash.

 DRUG INTERACTIONS/FOOD INTERACTIONS

Unknown.

 DOSING

Administered as 30 and 120 mg tablets.

T. cruzi: 8 to 10 mg/kg daily in 4 divided doses for 90–120 days.

T. brucei gambiense: 15 mg/kg/d PO in 3 doses × 10 days.

 SPECIAL POPULATIONS

RENAL IMPAIRMENT: Should not be administered.

HEPATIC DYSFUNCTION: Should not be administered.

PEDIATRICS:

T. cruzi: For children 1–10 years of age the dosage is 15–20 mg/kg per day in 4 divided doses for 90–120 days.

For adolescents, the daily dose is 12.5–15 mg/kg daily in 4 divided doses for 90–120 days.

 THE ART OF ANTIMICROBIAL THERAPY

Clinical Pearls

1. Nifurtimox may be obtained in the United States and is available from the CDC Drug Service, 404-639-3670. Evenings, weekends and holidays: 770-488-7100; FAX 404-639-3717.

2. The clinical efficacy of niturtimox is limited, especially with chronic *T. cruzi* infection, which has only a 20 % parasitologic cure rate.

Antibiotics Manual: A Guide to Commonly Used Antimicrobials, Second Edition. David Schlossberg and Rafik Samuel.
© 2017 John Wiley & Sons Ltd. Published 2017 by John Wiley & Sons Ltd.

■ LAMPRENE (Clofazimine)

 BASIC CHARACTERISTICS

Class: Iminophenzine.

Mechanisms of Action: Inhibits mycobacterial growth and binds preferentially to mycobacterial DNA.

Mechanisms of Resistance: Incompletely understood.

Metabolic Route: Partially metabolized with over 50 % excreted unchanged in feces.

 FDA-APPROVED INDICATIONS

(Clofazimine is not available through traditional pharmaceutical distribution. Application for use should be made through a hospital IRB and submission to the **FDA for an individual IND**).

Second-line treatment of lepromatous leprosy, including dapsone-resistant lepromatous leprosy.

Initial treatment of multibacillary leprosy, in combination with one or more other antileprosy agents

Treatment of lepromatous leprosy complicated by erythema nodosum leprosum reactions.

Also Used for: Resistant *M. tuberculosis* infection, in combination with other antituberculosis agents.

 SIDE EFFECTS/TOXICITY

Rash, photosensitivity, splenic infarction, abdominal pain, nausea, vomiting, bowel obstruction, hepatitis, jaundice, gastrointestinal bleeding, eosinophilic enteritis, retinopathy, pink or red to brownish-black discoloration of the skin, cornea, conjunctiva and body fluids, and QTc prolongation.

 DRUG INTERACTIONS/FOOD INTERACTIONS

Most patients tolerate it better when taken with food, and absorption is improved.

 DOSING

Clofazimine is supplied in 50 mg and 100 mg tablets. The usual adult dose is 200 mg daily for 2 months followed by 100 mg daily.

 SPECIAL POPULATIONS

RENAL IMPAIRMENT: No dose adjustment is necessary.

HEPATIC DYSFUNCTION: Use with caution.

PEDIATRICS: The accepted dose is 1 mg/kg/day but data are limited.

Antibiotics Manual: A Guide to Commonly Used Antimicrobials, Second Edition. David Schlossberg and Rafik Samuel.
© 2017 John Wiley & Sons Ltd. Published 2017 by John Wiley & Sons Ltd.

THE ART OF ANTIMICROBIAL THERAPY

Clinical Pearls

1. Clofazimine should never be used alone in the treatment of active mycobacterial infections.

2. Food increases the levels of clofazimine.

3. Although clofazimine demonstrates *in vitro* activity against MAC, disseminated MAC has shown increased mortality when treated with clofazimine, and clofazimine is not recommended for this indication.

LARIAM (Mefloquine Hydrochloride)

BASIC CHARACTERISTICS

Class: Antimalarial agent.

Mechanism of Action: Mefloquine is active against the schizont (erythrocytic stage) of *Plasmodium* species.

Mechanism of Resistance: Resistance has been reported in Southeast Asia.

Metabolic Route: Mefloquine is carboxylated and excreted in the feces.

FDA-APPROVED INDICATIONS

Treatment of mild to moderate acute malaria due to susceptible strains of *P. falciparum* and *P. vivax*, including chloroquine-resistant *P. falciparum*.

Prophylaxis of *P. falciparum* and *P. vivax* malaria infections, including prophylaxis of chloroquine-resistant *P. falciparum*.

SIDE EFFECTS/TOXICITY

> **WARNING:** Mefloquine may cause neuropsychiatric adverse reactions that can persist after mefloquine has been discontinued. Mefloquine should not be prescribed for prophylaxis in patients with major psychiatric disorders. During prophylactic use, if psychiatric or neurologic symptoms occur, the drug should be discontinued and an alternative medication should be substituted.

Other toxicities: Hypersensitivity; psychiatric symptoms including anxiety, paranoia, depression, hallucinations and psychosis; diarrhea, nausea, and vomiting; circulatory disturbances such as hypotension, tachycardia, bradycardia, A-V block or other transient conduction alterations, anemia, leucopenia, and thrombocytopenia.

DRUG INTERACTIONS/FOOD INTERACTIONS

Halofantrine and ketoconazole use after mefloquine has been associated with fatal prolongation of the QTc and should be avoided.

Concomitant use of mefloquine and other quinine medications should be avoided because of risk of electrocardiographic abnormalities and increased risk of convulsions.

Mefloquine may lower serum levels of anticonvulsants, which should be monitored during concomitant therapy with mefloquine.

DOSING

For malaria prophylaxis: 250 mg once weekly for prophylaxis. It should be started 1 week prior to arrival in endemic areas and continued for 4 weeks after leaving the endemic area. It should be taken with a full glass of water and with food.

For malaria treatment: 750 mg PO followed 12 hours later by 500 mg.

Antibiotics Manual: A Guide to Commonly Used Antimicrobials, Second Edition. David Schlossberg and Rafik Samuel.
© 2017 John Wiley & Sons Ltd. Published 2017 by John Wiley & Sons Ltd.

SPECIAL POPULATIONS

RENAL IMPAIRMENT: There is no adjustment needed.

HEPATIC DYSFUNCTION: There is no adjustment needed, but levels may increase in those with hepatic dysfunction.

PEDIATRICS:

For treatment: 15 mg/kg PO followed 12 hours later by 10 mg/kg.

For prophylaxis (begin 1–2 weeks before and continue for 4 weeks after leaving the malarious area):

<9 kg: 5 mg/kg salt once/week

9–19 kg: ¼ tab once/week

>19–30 kg: ½ tab once/week

>31–45 kg: ¾ tab once/week

>45 kg: 1 tab once/week

 THE ART OF ANTIMICROBIAL THERAPY

Clinical Pearls

1. Mefloquine should not be given to those with depression, anxiety disorders, psychosis, or schizophrenia.
2. Mefloquine resistance is seen in Southeast Asia and it therefore should not be used for prophylaxis.
3. Mefloquine does not eliminate hepatic phase parasites, and patients with acute *P. vivax* malaria are at high risk of relapse; to avoid relapse, after initial treatment of the acute infection, patients should subsequently be treated with an 8-amino-quinoline derivative (e.g., primaquine).
4. Mefloquine can induce hemolysis in patients with G6PD deficiency.
5. Because of the long half-life of mefloquine, adverse effects can persist for weeks after discontinuation of therapy.

■ LEVAQUIN (Levofloxacin)

 BASIC CHARACTERISTICS

Class: Fluoroquinolone.

Mechanism of Action: Inhibition of bacterial topoisomerase IV and DNA gyrase.

Mechanisms of Resistance: Mutations in DNA gyrase and/or topoisomerase IV, or through altered efflux.

Metabolic Route: Levofloxacin is predominantly excreted in the urine.

 FDA-APPROVED INDICATIONS

Levofloxacin is indicated for the treatment of serious infections caused by susceptible strains of microorganisms in the diseases listed below:

Pneumonia: nosocomial and community acquired

Acute bacterial sinusitis

Acute bacterial exacerbation of chronic bronchitis

Skin and skin structure infections: complicated and uncomplicated

Chronic bacterial prostatitis

Urinary tract infections: complicated and uncomplicated

Acute pyelonephritis

Inhalational anthrax, post-exposure

Also Used for the treatment of *Mycobacterium tuberculosis* and nontuberculous mycobacteria in combination with other medications, as well as *C. trachomatis* infection.

 SIDE EFFECTS/TOXICITY

> **WARNING:** Serious adverse reactions including tendinitis, tendon rupture, peripheral neuropathy, central nervous system effects, and exacerbation of myasthenia gravis. Fluoroquinolones, including levofloxacin, have been associated with disabling and potentially irreversible serious adverse reactions that have occurred together, including tendinitis and tendon rupture, and peripheral neuropathy and central nervous system effects.
>
> Discontinue levofloxacin immediately and avoid the use of fluoroquinolones, including levofloxacin, in patients who experience any of these serious adverse reactions. Fluoroquinolones, including levofloxacin, may exacerbate muscle weakness in patients with myasthenia gravis. Avoid levofloxacin in patients with a known history of myasthenia gravis.
>
> Because fluoroquinolones, including levofloxacin, have been associated with serious adverse reactions, reserve levofloxacin for use in patients who have no alternative treatment options for the following indications: uncomplicated urinary tract infection, acute bacterial exacerbation of chronic bronchitis, and acute bacterial sinusitis.

Levofloxacin is **contraindicated** in persons with a history of hypersensitivity associated with the use of levofloxacin or any quinolone.

The most common reactions are nausea, headache, diarrhea, insomnia, constipation and dizziness. Also reported are anaphylactic reactions and allergic skin reactions, occasionally fatal, which may occur after the first dose, photosensitivity, tendinitis

Antibiotics Manual: A Guide to Commonly Used Antimicrobials, Second Edition. David Schlossberg and Rafik Samuel.
© 2017 John Wiley & Sons Ltd. Published 2017 by John Wiley & Sons Ltd.

and tendon rupture, and renal toxicity, hepatotoxicity, sometimes fatal, central nervous system effects including convulsions, anxiety, confusion, depression, and insomnia (use with caution in patients at risk seizures), peripheral neuropathy, *Clostridium difficile*-associated colitis, prolongation of the QT interval and torsade de pointes (avoid use in patients with known prolongation of QT, hypokalemia, and with other drugs that prolong the QT interval), agranulocytosis, and thrombocytopenia.

 ## DRUG INTERACTIONS/FOOD INTERACTIONS

Levofloxacin tablets can be administered without regard to food. Levofloxacin oral solution should be taken 1 hour before or 2 hours after eating.

1. Antacids containing calcium, magnesium, or aluminum; sucralfate; divalent or trivalent cations such as iron; or multivitamins containing zinc should not be taken within the two-hour period before or within the two-hour period after taking levofloxacin.
2. Levofloxacin may enhance the effects of warfarin. However, no dosage adjustments are necessary for concomitantly administered probenecid, cimetidine, digoxin, or cyclosporine.
3. The concomitant administration of a nonsteroidal anti-inflammatory drug with a quinolone may increase the risk of CNS stimulation and convulsive seizures.
4. Disturbances of blood glucose, including hyperglycemia and hypoglycemia, may be seen in patients treated concurrently with antidiabetic agents.
5. Levofloxacin may produce false-positive urine screening results for opiates.

 ## DOSING

Levofloxacin is supplied in 250 mg, 500 mg, and 750 mg tablets and an oral solution containing 25 mg/mL. Levofloxacin is also available for intravenous administration.

Type of infection	Dose every 24 hours (IV or PO)	Duration (days)
Nosocomial pneumonia	750 mg	7–14
Community acquired pneumonia	500 mg	7–14
	750 mg	5
Acute bacterial sinusitis	750 mg	5
	500 mg	10–14
Acute exacerbation of chronic bronchitis	500 mg	7
Complicated skin and skin structure infections	750 mg	7–14
Uncomplicated SSSI	500 mg	7–10
Chronic bacterial prostatitis	500 mg	28
Complicated urinary tract infection or acute pyelonephritis	750 mg	5
Complicated urinary tract infection or acute pyelonephritis	250 mg	10
Uncomplicated urinary tract infection	250 mg	3
Inhalational anthrax (postexposure)		
Adults and pediatric patients >50 kg and ≥6 months of age	500 mg	60
Pediatric patients < 50 kg and ≥ 6 months of age	8 mg/kg BID	60
M. tuberculosis	500–1000 mg	Varies with anti-TB regimen used

SPECIAL POPULATIONS

RENAL IMPAIRMENT:

Normal renal function	Creatinine clearance, 20 to 49 mL/min	Creatinine clearance, 10 to 19 mL/min	Hemodialysis, CAPD or CRRT
750 mg daily	750 mg q 48 h	750 mg, then 500 mg q 48 h	750 mg, then 500 mg q 48 h
500 mg daily	500 mg, then 250 mg q 24 h	500 mg, then 250 mg q 48 h	500 mg then 250 mg q 48 h
250 mg daily	No dosage adjustment	250 mg every 48 hours	No information

HEPATIC DYSFUNCTION: A maximum dose of 400 mg of levofloxacin per day should not be exceeded.

PEDIATRICS: Levofloxacin is indicated in pediatric patients for the prophylaxis of inhalational anthrax. Prolonged therapy has not been studied in children.

 THE ART OF ANTIMICROBIAL THERAPY

Clinical Pearls

1. Levofloxacin should be given 2 hours before or after cations.
2. All fluoroquinolones can lead to tendon rupture, especially in patients over 65 years of age.
3. All fluoroquinolones can prolong QT intervals and caution should be used when given with medications that affect QT intervals.
4. All fluoroquinolones can cause phototoxicity.
5. All fluoroquinolones can lower the seizure threshold.
6. Levofloxacin should be avoided, if possible, in children, pregnant women, and nursing mothers because of concern for cartilage developmental problems.
7. Levofloxacin has activity against *Mycobacteria*; therefore levofloxacin monotherapy should be avoided if mycobacterial infection is possible.
8. Treatment of gonorrhea with fluoroquinolones should be undertaken with caution because of rising resistance.
9. In 2016, an FDA Safety Communication advised that the serious side effects associated with fluoroquinolones generally outweigh the benefits for patients with sinusitis, bronchitis, and uncomplicated urinary tract infections who have other treatment options.

BASIC CHARACTERISTICS

Class: Protease inhibitor.

Mechanism of Action: Amprenavir, the active drug, reversibly binds the active site of the enzyme protease. Inhibition of protease prevents cleavage of the *gag* and *gag-pol* polyprotein, resulting in the production of immature, noninfectious virus.

Mechanism of Resistance: Development of mutations on the enzyme protease causes a conformational change that prevents amprenavir from binding the active site, allowing protease activity to continue. The most frequent resistance mutations include I50V, I54 L/M, and I84V.

Metabolic Route: After oral administration, fosamprenavir is hydrolyzed to amprenavir and inorganic phosphate. Amprenavir is metabolized in the liver and excreted.

 FDA-APPROVED INDICATIONS

Treatment of HIV-1 in combinations with other antiretroviral agents.

 SIDE EFFECTS/TOXICITY

New onset diabetes mellitus, exacerbation of pre-existing diabetes mellitus, hyperglycemia, increased bleeding, including spontaneous skin hematomas and hemarthrosis, in patients with hemophilia type A and B, redistribution/accumulation of body fat including central obesity, dorsocervical fat enlargement (buffalo hump), peripheral wasting, facial wasting, breast enlargement, "cushingoid appearance", immune reconstitution syndrome, mouth ulceration, diarrhea, nausea, vomiting, anorexia, dyspepsia, epigastric pain, hepatitis, pancreatitis, headache, QTc prolongation and torsades de pointes, (hemolytic) anemia, leucopenia, thrombocytopenia, increased amylase, CPK, hyperlipemia, hyperuricemia, hyperglycemia, hypoglycemia, and dehydration.

 DRUG INTERACTIONS/FOOD INTERACTIONS

Fosamprenavir tablets may be taken with or without food. The oral suspension must be taken without food.

Drugs that **should not be coadministered** with fosamprenavir include alfuzosin, flecainide, propafenone, lurasidone, rifampin, ergot derivatives, St John's wort, simvastatin or lovastatin, pimozide, cisapride, midazolam, triazolam, oral contraceptives, salmeterol, fluticasone, lopinavir/ritonavir, tipranavir, nefirapine, delavirdine, etravirine, simeprevir, paritepravir.

Fosamprenavir is an inhibitor of the CYP3A enzyme; coadministration of fosamprenavir and drugs primarily metabolized by CYP3A may result in increased plasma concentrations of the other drug that could increase or prolong its therapeutic and adverse effects.

Fosamprenavir is metabolized by CYP3A; coadministration of fosamprenavir and drugs that induce CYP3A may decrease fosamprenavir plasma concentrations and reduce its therapeutic effect. Coadministration of fosamprenavir and drugs that inhibit

Antibiotics Manual: A Guide to Commonly Used Antimicrobials, Second Edition. David Schlossberg and Rafik Samuel.
© 2017 John Wiley & Sons Ltd. Published 2017 by John Wiley & Sons Ltd.

CYP3A may increase fosamprenavir plasma concentrations. Because of these metabolic effects, potential drug interactions that may require dosage change or clinical/laboratory monitoring are listed below:

Medication	Adjustment or action
Itraconzole	Dose adjustments for those taking >400 mg/day
Ketoconazole	Do not exceed 200 mg daily
Voriconazole	Monitor for toxicity
Rifabutin	Decrease rifabutin to 150/qod or 3 ×/week
Atorvastatin or rosuvastatin	Use lowest possible dose with close monitoring
Phenobarbital, phenytoin, or carbamazepine	Monitor anticonvulsant level; consider alternative
Methadone	Monitor; may require higher methadone dose
Sildenafil	25 mg every 48 hours
Tadalafil	5 mg, no more than 10 mg in 72 hours
Vardenafil	No more than 2.5 mg in 24 hours
Maraviroc	Maraviroc dose of 150 mg bid
Efavirenz	An additional dose of ritonavir 100 mg twice daily
Dolutegravir	Increase dolutegravir to 50 mg twice daily
Colchicine	Do not coadminister in renal or hepatic impairment
Quetiapine	Administer one-sixth of the quetiapine dose
Bosentan	Bosentan dose 62.5 mg daily

 DOSING

Fosamprenavir is supplied as 700 mg tablets and a white to off-white grape-bubblegum-peppermint flavored suspension that contains 50 mg/cc.

For therapy-naïve patients, fosamprenavir can be administered 1400 mg twice daily (without ritonavir), 1400 mg once daily plus ritonavir 200 mg once daily, or 1400 mg once daily plus ritonavir 100 mg once daily.

For protease inhibitor-experienced patients, the dose is 700 mg twice daily plus ritonavir 100 mg twice daily.

 SPECIAL POPULATIONS

RENAL IMPAIRMENT: There is no adjustment needed.

HEPATIC DYSFUNCTION: For Child Pugh class A*, fosamprenavir should be used with caution. Some recommend administering fosamprenavir at a reduced dosage of 700 mg twice daily without ritonavir (therapy-naive) or 700 mg twice daily plus ritonavir 100 mg once daily (therapy-naive or protease inhibitor-experienced).

For Child Pugh class B*, fosamprenavir should be used with caution at a reduced dosage of 700 mg twice daily (therapy-naive) without ritonavir, or 450 mg twice daily plus ritonavir 100 mg once daily (therapy-naive or protease inhibitor-experienced).

In those with Child Pugh class C*, fosamprenavir should be used with caution at a reduced dosage of 350 mg twice daily without ritonavir (therapy-naive) or 300 mg once daily with ritonavir 100 mg daily.

*See Helpful Formulas, Equations, and Definitions for Child Pugh classification.

PEDIATRICS: The recommended dosage of fosamprenavir in patients 4 weeks and older is as follows:

Weight	Twice daily regimen
<11 kg	Fosamprenavir 45 mg/kg plus ritonavir 7 mg/kg
11 kg to <15 kg	Fosamprenavir 30 mg/kg plus ritonavir 3 mg/kg
15 kg to <20 kg	Fosamprenavir 23 mg/kg plus ritonavir 3 mg/kg
>20 kg	Fosamprenavir 18 mg/kg plus ritonavir 3 mg/kg

Do not exceed the dose of 700 mg/100 mg.

Therapy-naive greater than 2 years of age: Oral suspension 30 mg/kg twice daily, not to exceed the adult dose of 1400 mg twice daily (no ritonavir).

 THE ART OF ANTIMICROBIAL THERAPY

Clinical Pearls

1. Fosamprenavir should always be used in combination with other antiretrovirals.
2. Fosamprenavir has a sulfa moiety and should be used with caution in patients with sulfa allergies.
3. Even though fosamprenavir can be taken with or without food, it is likely that taking boosted fosamprenavir with food may decrease gastrointestinal side effects.
4. When initiating boosted fosamprenavir in experienced patients, it must be given twice daily.
5. When assessing for resistance to fosamprenavir, a phenotype assay may be helpful.
6. Whenever initiating fosamprenavir, make sure to review all medications the patient is receiving to minimize drug interactions.

■ MALARONE (Atovaquone/Proguanil)

 BASIC CHARACTERISTICS

Class: Antimetabolite.

Mechanism of Action: Atovaquone is a selective inhibitor of parasite mitochondrial electron transport. Proguanil hydrochloride primarily exerts its effect by means of the metabolite cycloguanil, a dihydrofolate reductase inhibitor. Inhibition of dihydrofolate reductase in the malaria parasite disrupts deoxythymidylate synthesis.

Atovaquone and cycloguanil (an active metabolite of proguanil) are active against the erythrocytic and exoerythrocytic stages of *Plasmodium* spp.

Metabolic Route: Atovaquone is excreted unchanged in feces. Proguanil is metabolized by the liver and renally excreted.

 FDA-APPROVED INDICATIONS

Indicated for the prophylaxis of *P. falciparum* malaria and for the treatment of acute, uncomplicated *P. falciparum* malaria.

 SIDE EFFECTS/TOXICITY

Atovaquone/proguanil is **contraindicated** in:

1. Individuals with known hypersensitivity to atovaquone or proguanil hydrochloride or any component of the formulation. Rare cases of anaphylaxis following treatment with atovaquone/proguanil have been reported.

2. Prophylaxis of *P. falciparum* malaria in patients with severe renal impairment (creatinine clearance <30 mL/min).

Toxicity includes fever, hypersensitivity, rash, angioedema, pruritus, vasculitis, headache, dizziness, insomnia, depression, psychotic events, seizures, cough, keratopathy, stomatitis, hepatotoxicity, anorexia nausea, vomiting diarrhea, abdominal pain, pancreatitis, myalgia, renal failure, asthenia, methemoglobinemia, and pancytopenia.

 DRUG INTERACTIONS/FOOD INTERACTIONS

Administering atovaquone/proguanil with food enhances its absorption.

Medications that can **decrease the levels of atovaquone**: tetracycline, metoclopramide, rifampin, or rifabutin.

Caution should be exercised when prescribing atovaquone with indinavir due to the decrease in trough levels of indinavir.

 DOSING

Prophylactic treatment with atovaquone/proguanil should be started 1 or 2 days before entering a malaria-endemic area and continued daily during the stay and for 7 days after return. Dosage is one atovaquone/proguanil tablet (adult strength = 250 mg atovaquone/100 mg proguanil hydrochloride) per day.

Treatment of acute malaria: Four tablets (1 g atovaquone/400 mg proguanil hydrochloride) as a single dose daily for 3 consecutive days.

SPECIAL POPULATIONS

RENAL IMPAIRMENT: Should not be used for malaria prophylaxis in patients with severe renal impairment (creatinine clearance <30 mL/min) but may be used with caution for the treatment of malaria if the benefits of the 3-day treatment regimen outweigh the potential risks associated with increased drug exposure. In this case, no dosage adjustment is needed if creatinine clearance is > 30 mL/min.

HEPATIC DYSFUNCTION: Not studied in patients with severe hepatic dysfunction.

PEDIATRICS: Treatment of malaria has not been studied in pediatric patients who weigh less than 5 kg and prophylaxis has not been studied in pediatric patients who weigh less than 11 kg.

The dosage for **prophylaxis** of malaria is based upon body weight:

Weight	Daily dose
11–20 kg	1 pediatric tablet daily (62.5 mg/25 mg)
21–30 kg	2 pediatric tablets daily
31–40 kg	3 pediatric tablets daily
>40 kg	1 adult tablet daily (250 mg/100 mg)

The dosage for **treatment** of acute malaria is based upon body weight:

Weight	Regimen
5–8 kg	2 pediatric tablets 62.5 mg/25 mg) daily for 3 days
9–10 kg	3 pediatric tablets daily for 3 days
11–20 kg	1 adult tablet daily (250 mg/100 mg) for 3 days
21–30 kg	2 adult tablets daily for 3 days
31–40 kg	3 adult tablets daily for 3 days
>40 kg	4 adult tablets daily for 3 days

 THE ART OF ANTIMICROBIAL THERAPY

Clinical Pearls

1. Atovaquone/proguanil is not recommended for treatment of severe malaria.
2. Atovaquone/proguanil should not be used for patients with renal failure.
3. Atovaquone should be administered with food to increase its absorption.
4. Absorption of atovaquone may be reduced in patients with diarrhea or vomiting.
5. Atovaquone/proguanil may be crushed and mixed with condensed milk just prior to administration for children who may have difficulty swallowing tablets.

■ MANDOL (Cefamandole)

 BASIC CHARACTERISTICS

Class: Second generation cephalosporin.

Mechanism of Action: Binds penicillin-binding protein, disrupting cell wall synthesis.

Mechanisms of Resistance:

1. The PBP can be altered, with reduced affinity.
2. Production of a beta-lactamase, resulting in hydrolysis of the beta-lactam ring.
3. Decreased ability of the antibiotic to reach the PBP when bacteria decrease porin production, resulting in a decrease of the drug concentration within the cell.

Metabolic Route: Cefamandole is excreted unchanged in the urine.

 FDA-APPROVED INDICATIONS

Lower respiratory infections

Urinary tract infections

Peritonitis

Septicemia

Skin and skin structure infections

Bone and joint infections

Cefamandole preoperatively, intraoperatively, and postoperatively may reduce the incidence of certain postoperative infections.

 SIDE EFFECTS/TOXICITY

Cefamandole is **contraindicated** in patients with a known allergy to cephalosporins.

Cefamandole should be used with caution if hypersensitivity exists to penicillin.

Toxicity includes phlebitis, fever, anaphylaxis, rash including Stevens–Johnson syndrome, erythema multiforme and toxic epidermal necrolysis, angioedema, flushing, serum-sickness-like reactions, encephalopathy, seizures, diarrhea, *Clostridium difficile*-associated diarrhea and pseudomembranous colitis, oral candidiasis, anorexia, taste perversion, nausea, vomiting, stomach cramps, flatulence, hepatitis, renal impairment, genital moniliasis, vaginitis, hemorrhage, prolonged prothrombin time, pancytopenia, hemolytic anemia, positive Coombs' test; cephalosporins may cause false-positive urine glucose determinations when using cupric sulfate solution (Benedict's solution, *Clinitest®*). Tests utilizing glucose oxidase (*Tes-Tape®*, *Clinistix®*) are not affected by cephalosporins.

 DRUG INTERACTIONS/FOOD INTERACTIONS

Concomitant administration of probenecid with cefamandole increases the serum concentration.

Cefamandole inhibits the enzyme acetaldehyde dehydrogenase in laboratory animals. This causes accumulation of acetaldehyde when ethanol is administered concomitantly.

Antibiotics Manual: A Guide to Commonly Used Antimicrobials, Second Edition. David Schlossberg and Rafik Samuel.
© 2017 John Wiley & Sons Ltd. Published 2017 by John Wiley & Sons Ltd.

DOSING

Cefamandole can be administered intravenously or intramuscularly:

Infection	Dose
Skin structures and in uncomplicated pneumonia	500 mg every 6 hours
Uncomplicated urinary tract infections	500 mg every 8 hours
Complicated urinary tract infections	1 g every 8 hours
*Severe infections	1 g every 4–6 hours
**Life-threatening infections of less susceptible organisms	2 g every 4 hours

Perioperative use: 1 or 2 g intravenously or intramuscularly ¹/₂ to 1 hour prior to the surgical incision followed by 1 or 2 g every 6 hours for 24 to 48 hours.

 SPECIAL POPULATIONS

RENAL IMPAIRMENT:

Creatinine clearance, mL/min	Life-threatening infections	Less severe infections
50–80	1.5 g q 4 h or 6 g q 6 h	0.75–1.5 g q 6 h
25–50	1.5 g q 6 h or 2 g q 8 h	0.75–1.5 g q 8 h
10–25	1 g q 6 h or 1.25 g q 8 h	0.5–1 g q 8 h
2–10	0.67 g q 8 h or 1 g q 12 h	0.5–0.75 g q 12 h
<2	0.5 g q 8 h or 0.75 g q 12 h	0.25–0.5 g q 12 h
Hemodialysis	1 gram after dialysis	
CAPD	1 gram daily	
CRRT	1 gram every 6 hours	

HEPATIC DYSFUNCTION: No dose adjustment is necessary.

PEDIATRICS: 50 to 100 mg/kg/day in equally divided doses every 4 to 8 hours and may be increased to a total daily dose of 150 mg/kg (not to exceed the maximum adult dose) for severe infections.

 THE ART OF ANTIMICROBIAL THERAPY

Clinical Pearls

1. Cefamandole must be adjusted for renal dysfunction.
2. Cross allergy with penicillins is <10 %.

MAXIPIME (Cefepime)

 ## BASIC CHARACTERISTICS

Class: Fourth generation cephalosporin.

Mechanism of Action: Binds penicillin-binding protein, disrupting cell wall synthesis.

Mechanisms of Resistance:

1. The PBP can be altered, with reduced affinity.
2. Production of a beta-lactamase, resulting in hydrolysis of the beta-lactam ring.
3. Decreased ability of the antibiotic to reach the PBP when bacteria decrease porin production, resulting in a decrease of the drug concentration within the cell.

Metabolic Route: Excreted unchanged in the urine.

 ## FDA-APPROVED INDICATIONS

Treatment of the following infections when caused by susceptible organisms:

Pneumonia

Empiric therapy for febrile neutropenic patients

Uncomplicated and complicated urinary tract infections

Uncomplicated skin and skin structure infections

Complicated intra-abdominal infections (used in combination with metronidazole)

 ## SIDE EFFECTS/TOXICITY

Cefepime is **contraindicated** in patients who have shown immediate hypersensitivity reactions to cefepime or cephalosporins, penicillins, or other beta-lactam antibiotics. If other forms of hypersensitivity to penicillin exist, cefepime should be used with caution.

Toxicity includes fever, anaphylaxis, rash including Stevens–Johnson syndrome, erythema multiforme and toxic epidermal necrolysis, angioedema, flushing, serum-sickness-like reactions, encephalopathy, seizures, myoclonus, diarrhea, *Clostridium difficile*-associated diarrhea and pseudomembranous colitis, oral candidiasis, anorexia, nausea, vomiting, stomach cramps, flatulence, hepatitis, renal impairment, genital moniliasis, vaginitis, hemorrhage, prolonged prothrombin time, hypercalcemia, hypocalcemia, pancytopenia, hemolytic anemia, positive Coombs' test; cephalosporins may cause false-positive urine glucose determinations when using cupric sulfate solution (Benedict's solution, *Clinitest®*). Tests utilizing glucose oxidase (*Tes-Tape®*, *Clinistix®*) are not affected by cephalosporins.

DRUG INTERACTIONS/FOOD INTERACTIONS

Renal function should be monitored carefully if high doses of aminoglycosides or diuretics are to be administered with cefepime because of the increased potential of nephrotoxicity and ototoxicity of aminoglycoside antibiotics.

Solutions containing dextrose may be contraindicated in patients with known allergy to corn or corn products.

Antibiotics Manual: A Guide to Commonly Used Antimicrobials, Second Edition. David Schlossberg and Rafik Samuel.
© 2017 John Wiley & Sons Ltd. Published 2017 by John Wiley & Sons Ltd.

DOSING

Type of infection	Dose	Duration
Moderate to severe pneumonia	1–2 g q 12 hours	10 days
Febrile neutropenia	2 g q 8 hours	Neutropenia resolution
Urinary tract infection	500 mg–1 g q 12 hours	7–10 days
Severe urinary tract infection	2 g q 12 hours	10 days
Skin and skin structure infection	2 g q 12 hours	10 days
Intraabdominal infection	2 g q 12 hours	7–10 days

 SPECIAL POPULATIONS

RENAL IMPAIRMENT:

Creatinine clearance	Doses			
>60 mL/min	500 mg q12 h	1 g q 12 h	2 g q 12 h	2 g q 8 h
30–60 mL/min	500 mg q day	1 g q day	2 g q day	2 g q 12 h
11–29 mL/min	500 mg q day	500 mg q day	1 g q day	2 g q day
<11 mL/min	250 mg q day	250 mg q day	500 mg q day	1 g q day
HD	1 g on day 1, then 500 mg every 24 hours			1 g q day
CAPD	500 mg q 48 h	1 g q 48 h	2 g q 48 h	2 g q 48 h
CRRT	Not recommended			

HEPATIC DYSFUNCTION: No dose adjustment is necessary.

PEDIATRICS: Safety and effectiveness in pediatric patients below the age of 2 months have not been established.

The dosage is 50 mg per kg per dose, administered every 12 hours (50 mg per kg per dose, every 8 hours for febrile neutropenic patients).

 THE ART OF ANTIMICROBIAL THERAPY

Clinical Pearls

1. Cefepime is dose adjusted for renal dysfunction.
2. Cross allergy with penicillins is <10 %.
3. Patients with creatinine clearance less than or equal to 60 mL/min must have dosage adjustment to avoid adverse reactions such as encephalopathy, myoclonus, and seizures.
4. Concomitant aminoglycosides increase the potential of nephrotoxicity and ototoxicity.
5. Nephrotoxicity has been reported with concomitant administration of other cephalosporins with potent diuretics such as furosemide.

■ MEFOXIN (Cefoxitin)

 ## BASIC CHARACTERISTICS

Class: Second generation cephalosporin.

Mechanism of Action: Binds penicillin-binding protein, disrupting cell wall synthesis.

Mechanisms of Resistance:

1. The PBP can be altered, with reduced affinity.
2. Production of a beta-lactamase, resulting in hydrolysis of the beta-lactam ring.
3. Decreased ability of the antibiotic to reach the PBP when bacteria decrease porin production, resulting in a decrease of the drug concentration within the cell.

Metabolic Route: Cefoxitin is predominantly excreted unchanged in the urine.

 ## FDA-APPROVED INDICATIONS

Treatment of serious infections caused by susceptible strains of microorganisms in the diseases listed below:

Lower respiratory tract infections

Urinary tract infections

Intra-abdominal infections

Gynecological infections

Septicemia

Bone and joint infections

Skin and skin structure

Prevention of infection in patients undergoing uncontaminated gastrointestinal surgery, vaginal hysterectomy, abdominal hysterectomy, or cesarean section.

 ## SIDE EFFECTS/TOXICITY

Cefoxitin is **contraindicated** in patients who have shown hypersensitivity to cefoxitin and the cephalosporin group of antibiotics. Cefoxitin should be used with caution if hypersensitivity exists to penicillins.

Toxicity includes fever, anaphylaxis, rash including Stevens–Johnson syndrome, erythema multiforme and toxic epidermal necrolysis, angioedema, flushing, hypotension, serum-sickness-like reactions, encephalopathy, seizures, possible exacerbation of myasthenia gravis, diarrhea, *Clostridium difficile*-associated diarrhea and pseudomembranous colitis, oral candidiasis, anorexia, nausea, vomiting, stomach cramps, flatulence, hepatitis, renal impairment, genital moniliasis, vaginitis, hemorrhage, prolonged prothrombin time, pancytopenia, hemolytic anemia, positive Coombs' test.

DRUG INTERACTIONS/FOOD INTERACTIONS

Increased nephrotoxicity has been reported following concomitant administration of cephalosporins and aminoglycoside antibiotics. Cephalosporins may cause false-positive urine glucose determinations when using cupric sulfate solution (Benedict's solution, *Clinitest®*). Tests utilizing glucose oxidase (*Tes-Tape®*, *Clinistix®*) are not affected by cephalosporins.

Solutions containing dextrose may be **contraindicated** in patients with hypersensitivity to corn products.

Antibiotics Manual: A Guide to Commonly Used Antimicrobials, Second Edition. David Schlossberg and Rafik Samuel.
© 2017 John Wiley & Sons Ltd. Published 2017 by John Wiley & Sons Ltd.

DOSING

Uncomplicated infections	1 g q 6–8 hours IV
Moderate to severe infections	1 g q 4 hours or 2 g q 6–8 hours IV
Prevention	2 g IV 30–60 min before incision followed by 2 g IV q 6 hours after first dose for no more than 24 hours

 SPECIAL POPULATIONS

RENAL IMPAIRMENT:

Creatinine clearance	Dose
30–50 mL/min	1–2 grams every 8–12 hours
10–29 mL/min	1–2 grams every 12–24 hours
5–10 mL/min	500 mg–1 gram every 12–24 hours
<5 mL/min	500 mg–1 gram every 24–48 hours
Hemodialysis	1 gram after dialysis
CAPD	1 gram daily
CRRT	1–2 grams every 8–12 hours

HEPATIC DYSFUNCTION: No dose adjustment is necessary.

PEDIATRICS: Safety and efficacy in pediatric patients less than three months of age have not yet been established. In patients three months of age and older, the dose is 80 to 160 mg/kg per day divided into four to six equal doses. The higher dosages should be used for more severe or serious infections. The total daily dosage should not exceed 12 grams.
Surgical prevention: 30 to 40 mg/kg doses may be given at the times designated above.

 THE ART OF ANTIMICROBIAL THERAPY

Clinical Pearls

1. Cefoxitin is dose adjusted for renal dysfunction.
2. Cross allergy with penicillins is <10%.
3. Cefoxitin may cause an exacerbation of myasthenia gravis.

■ MEL-B (Melarsoprol B)

 BASIC CHARACTERISTICS

Class: Aromatic arsenicals.

Mechanism of Action:

1. Inhibitor of glycolytic kinases.
2. A potent inhibitor of trypanothione reductase.
3. Interaction with lipoic acid.

Metabolic Route: Oxidized in the liver and is excreted in the urine and feces.

Used for: Treatment of African trypanosomiasis in the late stages (with CNS involvement).

 SIDE EFFECTS/TOXICITY

Life threatening encephalopathy may occur in up to 20 % of patients receiving melarsoprol. It is more common with Rhodesian than Gambian sleeping sickness and may be an immune mediated reaction. If this occurs, IV dexamethasone and anticonvulsants may be beneficial and therapy should be switched to eflornithine.

Other toxic effects include fever, rash, polyneuropathy (possibly ameliorated by thiamine), tremors, phlebitis, cellulitis, and abdominal pain.

 DRUG INTERACTIONS/FOOD INTERACTIONS

Unknown.

 DOSING

T. brucei gambiense and *T. brucei rhodesiense*:

2.2 mg/kg/d IV × 10 days after 2 or 3 doses of suramin as pretreatment (to decrease the possibility of encephalopathy).

 SPECIAL POPULATIONS

RENAL IMPAIRMENT: There is no dose adjustment for renal insufficiency.

HEPATIC DYSFUNCTION: There is no dose adjustment for hepatic dysfunction.

PEDIATRICS: As for adults.

 THE ART OF ANTIMICROBIAL THERAPY

Clinical Pearls

1. Melarsoprol can be obtained from the CDC Drug Service (404-639-3670). Evenings, weekends, and holidays: (770-488-7100; FAX 404-639-3717).

Antibiotics Manual: A Guide to Commonly Used Antimicrobials, Second Edition. David Schlossberg and Rafik Samuel.
© 2017 John Wiley & Sons Ltd. Published 2017 by John Wiley & Sons Ltd.

2. For late-stage Rhodesian trypanosomiasis eflornithine is ineffective; thus, melarsoprol is the only option.

3. Corticosteroids may prevent treatment-associated encephalopathy.

4. Pretreatment with suramin or pentamidine may decrease the toxicity of melarsoprol, but its beneficial effect has never been documented.

5. Thiamine may be helpful for the polyneuropathy.

■ MEPRON (Atovaquone)

 BASIC CHARACTERISTICS

Class: Antimetabolite.

Mechanism of Action: Atovaquone is an analog of ubiquinone. The mechanism of action against *Pneumocystis jirovecii* has not been fully elucidated.

In *Plasmodium* species, the site of action appears to be the cytochrome bc1 complex (Complex III). Inhibition of electron transport by atovaquone results in indirect inhibition of these enzymes. The ultimate metabolic effect of such a blockade includes inhibition of nucleic acid and ATP synthesis.

Metabolic Route: Excreted unchanged in feces.

 FDA-APPROVED INDICATIONS

Prevention of *Pneumocystis jirovecii* pneumonia in patients 13 years and older who are intolerant to trimethoprim-sulfamethoxazole (TMP-SMX).

Treatment of mild-to-moderate PCP in patients 13 years and older who are intolerant to TMP-SMX.

Also Used for: Alternative therapy for toxoplasmosis (in combination with pyrimethamine), babesiosis, malaria therapy, and malaria prophylaxis.

 SIDE EFFECTS/TOXICITY

Atovaquone is **contraindicated** for patients who develop or have a history of potentially life-threatening allergic reactions to any of the components of the formulation. Toxic effects include fever, hypersensitivity, rash, insomnia, headache, depression, keratopathy, cough, diarrhea, nausea, pancreatitis, hepatotoxicity, myalgia, renal failure leucopenia, thrombocytopenia, and methemoglobinemia.

 DRUG INTERACTIONS/FOOD INTERACTIONS

Administering atovaquone with food enhances its absorption.

Rifampin lowers atovaquone levels.

 DOSING

Prevention of PCP: 1500 mg (10 mL) once daily.

Treatment of mild-to-moderate PCP: 750 mg (5 mL) administered with meals twice daily for 21 days.

 SPECIAL POPULATIONS

RENAL IMPAIRMENT: Unknown.

HEPATIC DYSFUNCTION: Unknown.

PEDIATRICS: Not studied in children.

Antibiotics Manual: A Guide to Commonly Used Antimicrobials, Second Edition. David Schlossberg and Rafik Samuel.
© 2017 John Wiley & Sons Ltd. Published 2017 by John Wiley & Sons Ltd.

THE ART OF ANTIMICROBIAL THERAPY

Clinical Pearls

1. Atovaquone is not recommended for treatment of moderate to severe PCP because of the unreliability of absorption.
2. Atovaquone should be administered with food to increase its absorption.

■ MERREM (Meropenem)

 BASIC CHARACTERISTICS

Class: Carbapenem.

Mechanism of Action: Binds penicillin-binding protein, disrupting cell wall synthesis.

Mechanisms of Resistance:

1. The PBP can be altered, with reduced affinity.
2. Production of beta-lactamases (carbapenemases, metallo-β-lactamases), resulting in hydrolysis of the beta-lactam ring.
3. Decreased ability of the antibiotic to reach the PBP when bacteria decrease porin production, resulting in a decrease of the drug concentration within the cell.
4. Increased expression of efflux pump components.

Metabolic Route: Meropenem is excreted in the urine.

 FDA-APPROVED INDICATIONS

Treatment of serious infections caused by susceptible strains of microorganisms in the conditions listed below:

1. **Complicated skin and skin structure infections** (adult patients and pediatric patients 3 months of age and older only).
2. **Intra-abdominal infections including complicated appendicitis and peritonitis** (adult and pediatric patients).
3. **Bacterial meningitis** (pediatric patients 3 months of age and older only).

 SIDE EFFECTS/TOXICITY

Meropenem is **contraindicated** in patients with known hypersensitivity to any component of this product or to other drugs in the same class or in patients who have demonstrated anaphylactic reactions to β-lactams. Before initiating therapy with meropenem, careful inquiry should be made concerning previous hypersensitivity reactions to penicillins, cephalosporins, other beta-lactams, and other allergens, because of the increased possibility of hypersensitivity.

Additional toxicity: phlebitis, fever, anaphylaxis, rash including Stevens–Johnson syndrome, erythema multiforme and toxic epidermal necrolysis, angioedema, hypotension, seizures, encephalopathy, hearing loss, diarrhea, *Clostridium difficile*-associated diarrhea and pseudomembranous colitis, oral candidiasis, glossitis, anorexia, nausea, vomiting, stomach cramps, hepatitis, renal impairment, pyuria, hematuria, genital pruritis, dyspnea, polyarthralgia, prolonged prothrombin time, pancytopenia, positive Coombs' test, increased ALT (SGPT), AST (SGOT), alkaline phosphatase, bilirubin and LDH, decreased serum sodium, and increased potassium and chloride.

 DRUG INTERACTIONS/FOOD INTERACTIONS

Meropenem may reduce serum valproic acid concentrations; levels should be monitored.

It is not recommended that probenecid be given with meropenem.

Antibiotics Manual: A Guide to Commonly Used Antimicrobials, Second Edition. David Schlossberg and Rafik Samuel.
© 2017 John Wiley & Sons Ltd. Published 2017 by John Wiley & Sons Ltd.

DOSING

The recommended dose of meropenem is 500 mg IV given every 8 hours for skin and skin structure infections and 1 g given every 8 hours for intra-abdominal infections.

 ## SPECIAL POPULATIONS

RENAL IMPAIRMENT:

Creatinine clearance	Skin	Abdominal
26–50 mL/min	500 mg q 12 hours	1 g q 12 hours
10–25 mL/min	250 mg q 12 hours	500 mg q 12 hours
<10 mL/min	250 mg q daily	500 mg daily
After hemodialysis or peritoneal dialysis		500 mg
CRRT		1 g q 12 hours

HEPATIC DYSFUNCTION: No dose adjustment is necessary.

PEDIATRICS:

Infection	Dose
Complicated skin and skin structure	10 mg/kg (up to 500 mg) every 8 hours
Intra-abdominal	20 mg/kg (up to 1 g) every 8 hours
Meningitis	40 mg/kg (up to 2 g) every 8 hours

 ## THE ART OF ANTIMICROBIAL THERAPY

Clinical Pearls

1. Meropenem must be dose-adjusted for renal dysfunction.
2. Cross allergy with penicillins is <10 %.
3. Risk for seizures is greatest in patients with CNS disorders or renal dysfunction.
4. Meropenem is active against organisms producing extended spectrum beta-lactamases.

■ MINTEZOLE (Thiabendazole)

 BASIC CHARACTERISTICS

Class: Broad-spectrum antihelminthic.

Mechanism of Action: Inhibits the helminth-specific enzyme fumarate reductase. Thiabendazole also suppresses egg and/or larval production.

Metabolic Route: Metabolized in the liver and excreted in the urine.

 FDA-APPROVED INDICATIONS

Treatment of strongyloidiasis (threadworm), cutaneous larva migrans (creeping eruption) and visceral larva migrans.

Also Used for (when preferred regimens cannot be used): hookworm (*Necator americanus* and *Ancylostoma duodenale*), whipworm (Trichuriasis) roundworm (Ascariasis), and trichinosis.

 SIDE EFFECTS/TOXICITY

Erythema multiforme and Stevens–Johnson syndrome, dizziness, weariness, drowsiness, giddiness, headache, numbness, hyperirritability, convulsions, collapse, confusion, depression, floating sensation, weakness, lack of coordination, jaundice, cholestasis, parenchymal liver damage, anorexia, nausea, vomiting, diarrhea, epigastric distress, abdominal pain, tinnitus, abnormal sensation in eyes, xanthopsia, blurred vision, drying of mucous membranes, Sicca syndrome, hypotension, hyperglycemia, leukopenia, hematuria, enuresis, malodorous urine, and crystalluria.

 DRUG INTERACTIONS/FOOD INTERACTIONS

Thiabendazole should be given after meals if possible.

When concomitant use of thiabendazole and xanthine derivatives (theophylline) is anticipated, it may be necessary to monitor blood levels and/or reduce the dosage of such compounds.

 DOSING

Administered as 500 mg chewable tablets or as a suspension, containing 500 mg thiabendazole per 5 mL.

The recommended maximum daily dose is 3 grams.

Tablets should be chewed before swallowing.

To determine the dose, see the following table:

Weight, lb	Tablet	mL
30	250 mg (0.5 tablet)	2.5
50	500 mg (1 tablet)	5
75	750 mg (1.5 tablets)	7.5
100	1000 mg (2 tablets)	10
125	1250 (2.5 tablets)	12.5
150 and over	1500 (3 tablets)	15

Antibiotics Manual: A Guide to Commonly Used Antimicrobials, Second Edition. David Schlossberg and Rafik Samuel.
© 2017 John Wiley & Sons Ltd. Published 2017 by John Wiley & Sons Ltd.

For frequency and duration, see the following table:

Indication	Regimen
Strongyloidiasis	2 doses per day for 2 days
Cutaneous larva migrans	2 doses per day for 2 days
Visceral larva migrans	2 doses per day for 7 days
Trichinosis	2 doses per day for 2–4 days
Intestinal roundworms	2 doses per day for 2 days

 ## SPECIAL POPULATIONS

RENAL IMPAIRMENT: There is no dose adjustment for renal insufficiency.

HEPATIC DYSFUNCTION: During therapy, monitoring of LFTs is suggested if prolonged therapy is given.

PEDIATRICS: The safety and effectiveness of thiabendazole in pediatric patients weighing less than 30 lb has been limited.

 ## THE ART OF ANTIMICROBIAL THERAPY

Clinical Pearls

1. Thiabendazole should be used only in patients in whom susceptible worm infestation has been diagnosed and should not be used prophylactically.
2. Because CNS side effects may occur quite frequently, activities requiring mental alertness should be avoided.

■ MONUROL (Fosfomycin)

 BASIC CHARACTERISTICS

Class: Phosphonic antibiotic.

Mechanism of Action: Inactivation of the enzyme enolpyruvyl transferase, thereby irreversibly blocking the condensation of uridine diphosphate-*N*-acetylglucosamine with *p*-enolpyruvate, one of the first steps in bacterial cell wall synthesis. It also reduces adherence of bacteria to uroepithelial cells.

Mechanisms of Resistance: Limited information.

Metabolic Route: Excreted in urine and feces.

 FDA-APPROVED INDICATIONS

Only for treatment of uncomplicated urinary tract infections (acute cystitis) in women due to susceptible strains of *Escherichia coli* and *Enterococcus faecalis*; not indicated for the treatment of pyelonephritis or perinephric abscess.

 SIDE EFFECTS/TOXICITY

Contraindicated in patients who have shown serious hypersensitivity to fosfomycin. Toxicity includes **diarrhea**, **headache**, **vaginitis**, **nausea**, **rhinitis**, **back pain**, **dysmenorrhea**, **pharyngitis**, **dizziness**, **abdominal pain**, **dyspepsia**, **asthenia**, **rash**, abnormal stools, CDAD, anorexia, constipation, dry mouth, dysuria, ear disorder, fever, flatulence, flu syndrome, hematuria, infection, insomnia, lymphadenopathy, menstrual disorder, migraine, myalgia, nervousness, paresthesia, pruritus, increased SGPT, skin disorder, somnolence, vomiting, optic neuritis, angioedema, aplastic anemia, asthma (exacerbation), cholestatic jaundice, hepatic necrosis, and toxic megacolon.

INTERACTIONS/FOOD INTERACTIONS

Metoclopramide lowers serum concentration and urinary excretion of fosfomycin. Other drugs that increase gastrointestinal motility may produce similar effects.

Can be taken with or without food.

 DOSING

The recommended dosage for women 18 years of age and older for uncomplicated urinary tract infection (acute cystitis) is one sachet of fosfomycin.

 SPECIAL POPULATIONS

RENAL IMPAIRMENT: Significantly decreases the excretion of fosfomycin.

HEPATIC DYSFUNCTION: Limited information.

PEDIATRICS: Safety and effectiveness in children under 12 not established.

Antibiotics Manual: A Guide to Commonly Used Antimicrobials, Second Edition. David Schlossberg and Rafik Samuel.
© 2017 John Wiley & Sons Ltd. Published 2017 by John Wiley & Sons Ltd.

THE ART OF ANTIMICROBIAL THERAPY

Clinical Pearls

1. Do not use more than one single dose to treat a single episode of acute cystitis. Repeated daily doses do not improve the clinical success or microbiological eradication rates but may increase the incidence of adverse events.

2. There is generally no cross-resistance between fosfomycin and other classes of antibacterial agents such as beta-lactams and aminoglycosides.

3. Fosfomycin is bactericidal.

4. Fosfomycin is active against ESBL-producing Enterobacteriaceae.

5. Fosfomycin should not be used to treat pyelonephritis or complicated UTI.

■ MYAMBUTOL (Ethambutol Hydrochloride)

 BASIC CHARACTERISTICS

Mechanism of Action: Inhibition of arabinosyl transferase enzymes involved in biosynthesis of mycobacterial cell wall.

Mechanism of Resistance: Point mutations in the arabinosyl transferase enzyme.

Metabolic Route: Approximately 50 % of ethambutol is excreted in the urine, 25 % is metabolized by in the liver, and 25 % is excreted in the feces unchanged.

 FDA-APPROVED INDICATIONS

Treatment of *Mycobacterium tuberculosis* in combination with other antimycobacterial agents.

Also Used for: Treatment of nontuberculous mycobacterial infection, including *Mycobacterium avium*-intracellulare complex, *M. kansasii*, *M. bovis*, and infection due to BCG.

 SIDE EFFECTS/TOXICITY

Optic neuritis, peripheral neuropathy, rash, thrombocytopenia, anaphylaxis, dermatitis, arthralgias, fever, and elevations of serum uric acid with precipitation of acute gout.

 DRUG INTERACTIONS/FOOD INTERACTIONS

Antacids may reduce absorption and should be separated from ethambutol administration by 2 hours.

 DOSING (DOSE SHOULD NEVER BE DIVIDED, BUT SHOULD BE GIVEN AS A SINGLE DOSE)

15–25 mg/kg/day in one daily dose. If the larger dose is initiated, reduce to 15 mg/kg after 60 days.
Twice weekly: 40–55 kg: 2000 mg; 56–75 kg: 2800 mg; 76–90 kg: 4000 mg (maximum).
Thrice weekly: 40–55 kg: 1200 mg; 56–75 kg: 2000 mg; 76–90 kg: 2400 mg (maximum).

 SPECIAL POPULATIONS

RENAL IMPAIRMENT: Renal failure (creatinine clearance <30) or hemodialysis: 15–25 mg/kg three times weekly; monitor assays in patients with renal failure (usual levels 2–5 mcg/mL).

HEPATIC DYSFUNCTION: No dose adjustment necessary.

PEDIATRICS: 15–20 mg/kg/day in one daily dose; maximum 1 g. Twice weekly: 50 mg/kg; maximum 4 g.

Antibiotics Manual: A Guide to Commonly Used Antimicrobials, Second Edition. David Schlossberg and Rafik Samuel.
© 2017 John Wiley & Sons Ltd. Published 2017 by John Wiley & Sons Ltd.

THE ART OF ANTIMICROBIAL THERAPY

Clinical Pearls

1. Ethambutol should always be used in combination with other antimycobacterial agents.
2. All patients receiving ethambutol should have evaluation of visual acuity and color vision at initiation of therapy and at least monthly during therapy.
3. Since the visual toxicity is dose-related, serum levels should be assayed in patients with renal impairment.
4. Visual toxicity is less common with intermittent therapy, e.g. twice or thrice-weekly administration.
5. Visual toxicity is uncommon at the lower dose of 15 mg/kg/day

■ MYCAMINE (Micafungin)

 ## BASIC CHARACTERISTICS

Class: Echinocandin.

Mechanism of Action: Inhibition of synthesis of 1,3-beta-D-glucan, an essential component of fungal cell walls.

Mechanism of Resistance: Data incomplete.

Metabolic Route: Slow chemical degradation to multiple products with the majority of them excreted in the feces. It is not metabolized by the cytochrome P450 enzymes.

 ## FDA-APPROVED INDICATIONS

Candidemia, acute disseminated candidiasis, candida peritonitis and abscess, and esophageal candidiasis in HIV infected patients. Prophylaxis of *Candida* infections in patients undergoing hematopoietic transplantation.

 ## SIDE EFFECTS/TOXICITY

Possible histamine-related syndrome, characterized by rash, urticaria, flushing, pruritus, injection site reactions when administered through peripheral lines, fever, rash, erythema multiforme, nausea, vomiting diarrhea, hepatitis with liver failure, renal failure, arrhythmia, arthralgia, seizure, encephalopathy, hyponatremia, hypokalemia, and pancytopenia.

DRUG INTERACTIONS

Patients receiving sirolimus, nifedipine, or itraconazole with micafungin should be monitored for toxicity due to sirolimus, nifedipine, or itraconazole, dosage reductions of which may be necessary.

 ## DOSING

Candidemia, acute disseminated candidiasis, peritonitis, or abscesses: 100 mg IV daily.

Esophageal candidiasis: 150 mg IV daily.

Prophylaxis for hematopoietic transplant recipients: 50 mg IV daily.

 ## SPECIAL POPULATIONS

RENAL IMPAIRMENT: There is no dose adjustment needed.

HEPATIC DYSFUNCTION: No dose adjustment needed.

PEDIATRICS: Indicated in children 4 months and older.

Indication	30 kg or less	>30 kg
Candidemia, candidiasis, peritonitis, abscesses	2 mg/kg	2 mg/kg (max. 100 mg)
Esophageal candidiasis	3 mg/kg	2.5 mg/kg (max. 150 mg)
Prophylaxis	1 mg/kg	1 mg/kg (max. 50 mg)

Antibiotics Manual: A Guide to Commonly Used Antimicrobials, Second Edition. David Schlossberg and Rafik Samuel.
© 2017 John Wiley & Sons Ltd. Published 2017 by John Wiley & Sons Ltd.

THE ART OF ANTIMICROBIAL THERAPY

Clinical Pearls

1. Echinocandins have activity only against *Candida* species, *Pneumocystis jirovecii* and *Aspergillus* species. They should not be used for other fungal infections.
2. Micafungin is active against all pathogenic *Candida* species, including those resistant to fluconazole.
3. Increasing resistance to echinocandins has been noted in *Candida glabrata* and *Candida parapsilosis*.

■ MYCOBUTIN (Rifabutin)

 ## BASIC CHARACTERISTICS

Class: Rifamycin.

Mechanisms of Action: Rifabutin inhibits DNA-dependent RNA polymerase activity in susceptible cells.

Mechanisms of Resistance: Resistance occurs as single-step mutations of the DNA-dependent RNA polymerase.

Metabolic Route: Metabolized in the liver into 5 products that are excreted in the feces and urine.

 ## FDA-APPROVED INDICATIONS

Prevention of disseminated *Mycobacterium avium* complex (MAC) disease in patients with advanced HIV infection.

Also Used for: Treatment of MAC in combination with other medications in both HIV infected and noninfected patients.

Rifabutin is commonly substituted for rifampin in the treatment of TB disease because it interacts with other medications less than rifampin (approximately 40 % of rifampin activity).

 ## SIDE EFFECTS/TOXICITY

Rifabutin is **contraindicated** in patients with a history of hypersensitivity to any of the rifamycins.

Adverse effects: anterior uveitis, liver dysfunction, both hepatocellular damage and jaundice, porphyria, reddish coloration of the urine, sweat, sputum, tears, "flu syndrome" (fever, chills, and malaise) when used intermittently, anaphylaxis, rash, flushing, epigastric distress, anorexia, nausea, vomiting, flatulence, *Clostridium difficile*-associated diarrhea, disseminated intravascular coagulation, visual disturbances, adrenal insufficiency, renal insufficiency, confusion, elevations in serum uric acid thrombocytopenia, leukopenia, and hemolytic anemia.

DRUG INTERACTIONS/FOOD INTERACTIONS

Absorption of rifabutin is reduced when the drug is ingested with food, but absorption is usually adequate and ingestion with food reduces GI intolerance.

Rifabutin is known to induce certain cytochrome P-450 enzymes. Administration of rifabutin with drugs that undergo biotransformation through these metabolic pathways may accelerate elimination and decrease the therapeutic effect of these coadministered drugs, many of which require monitoring and possible adjustment during and following coadministration with rifabutin. The list of drugs so affected includes the following drugs/classes: anticonvulsants, antiarrhythmics, oral anticoagulants, antifungals, barbiturates, beta-blockers, calcium channel blockers, chloramphenicol, clarithromycin, corticosteroids, cyclosporine, cardiac glycoside preparations, clofibrate, hormonal contraceptives (patients should be advised to use nonhormonal methods of birth control during rifabutin therapy), dapsone, diazepam, doxycycline, enalapril, fluoroquinolones, haloperidol, oral hypoglycemic agents, levothyroxine, methadone, narcotic analgesics, nortriptyline, progestins, quinine, tacrolimus, sulfapyridine, theophylline, tricyclic antidepressants, protease inhibitors, nonnucleoside reverse transcriptase inhibitors, CCR5 inhibitors, and zidovudine.

Rifabutin levels may increase when coadministered with atovaquone, probenecid, and cotrimoxazole, and may decrease when given with ketoconazole and antacids (give rifabutin at least 1 hour before the ingestion of antacids).

When rifabutin is given concomitantly with either halothane or isoniazid, the potential for hepatotoxicity is increased and concomitant use of rifabutin and halothane should be avoided.

Antibiotics Manual: A Guide to Commonly Used Antimicrobials, Second Edition. David Schlossberg and Rafik Samuel.
© 2017 John Wiley & Sons Ltd. Published 2017 by John Wiley & Sons Ltd.

Drug/laboratory interactions

Cross-reactivity and false-positive urine screening tests for opiates have been reported in patients receiving rifampin.

Therapeutic levels of rifabutin have been shown to inhibit standard microbiological assays for serum folate and vitamin B12.

Dosage adjustment is frequently necessary with antiretroviral drugs and updated recommendations may be found at www. cdc.gov/TB/TB_HIV_Drugs/default.htm. Current recommendations:

Rifabutin

450–600/d or 600 3 × /week	Efavirenz (usual dose)
300/d or 300 3 × /week	Nevirapine (standard dose)
150/d or 300 3 × /week	Fosamprenavir (usual dose)
	Atazanavir (usual dose)
	RTV-boosted PI
	Evotaz
150 qod	Cobicistat
Avoid	Stribild, Genvoya, Descovy, elvitegravir
Usual dose	Maraviroc (usual dose)
Usual dose	Raltegravir, dolutegravir (usual dose)
Usual dose	Etravirine (usual dose)
Usual dose	Triumeq

 ## DOSING

Rifabutin is supplied as 150 mg tablets. Standard dose is 300 mg daily. For intermittent dosing, the same dose can be given twice or thrice weekly.

 ## SPECIAL POPULATIONS

RENAL IMPAIRMENT: If creatinine clearance < 30 mL/minute, decrease dose by 50 %.

HEPATIC DYSFUNCTION: Patients with impaired liver function should be given rifabutin only in cases of necessity and then with caution and monitoring of liver function.

PEDIATRICS: Not studied; however, 5–10 mg/kg/day is used.

 ## THE ART OF ANTIMICROBIAL THERAPY

Clinical Pearls

1. Rifabutin should never be used for prophylaxis of MAC in the setting of active tuberculosis, since resistance may develop.
2. Liver function tests and symptoms of gastrointestinal intolerance should be monitored in all patients receiving rifabutin.

3. Rifabutin is a potent inducer of the p450 cytochrome system, and coadministered medications may require discontinuation or monitoring for possible dosage adjustment. However, the interactions are less than those seen with rifampin.

4. Rifabutin can enhance the metabolism of endogenous substrates including adrenal hormones, thyroid hormones, and vitamin D.

5. Soft contact lenses can be permanently stained.

BASIC CHARACTERISTICS

Class: Semisynthetic penicillin.

Mechanism of Action: Binds penicillin-binding protein, disrupting cell wall synthesis.

Mechanisms of Resistance:

1. The PBP can be altered, with reduced affinity.
2. Production of a beta-lactamase, resulting in hydrolysis of the beta-lactam ring.
3. Decreased ability of the antibiotic to reach the PBP when bacteria decrease porin production, resulting in a decrease of the drug concentration within the cell.

Metabolic Route: The majority of nafcillin is inactivated by the liver and excreted in the bile. The remaining 30 % is excreted unchanged in the urine.

 FDA-APPROVED INDICATIONS

Nafcillin is indicated in the treatment of infections caused by susceptible penicillinase-producing staphylococci.

 SIDE EFFECTS/TOXICITY

A history of allergic reaction to any of the penicillins is a **contraindication.**

Side effects include *Clostridium difficile*-associated diarrhea (CDAD), interstitial nephritis including rash, fever, eosinophilia, hematuria, proteinuria, and renal insufficiency, thrombophlebitis, hypersensitivity reactions including rash, erythema multiforme, and Stevens–Johnson syndrome, hepatitis, nausea, vomiting, diarrhea, stomatitis, black or hairy tongue, hyperactivity and seizures, anemia, thrombocytopenia, neutropenia, and eosinophilia.

 DRUG INTERACTIONS/FOOD INTERACTIONS

Chloramphenicol, macrolides, sulfonamides, and tetracyclines may interfere with the bactericidal effects of penicillins.

When nafcillin and warfarin are used concomitantly, the prothrombin time should be closely monitored.

When cyclosporine and nafcillin are used concomitantly in organ transplant patients, the cyclosporine levels should be monitored. High urine concentrations of nafcillin may result in false-positive reactions when testing for the presence of glucose in urine using *Clinitest®*. It is recommended that glucose tests based on enzymatic glucose oxidase reactions (such as *Clinistix®*) be used. Nafcillin may cause false-positive urine reaction for protein.

 DOSING

The usual IV or IM dosage for adults is 500 mg every 4 hours.

For severe infections, 1 g IM or IV every 4 hours is recommended.

Antibiotics Manual: A Guide to Commonly Used Antimicrobials, Second Edition. David Schlossberg and Rafik Samuel.
© 2017 John Wiley & Sons Ltd. Published 2017 by John Wiley & Sons Ltd.

SPECIAL POPULATIONS

RENAL IMPAIRMENT: No dose adjustment is necessary.

HEPATIC DYSFUNCTION: No dose adjustment is necessary.

Combined renal and hepatic insufficiency: Measurement of nafcillin serum levels should be performed and dosage adjusted accordingly.

PEDIATRICS: Infants and children <40 kg: 25 mg/kg IM twice daily.

Neonates: 10 mg/kg IM twice daily.

 THE ART OF ANTIMICROBIAL THERAPY

Clinical Pearls

1. Nafcillin does not need dosage adjustment for renal dysfunction.
2. Occasional skin sloughing at the injection site has been reported.
3. Nafcillin should be used with caution in patients with both renal and hepatic insufficiency.

BASIC CHARACTERISTICS

Class: Aromatic diamidine.

Mechanism of Action: It inhibits putrescine and spermidine uptake competitively.

Metabolic Route: Pentamidine is hydroxylated by the liver and subsequently excreted.

 FDA-APPROVED INDICATIONS

IV pentamidine is indicated for the treatment for pneumonia due to *Pneumocystis jirovecii*.

Inhaled pentamidine is indicated for prophylaxis of *P. jirovecii* pneumonia in patients with AIDS who have a history of *P. jirovecii* pneumonia and CD4 count <200.

Also Used for: Granulomatous amebic encephalitis due to Acanthamoeba and *Balamuthia mandrillaris* spp. (IV).

Cutaneous leishmaniasis (IV).

Inhaled pentamidine is also used for treatment of mild infection due to *P. jirovecii*.

Early-stage *Trypanosoma gambiense* (IV).

 SIDE EFFECTS/TOXICITY

Intravenous pentamadine can cause hypotension, especially if given in less than one hour, renal failure, hypocalcemia, hypomagnesemia, hyperkalemia and hyponatremia, hypoglycemia, fatal pancreatitis, diabetes, neutropenia, anemia and thrombocytopenia, nausea, vomiting, abnormal liver function tests, ventricular arrhythmias, as well as QT interval prolongation and changes in ST segment and T waves.

Intramuscular pentamidine may also result in sterile abscesses.

Aerosolized pentamidine can cause coughing and bronchospasm.

 DRUG INTERACTIONS/FOOD INTERACTIONS

Data incomplete.

 DOSING

Should be given IV if possible, due to pain and abscess formation from IM administration.

Disease	Dose and duration
P. jirovecii pneumonia in AIDS patients	4 mg/kg daily for 21 days
P. jirovecii pneumonia for non-HIV infected patients	4 mg/kg daily for 14 days
P. jirovecii pneumonia prophylaxis	300 mg aerosol inhaled monthly
T. brucei gambiense trypanosomiasis	4 mg/kg/d IM or IV × 7 days
Cutaneous leishmaniasis	2–3 mg/kg IV or IM daily or every second day × 4–7 doses
Amebic encephalitis	4 mg/kg IV once/day

Antibiotics Manual: A Guide to Commonly Used Antimicrobials, Second Edition. David Schlossberg and Rafik Samuel.
© 2017 John Wiley & Sons Ltd. Published 2017 by John Wiley & Sons Ltd.

SPECIAL POPULATIONS

RENAL IMPAIRMENT: No dose adjustment for renal insufficiency, however, if creatinine increases by 1 mg/dL or more, the daily dosage should be decreased to 2–3 mg/kg.

HEPATIC DYSFUNCTION: No dose adjustment is necessary.

PEDIATRICS: The same dose as in adults.

 THE ART OF ANTIMICROBIAL THERAPY

Clinical Pearls

1. Although inhaled pentamidine is used for mild PCP, other agents are preferable (TMP/SMX, clindamycin + primaquine).
2. Although inhaled pentamidine is recommended for prophylaxis for PCP, other agents are more effective (TMP/SMX, dapsone, atovaquone).
3. Severe complications may occur in patients receiving pentamidine, including hypotension, hypoglycemia, pancreatitis, and renal failure. Close monitoring is necessary.

BASIC CHARACTERISTICS

Class: Poorly absorbed oral aminoglycoside.

Mechanism of Action: Inhibits the synthesis of protein in susceptible bacterial cells.

Metabolic Route: Neomycin is poorly absorbed and is excreted in the feces.

 FDA-APPROVED INDICATIONS

Hepatic coma.

Also Used for: Suppression of intestinal bacteria in a preoperative bowel preparation.

 SIDE EFFECTS/TOXICITY

WARNING: Systemic absorption of neomycin occurs following oral administration and toxic reactions may occur.

Neurotoxicity (including ototoxicity) and nephrotoxicity following the oral use of neomycin sulfate have been reported. Serial, vestibular, and audiometric tests, as well as tests of renal function, should be performed (especially in high-risk patients).

The risk of nephrotoxicity and ototoxicity is greater in patients with impaired renal function. Ototoxicity is often delayed in onset and patients developing cochlear damage will not have symptoms during therapy to warn them of developing eighth nerve destruction and total or partial deafness may occur long after neomycin has been discontinued.

Neuromuscular blockage and respiratory paralysis have been reported following the oral use of neomycin. The possibility of the occurrence of neuromuscular blockage and respiratory paralysis should be considered if neomycin is administered, especially to patients receiving anesthetics, neuromuscular blocking agents such as tubocurarine, succinylcholine, or decamethonium, or in patients receiving massive transfusions of citrate anticoagulated blood. If blockage occurs, calcium salts may reverse these phenomena but mechanical respiratory assistance may be necessary.

Concurrent and/or sequential systemic, oral, or topical use of other aminoglycosides including paromomycin and other potentially nephrotoxic and/or neurotoxic drugs such as bacitracin, cisplatin, vancomycin, amphotericin B, polymyxin B, colistin, and viomycin should be avoided because the toxicity may be additive.

Other factors that increase the risk of **toxicity** are advanced age and dehydration.

The concurrent use of neomycin with potent diuretics such as ethacrynic acid or furosemide should be avoided since certain diuretics by themselves may cause ototoxicity. In addition, when administered intravenously, diuretics may enhance neomycin toxicity by altering the antibiotic concentration in serum and tissue.

Contraindicated

1. In the presence of intestinal obstruction.
2. In individuals with a history of hypersensitivity to the drug.
3. Patients with a history of hypersensitivity to other aminoglycosides.
4. In patients with inflammatory or ulcerative gastrointestinal disease.

Antibiotics Manual: A Guide to Commonly Used Antimicrobials, Second Edition. David Schlossberg and Rafik Samuel.
© 2017 John Wiley & Sons Ltd. Published 2017 by John Wiley & Sons Ltd.

Side effects include: numbness, skin tingling, muscle twitching, convulsions, nausea, vomiting, diarrhea, nephrotoxicity, ototoxicity, neuromuscular blockade, and malabsorption.

 DRUG INTERACTIONS/FOOD INTERACTIONS

Caution should be taken in concurrent or serial use of other neurotoxic and/or nephrotoxic drugs including aminoglycosides and polymyxins.

Oral neomycin inhibits the gastrointestinal absorption of penicillin V, oral vitamin B-12, methotrexate, 5-fluorouracil, and digoxin.

Oral neomycin sulfate may enhance the effect of coumarin anticoagulants by decreasing vitamin K availability.

 DOSING

Neomycin sulfate is supplied as 500 mg tablets or as an oral solution (Neo-Fradin) containing 125 mg/mL.

Hepatic coma

The recommended dose is 4–12 grams per day given in divided doses.

Preoperative prophylaxis for elective colorectal surgery

Neomycin sulfate 1 g and erythromycin base 1 g orally three times the day prior to surgery.

 SPECIAL POPULATIONS

RENAL IMPAIRMENT: No dose adjustment is necessary.

HEPATIC DYSFUNCTION: No dose adjustment is necessary.

PEDIATRICS: The safety and efficacy of oral neomycin sulfate in patients less than 18 years of age have not been established. If treatment of a patient less than 18 years of age is necessary, neomycin should be used with caution and the period of treatment should not exceed two weeks because of absorption from the gastrointestinal tract.

 THE ART OF ANTIMICROBIAL THERAPY

Clinical Pearls

1. Small amounts of orally administered neomycin are absorbed through intact intestinal mucosa.
2. Neomycin irrigation of absorptive surfaces, e.g., pleura, has resulted in systemic absorption and neurotoxicity.

BASIC CHARACTERISTICS

Class: Protease inhibitor.

Mechanism of Action: Ritonavir reversibly binds the active site of the enzyme protease. Inhibition of protease prevents cleavage of the *gag* and *gag-pol* polyprotein, resulting in the production of immature, noninfectious virus.

Mechanism of Resistance: Development of mutations on the enzyme protease causes a conformational change that prevents ritonavir from binding the active site, allowing protease activity to continue. The most frequent resistance mutations include 46I, 71V, 82A, and 84V.

Metabolic Route: Ritonavir is metabolized by the liver.

FDA-APPROVED INDICATIONS

Treatment of HIV-1 in combinations with other antiretroviral agents.

SIDE EFFECTS/TOXICITY

> **WARNING:** Coadministration of ritonavir with several classes of drugs including sedative hypnotics, antiarrhythmics, or ergot alkaloid preparations may result in potentially serious and/or life-threatening adverse events due to possible effects of ritonavir on the hepatic metabolism of certain drugs. Review medications taken by patients prior to prescribing ritonavir or when prescribing other medications to patients already taking ritonavir.

Other adverse effects: Diarrhea, new-onset diabetes mellitus, exacerbation of preexisting diabetes mellitus and hyperglycemia, increased bleeding, including spontaneous skin hematomas and hemarthrosis, in patients with hemophilia types A and B, redistribution/accumulation of body fat including central obesity, dorsocervical fat enlargement (buffalo hump), peripheral wasting, facial wasting, breast enlargement, "cushingoid appearance", immune reconstitution syndrome, QTc prolongation, torsades de pointes, abdominal pain, headache, anorexia, dyspepsia, epigastric pain, hepatitis, mouth ulceration, pancreatitis vomiting, anemia, leucopenia, thrombocytopenia, increases in alkaline phosphatase, amylase, creatine phosphokinase, lactic dehydrogenase, SGOT, SGPT, gamma glutamyl transpeptidase, hyperlipemia, hyperuricemia, hyperglycemia, hypoglycemia, and dehydration.

DRUG INTERACTIONS/FOOD INTERACTIONS

Ritonavir tablets should be taken with a meal; ritonavir capsules may be taken with or without meals.

Drugs that **should not be coadministered** with ritonavir include amiodarone, quinidine, flecainide, propafenone, alfuzosin, voriconazole, astemizole, terfenidine, ergot derivatives, St John's wort, simvastatin, lovastatin, lurasidone, pimozide, cisapride, meperidine, benzodiazepines, rivaroxaban, fluticasone, butesonide, salmeterol, and rifampin.

Ritonavir is an inhibitor of the CYP3A enzyme; coadministration of ritonavir and drugs primarily metabolized by CYP3A may result in increased plasma concentrations of the other drug that could increase or prolong its therapeutic and adverse effects.

Ritonavir is metabolized by CYP3A and CYP2C19; coadministration of ritonavir and drugs that induce CYP3A or CYP2C19 may decrease ritonavir plasma concentrations and reduce its therapeutic effect. Coadministration of ritonavir and drugs that inhibit

Antibiotics Manual: A Guide to Commonly Used Antimicrobials, Second Edition. David Schlossberg and Rafik Samuel.
© 2017 John Wiley & Sons Ltd. Published 2017 by John Wiley & Sons Ltd.

CYP3A or CYP2C19 may increase ritonavir plasma concentrations. Because of these metabolic affects, potential drug interactions that may require dosage change or clinical/laboratory monitoring are listed below:

Medication	Adjustment or action
Itraconzole	Monitor for toxicity
Ketoconazole	Use with caution
Voriconazole	Monitor for toxicity
Rifabutin	Decrease rifabutin to 150/qod or 3 ×/week
Contraceptives	Use alternative or additional method
Atorvastatin, rosuvastatin	Use lowest possible dose with close monitoring
Phenobarbital, phenytoin, or carbamazepine	Monitor anticonvulsant level, consider alternative
Methadone	Monitor, may require higher methadone dose
Sildenafil	25 mg every 48 hours
Tadalafil	5 mg, no more than 10 mg in 72 hours
Vardenafil	2.5 mg in 24 hours
Colchicine	Do not coadminister in renal or hepatic impairment
Quetiapine	Administer one-sixth of the quetiapine dose
Bosentan	Dose is 62.5 mg daily

 ## DOSING

Ritonavir is supplied as a 100 mg tablet and a liquid containing 600 mg/7.5 mL. Although the recommended dosage of ritonavir is 600 mg twice daily by mouth it is rarely used in this fashion. It is primarily dosed as a booster of the other protease inhibitors as follows:

	Dosing options
Atazanavir	Atazanavir 300 mg daily + ritonavir 100 mg daily
Darunavir	Darunavir 600 mg bid + ritonavir 100 mg bid or darunavir 800 mg daily + ritonavir 100 mg daily (naïve)
Fosamprenavir	Fosamprenavir 700 mg bid + ritonavir 100 bid
	Fosamprenavir 1400 q d + ritonavir 200 or 100 q d (naive)
Indinavir	Indinavir 800 bid + ritonavir 100 bid
Nelfinavir	Not recommended
Saquinavir	Saquinavir 1000 bid + ritonavir 100 bid
Tipranavir	Tipranavir 500 bid + ritonavir 200 bid

 ## SPECIAL POPULATIONS

RENAL IMPAIRMENT: There is no adjustment needed.

HEPATIC DYSFUNCTION: Do not administer in patients with severe hepatic dysfunction.

PEDIATRICS: In children older than 1 month, the recommended dose is 400 mg/m^2 but should be initiated at 250 mg/m^2 and titrated by 50 mg/m^2 every 3 days until the recommended dose is reached.

 ## THE ART OF ANTIMICROBIAL THERAPY

Clinical Pearls

1. Ritonavir should always be used in combination with other antiretrovirals.
2. Ritonavir should be taken with food to decrease side effects.
3. Ritonavir is mainly used as a booster of other protease inhibitors except nelfinavir.
4. The protease inhibitors saquinavir, darunavir, and tipranavir **must** be administered with ritonavir.
5. Whenever initiating ritonavir, make sure to review all medications the patient is receiving to minimize drug interactions.

■ NOXAFIL (Posaconazole)

 BASIC CHARACTERISTICS

Class: Triazole.

Mechanism of Action: Inhibition of lanosterol 14-α-demethylase, which is involved in the synthesis of ergosterol, an essential component of fungal cell membranes.

Mechanisms of Resistance:

1. Point mutations in the gene (*ERG11*) encoding for the target enzyme lead to an altered target with decreased affinity for azoles.
2. Overexpression of *ERG11* results in the production of high concentrations of the target enzyme, creating the need for higher intracellular drug concentrations to inhibit all of the enzyme molecules in the cell.
3. Active efflux of itraconazole out of the cell through the activation of two types of multidrug efflux transporters.

Metabolic Route: Posaconazole is predominantly eliminated unchanged in the feces.

 FDA-APPROVED INDICATIONS

Prophylaxis of invasive *Aspergillus* and *Candida* infections in patients who are at high risk of developing these infections due to being severely immunocompromised, such as hematopoietic stem cell transplant (HSCT) recipients with graft-versus-host disease (GVHD) or those with hematologic malignancies with prolonged neutropenia from chemotherapy.

Treatment of oropharyngeal candidiasis, including oropharyngeal candidiasis refractory to itraconazole and/or fluconazole.

Also Used for: Posaconazole has activity against *Zygomycete* sp.

 SIDE EFFECTS/TOXICITY

Caution should be used when prescribing posaconazole to patients with hypersensitivity to other azoles.

Posaconazole should be administered with caution to patients with potentially proarrhythmic conditions and should not be administered with drugs that are known to prolong the QTc interval and are metabolized through CYP3A4.

Other adverse events include fever, neutropenia, thrombocytopenia, abdominal pain, hepatotoxicity, nausea, vomiting, diarrhea, rash, adrenal insufficiency, thrombocytopenia, and hypokalemia.

 DRUG INTERACTIONS/ADMINISTRATION

Administer posaconazole tablets or solution with food. In those who cannot eat a meal, the oral solution can be given with an acidic beverage. Since posaconazole is a strong inhibitor of CYP3A4, plasma concentrations of drugs predominantly metabolized by CYP3A4 may be increased by posaconazole.

The following medications are **contraindicated** with posaconazole: astemizole, cisapride, sirolimus, terfenadine, halofantrane, pimozide, quinidine, simvastatin, lovastatin, ergot alkaloids, and efavirenz.

The following drug interactions may be seen and may require dosage adjustment when appropriate:

Benzodiazepines: may see increased levels of benzodiazepines.
Calcium channel blockers: may increase levels of calcium channel blockers.
Cyclosporine: reduce cyclosporine dose to approximately three-fourths of the original dose and monitor cyclosporine levels.
Digoxin: may increase levels of digoxin.

Antibiotics Manual: A Guide to Commonly Used Antimicrobials, Second Edition. David Schlossberg and Rafik Samuel.
© 2017 John Wiley & Sons Ltd. Published 2017 by John Wiley & Sons Ltd.

H2 blockers and proton pump inhibitors: will decrease levels of the oral solution but have no effect on the delayed release tablet or IV formulations.

Metaclopromide: may decrease levels of the oral solution; no effect on the delayed release tablets or IV formulations.

Phenytoin: may lower levels of posaconazole; levels of phenytoin may increase. Avoid unless benefit outweighs risk.

Protease inhibitors: may increase levels of PIs.

Rifabutin: may lower levels of posaconazole; also, levels of rifabutin may increase. Avoid unless benefit outweighs risk.

Rifampin: may lower levels of posaconazole.

Tacrolimus: reduce tacrolimus dose to approximately one-third of the original dose and monitor tacrolimus levels.

Vinca alkaloids: may increase levels of vinca alkaloids.

DOSING

Posaconazole is available in a solution containing 40 mg/mL, 100 mg delayed release tablets, and a solution for injection.

Dosing of the IV and delayed release tablet formulations

Prophylaxis of candida or aspergillus: loading dose of 300 mg twice daily for one day followed by 300 mg daily.

Dosing of the oral solution

Prophylaxis of candida or aspergillus: 200 mg three times daily.

Oropharyngeal candidiasis: 100 mg loading dose twice daily for one day followed by 100 mg daily.

Oropharyngeal candidiasis refractory to fluconazole: 400 mg twice daily.

SPECIAL POPULATIONS

RENAL IMPAIRMENT: In patients with a creatinine clearance <50 mL/min, accumulation of the intravenous vehicle, Betadex sulfobutyl ether sodium (SBECD), is expected to occur. Serum creatinine levels should be closely monitored in these patients and, if increases occur, consideration should be given to changing to oral posaconazole therapy. No dose adjustment is needed for the oral formulations.

HEPATIC DYSFUNCTION: No dose adjustment is necessary.

PEDIATRICS: Safety and effectiveness of posaconazole in pediatric patients below the age of 13 years have not been established. For pediatric patients over 13 years of age, the adult dose of the delayed release tablet or oral solution should be used. The IV formulation should not be used in those under the age of 18 years of age.

THE ART OF ANTIMICROBIAL THERAPY

Clinical Pearls

1. Dosing of the delayed release tablet and oral solution are not interchangeable.
2. Do not chew, crush, or divide the delayed release tablets.
3. Posaconazole delayed release tablets and oral solution should be administered with food.
4. In all studies, the delayed release tablet resulted in much higher levels than the oral solution.
5. Posaconazole has activity against Zygomycetes and has been used in cases refractory to amphotericin.
6. Posaconazole is an inhibitor of cytochrome P450 and can enhance the activity of many commonly used drugs.
7. Liver function tests should be evaluated at the start of and during the course of posaconazole therapy.

BASIC CHARACTERISTICS

Class: Nucleotide reverse transcriptase inhibitor, nucleoside reverse transcriptase inhibitor, and nonnucleoside reverse transcriptase inhibitor.

Mechanism of Action: Tenofovir and emtricitabine are converted by cellular enzymes to their active drugs tenofovir biphosphate (an analog of adenosine triphosphate) and emtricitabine triphosphate (an analog of cytosine triphosphate). These drugs compete with the naturally occurring nucleotides for incorporation in newly forming HIV DNA. Since they do not have a terminal hydroxyl group, they halt transcription and replication of the virus.

Rilpivirine inhibits reverse transcriptase activity by binding the enzyme.

Mechanism of Resistance: Changes in the structure of HIV reverse transcriptase leads to preferred incorporation of adenosine triphosphate and decreased incorporation of tenofovir biphosphate, which allows transcription of DNA to continue. Resistance mutations include K65R, M184V, and "TAMS": 41 L, 67 N, 70R, 210 W, 215 F, and 219E.

Changes in the structure of reverse transcriptase prevents rilpivirine from binding the enzyme and allowing transcription to continue. The most frequent resistance mutation is E138K.

Metabolic Route: Tenofovir and emtricitabine are excreted in the urine unchanged.

Rilpivirine primarily undergoes oxidative metabolism mediated by the cytochrome P450 CYP 3A.

 FDA-APPROVED INDICATIONS

Odefsey is indicated as a complete regimen for the treatment of HIV-1 infection in patients 12 years of age and older as initial therapy in those with no antiretroviral treatment history with HIV-1 RNA less than or equal to 100 000 copies per mL, or to replace a stable antiretroviral regimen in those who are virologically suppressed (HIV-1 RNA less than 50 copies per mL) for at least six months with no history of treatment failure and no known substitutions associated with resistance to the individual components of Odefsey.

 SIDE EFFECTS/TOXICITY

> **WARNING: Lactic acidosis and severe hepatomegaly with steatosis,** including fatal cases, have been reported with the use of nucleoside analogs in combination with other antiretrovirals.
>
> Odefsey is not approved for the treatment of chronic hepatitis B virus (HBV) infection, and the safety and efficacy of Odefsey have not been established in patients coinfected with human immunodeficiency virus-1 (HIV-1) and HBV. Severe acute exacerbations of hepatitis B have been reported in patients who are coinfected with HIV-1 and HBV and have discontinued products containing emtricitabine (FTC) and/or tenofovir disoproxil fumarate (TDF), and may occur with discontinuation of Odefsey.
>
> Hepatic function should be monitored closely with both clinical and laboratory follow-up for at least several months in patients who are coinfected with HIV-1 and HBV and discontinue Odefsey. If appropriate, initiation of anti-hepatitis B therapy may be warranted.

Antibiotics Manual: A Guide to Commonly Used Antimicrobials, Second Edition. David Schlossberg and Rafik Samuel.
© 2017 John Wiley & Sons Ltd. Published 2017 by John Wiley & Sons Ltd.

Other adverse events: Immune reconstitution inflammatory syndrome, fat redistribution including central obesity and dorso-cervical fat enlargement, peripheral wasting, facial wasting, breast enlargement, rash, renal impairment, including acute renal failure and Fanconi syndrome, decreased bone mineral density, and depression.

 ## DRUG INTERACTIONS/FOOD INTERACTIONS

Odefsey should be administered with at least a 533 calorie meal.

Rilpivirine is primarily metabolized by cytochrome P450 (CYP)3A, and drugs that induce or inhibit CYP3A may affect the clearance of rilpivirine.

Do not administer Odefsey with carbamazepine, oxcarbazepine, phenobarbital, phenytoin, rifampin, rifabutin, rifapentine, dexlansoprazole, esomeprazole, lansoprazole, omeprazole, pantoprazole, rabeprazole, dexamethasone, or St John's wort.

Odefsey should not be administered with any medication containing lamivudine because lamivudine and emtricitabine are both cytosine analogs and may be antagonistic.

Odefsey should not be administered with any medications that contain tenofovir, emtricitabine or rilpivirine: Viread, Emtriva, Atripla, Descovy, Stribild, Genvoya, Edurant, or Complera.

If administered with antacids, Odefsey should be given 4 hours before or 2 hours after.

If administered with H2 blockers, they should be given 12 hours apart.

 ## DOSING

Fixed dose combination of tenofovir alafenamide 25 mg + emtricitabine 200 mg + rilpivirine 25 mg given once daily.

 ## SPECIAL POPULATIONS

RENAL IMPAIRMENT: Do not administer for estimated creatinine clearance below 30 mL per minute.

HEPATIC DYSFUNCTION: Not studied in those with Child Pugh class C hepatic impairment.

PEDIATRICS: **for treatment:** Recommended for those over 12 years of age.

 ## THE ART OF ANTIMICROBIAL THERAPY

Clinical Pearls

1. Odefsey should not be used with other agents containing tenofovir, emtricitabine or rilpivirine: Viread, Emtriva, Atripla, Descovy, Stribild, Genvoya, Edurant, or Complera.
2. Odefsey should not be used with other nonnucleoside reverse transcriptase inhibitors such as efavirenz, nevirapine, etravirine, or delavirdine.
3. Complera must be given with a meal of at least 533 calories.
4. Protein supplement drinks are not sufficient to ensure adequate levels of rilpivirine.
5. Do not initiate Odefsey in patients who have a viral load of > 100 000 copies.
6. Do not administer Odefsey with a proton pump inhibitor.

OLYSIO (Simeprevir)

BASIC CHARACTERISTICS

Class: Simeprevir is an inhibitor of the HCV NS3/4A protease.

Mechanism of Action: Simeprevir binds to the protease enzyme terminating replication of the virus.

Mechanism of Resistance: Resistance to simeprevir was characterized by one or multiple amino acid substitutions at NS3 protease positions F43, Q80, R155, A156, and/or D168. These mutations allow protease to continue working in the presence of simeprevir.

Metabolic Route: Simeprevir is metabolized in the liver by undergoing oxidative metabolism by the hepatic CYP3A system.

FDA-APPROVED INDICATIONS

Simperevir is indicated for:

1. The treatment of adults with chronic hepatitis C virus (HCV) infection in combination with sofosbuvir in patients with HCV genotype 1 without cirrhosis or with compensated cirrhosis.

2. The treatment of adults with chronic hepatitis C virus (HCV) infection in combination with peginterferon alfa (Peg-IFN-alfa) and ribavirin (RBV) in patients with HCV genotype 1 or 4 without cirrhosis or with compensated cirrhosis.

SIDE EFFECTS/TOXICITY

Serious symptomatic bradycardia when coadministered with sofosbuvir and amiodarone.

Hepatic decompensation and hepatic failure, including fatal cases, have been reported in patients treated with simeprevir in combination with Peg-IFN-alfa and RBV or in combination with sofosbuvir.

Other side effects include photosensitivity reactions, rash, headache, fatigue, nausea, diarrhea, dizziness, dyspnea, and elevated amylase and lipase.

DRUG INTERACTIONS/FOOD INTERACTIONS

Contraindications to other drugs also apply to the combination regimen. Refer to the respective prescribing information for a list of **contraindications**.

Simeprevir should not be administered with amiodarone, carbamazepine, oxcarbazepine, phenobarbital, phenytoin, erythromycin, clarithromycin, itraconazole, ketoconazole, posaconazole, fluconazole, voriconazole, rifampin, rifabutin, rifapentine, dexamethasone, cisapride, milk thistle, St John's wort, cobicistat, efavirenz, nevirapine, etravirine, delavirdine, darunavir, nelfinavir, saquinavir, fosamprenavir, atazanavir, Kaletra, indinavir, tipranavir, ritonavir, or cyclosporine.

Medication	Adjustment or action
Digoxin	Monitor levels
Antiarrhythmics	Monitor levels
Calcium channel blockers	Clinically monitor
HMG CoA reductase inhibitors	Administer the lowest possible dose and monitor
Sirolimus	Monitor levels
Midazolam, triazolam	Monitor closely

Antibiotics Manual: A Guide to Commonly Used Antimicrobials, Second Edition. David Schlossberg and Rafik Samuel.
© 2017 John Wiley & Sons Ltd. Published 2017 by John Wiley & Sons Ltd.

DOSING

The recommended dosage of simeprevir is one 150 mg capsule taken orally once daily with food.

Patient population	Medication	Duration
Genotype 1 without cirrhosis	Simeprevir + sofosbuvir	12 weeks
Genotype 1 with compensated cirrhosis	Simeprevir + sofosbuvir	24 weeks
Genotype 1 or 4 without cirrhosis or with compensated cirrhosis	Simeprevir + Peg-IFN-alfa and RBV	12 weeks
	then	
	Peg-IFN-alfa and RBV	12 weeks
Genotype 1 or 4 prior nonresponders	Simeprevir + Peg-IFN-alfa and RBV	12 weeks
without cirrhosis or	**then**	
with compensated cirrhosis	Peg-IFN-alfa and RBV	36 weeks

 ## SPECIAL POPULATIONS

RENAL IMPAIRMENT: No dosage adjustment.

HEPATIC DYSFUNCTION: Not recommended for patients with moderate or severe hepatic impairment.

PEDIATRICS: Do not use in patients under 18 years of age.

 ## THE ART OF ANTIMICROBIAL THERAPY

Clinical Pearls

1. Simeprevir is active against HCV genotypes 1 and 4 only.
2. All patients should have HCV resistance testing prior to initiation of simeprevir. An alternative therapy should be considered for patients who have the Q80K mutation.
3. Monitor liver chemistry tests before and during simeprevir therapy.
4. Simeprevir can be combined with sofosbuvir for the treatment of HCV genotype 1.
5. Simeprevir can be combined with Peg-IFN-alfa and RBV for the treatment of HCV genotype 1 or 4.
6. Significant bradycardia has been reported if simeprevir is coadministered with sofosbuvir and amiodarone.
7. Simeprevir can be used in HIV coinfected patients.
8. Review the most current hepatitis C treatment guidelines because they are changing rapidly: http://www.cdc.gov/hepatitis/HCV/index.htm.

OMNICEF (Cefdinir)

 ## BASIC CHARACTERISTICS

Class: Third generation cephalosporin.

Mechanism of Action: Binds penicillin-binding protein, disrupting cell wall synthesis.

Mechanisms of Resistance:

1. The PBP can be altered, with reduced affinity.
2. Production of a beta-lactamase, resulting in hydrolysis of the beta-lactam ring.
3. Decreased ability of the antibiotic to reach the PBP when bacteria decrease porin production, resulting in a decrease of the drug concentration within the cell.

Metabolic Route: Cefdinir is excreted unchanged in the urine.

 ## FDA-APPROVED INDICATIONS

Treatment of the following infections when caused by susceptible organisms:

Adults

Community-acquired pneumonia

Acute exacerbations of chronic bronchitis

Acute maxillary sinusitis

Pharyngitis/tonsillitis

Uncomplicated skin and skin structure infections

Pediatrics

Acute bacterial otitis media

Pharyngitis/tonsillitis

Uncomplicated skin and skin structure infections

 ## SIDE EFFECTS/TOXICITY

Cefdinir is **contraindicated** in patients with allergy to cephalosporins. Cefdinir should be used with caution if hypersensitivity exists to penicillins.

Toxicity includes fever, anaphylaxis, rash including Stevens–Johnson syndrome, erythema multiforme and toxic epidermal necrolysis, angioedema, flushing, serum-sickness-like reactions, encephalopathy, seizures, diarrhea, *Clostridium difficile*-associated diarrhea and pseudomembranous colitis, oral candidiasis, anorexia, nausea, vomiting, stomach cramps, flatulence, hepatitis, renal impairment, genital moniliasis, vaginitis, hemorrhage, prolonged prothrombin time, pancytopenia, hemolytic anemia, and positive Coombs' test.

DRUG INTERACTIONS/FOOD INTERACTIONS

Cefdinir can be taken with or without food.

Cefdinir should be taken at least 2 hours before or after an antacid or iron supplement.

Probenecid inhibits the renal excretion of cefdinir.

There have been reports of reddish stools in patients receiving cefdinir.

Antibiotics Manual: A Guide to Commonly Used Antimicrobials, Second Edition. David Schlossberg and Rafik Samuel.
© 2017 John Wiley & Sons Ltd. Published 2017 by John Wiley & Sons Ltd.

Cephalosporins may cause false-positive urine glucose determinations when using cupric sulfate solution (Benedict's solution, *Clinitest®*). Tests utilizing glucose oxidase (*Tes-Tape®*, *Clinistix®*) are not affected by cephalosporins. False-positive reaction for ketones in the urine may occur with tests using nitroprusside, but not with those using nitroferricyanide.

 ## DOSING

Cefdinir is supplied as 300 mg capsules and a cream-colored powder formulation containing 125 mg/5 mL or 250 mg/5 mL. The doses for patients over 13 years of age:

Infection	Dosage	Duration
Community acquired pneumonia	300 mg q 12 h	10 days
Acute exacerbations of chronic bronchitis	300 mg q 12 or 600 mg daily	5–10 days
Acute sinusitis	300 mg q 12 or 600 mg daily	10 days
Pharyngitis	300 mg q 12 or 600 mg daily	5–10 days
Uncomplicated skin and skin structure	300 mg q 12 h	10 days

 ## SPECIAL POPULATIONS

RENAL IMPAIRMENT:

Creatinine clearance, mg/mL	Dose
<30	300 mg once daily
Hemodialysis	300 mg after dialysis
CAPD	N/A
CRRT	N/A

HEPATIC DYSFUNCTION: No dose adjustment is necessary.

PEDIATRICS: Safety and efficacy in neonates and infants less than 6 months of age have not been established.

Infection	Dose	Duration
Otitis media	7 mg/kg q 12 h or 14 mg/kg/day	5–10 days
Acute maxillary sinusitis	7 mg/kg q 12 h or 14 mg/kg/day	10 days
Pharyngitis/tonsillitis	7 mg/kg q 12 h or 14 mg/kg/day	5–10 days
Skin and skin structure	7 mg/kg q 12 h	10 days

For pediatric patients with a creatinine clearance of $<30 \, mL/min/1.73 \, m^2$, the dose of cefdinir should be 7 mg/kg (up to 300 mg) given once daily.

 ## THE ART OF ANTIMICROBIAL THERAPY

Clinical Pearls
1. Cefdinir must be adjusted for renal insufficiency.
2. Cross allergy with penicillins is <10 %.

ORBACTIVE (Oritavancin)

 BASIC CHARACTERISTICS

Class: Lipoglycopeptide.

Mechanism of Action:

1. Inhibition of the transglycosylation (polymerization) step of cell wall biosynthesis by binding to the stem peptide of peptidoglycan precursors.
2. Inhibition of the transpeptidation (crosslinking) step of cell wall biosynthesis by binding to the peptide bridging segments of the cell wall.
3. Disruption of bacterial membrane integrity.

Mechanisms of Resistance: Limited data. Resistance was not observed in clinical studies.

Metabolic Route: Not metabolized; slowly excreted in feces and urine.

 FDA-APPROVED INDICATIONS

Acute bacterial skin and skin structure infections (ABSSSI) caused by susceptible isolates of staphylococci (including MRSA) and streptococci.

 SIDE EFFECTS/TOXICITY

Headache, nausea, vomiting, limb and subcutaneous abscesses, and diarrhea.

Hypersensitivity, cellulitis, osteomyelitis, anemia, eosinophilia, infusion site erythema, extravasation, pruritis, rash, edema, elevated bilirubin, hyperuricemia, tenosynovitis, myalgia, bronchospasm, wheezing, urticaria, angioedema, erythema multiforme, pruritis, leucocytoclastic vasculitis, rash, which may have cross-sensitivity with other glycopeptides, and *Clostridium difficile*-associated diarrhea.

 DRUG INTERACTIONS/FOOD INTERACTIONS

Weak inducer or inhibitor of several CYP450 enzymes.

Coadministration of oritavancin and warfarin may result in higher exposure of warfarin, which may increase the risk of bleeding.

 DOSING

A 1200 mg single dose is administered by intravenous infusion over 3 hours.

SPECIAL POPULATIONS

RENAL IMPAIRMENT: No dosage adjustment is needed with mild or moderate renal impairment. The pharmacokinetics in severe renal impairment have not been evaluated. Not removed from blood by hemodialysis.

Antibiotics Manual: A Guide to Commonly Used Antimicrobials, Second Edition. David Schlossberg and Rafik Samuel.
© 2017 John Wiley & Sons Ltd. Published 2017 by John Wiley & Sons Ltd.

HEPATIC DYSFUNCTION: Dosage adjustment is not needed in patients with mild or moderate hepatic impairment. The pharmacokinetics in patients with severe hepatic insufficiency has not been studied.

PEDIATRICS: Safety and effectiveness in pediatric patients younger than 18 years have not been studied.

 THE ART OF ANTIMICROBIAL THERAPY

Clinical Pearls

1. Use of intravenous unfractionated heparin sodium is **contraindicated** for 120 hours (5 days) after oritavancin administration because the activated partial thromboplastin time (aPTT) test results may remain falsely elevated for up to 120 hours (5 days) after oritavancin administration.

2. Oritavancin has been shown to artificially prolong prothrombin time (PT) and international normalized ratio (INR) for up to 12 hours, making the monitoring of the anticoagulation effect of warfarin unreliable up to 12 hours after an oritavancin dose.

■ ORNIDYL (Eflornithine)

 BASIC CHARACTERISTICS

Class: Fluorinated analog of ornithine.

Mechanism of Action: Inhibitor of ornithine decarboxylase, resulting in a decrease in spermidine and trypanothione.

Metabolic Route: Excreted unchanged in the urine.

Used for: Active against *Trypanosoma brucei gambiense* trypanosomiasis. Used in late disease with CNS involvement.

 SIDE EFFECTS/TOXICITY

Anemia, leukopenia and thrombocytopenia, seizures, diarrhea, hearing loss, alopecia.

 DRUG INTERACTIONS/FOOD INTERACTIONS

Data incomplete.

 DOSING

New cases of late-stage Gambian trypanosomiasis: 100 mg/kg q 6 h IV for 14 days.

Relapse: same dose for 7 days.

 SPECIAL POPULATIONS

RENAL IMPAIRMENT: The dose should be reduced in renal insufficiency.

HEPATIC DYSFUNCTION: No dose adjustment is necessary.

PEDIATRICS: Children less than 12 years old should receive 125 mg/kg q 6 h IV for 14 days. Older children should receive 100 mg/kg q 6 h for 14 days.

 THE ART OF ANTIMICROBIAL THERAPY

Clinical Pearls

1. Patients treated with eflornithine should be followed for 2 years, with a lumbar puncture every 6 months.
2. Eflornithine monotherapy should not be used to treat *T. b. rhodesiense* trypanosomiasis since it is much less active.
3. Eflornithine and melarsoprol may be synergistic for the treatment of Old World trypanosomiasis.
4. Eflornithine is available from the CDC Drug Service, 404-639-3670. Evenings, weekends, and holidays: 770-488-7100; FAX 404-639-3717.

Antibiotics Manual: A Guide to Commonly Used Antimicrobials, Second Edition. David Schlossberg and Rafik Samuel.
© 2017 John Wiley & Sons Ltd. Published 2017 by John Wiley & Sons Ltd.

BASIC CHARACTERISTICS

Class: Semisynthetic penicillin.

Mechanism of Action: Binds penicillin-binding protein, disrupting cell wall synthesis.

Mechanisms of Resistance:

1. The PBP can be altered, with reduced affinity.
2. Production of a beta-lactamase, resulting in hydrolysis of the beta-lactam ring.
3. Decreased ability of the antibiotic to reach the PBP when bacteria decrease porin production, resulting in reduced drug concentration within the cell.

Metabolic Route: Oxacillin is excreted unchanged in the urine.

 FDA-APPROVED INDICATIONS

Oxacillin is indicated in the treatment of infections caused by susceptible penicillinase-producing staphylococci.

 SIDE EFFECTS/TOXICITY

A history of allergic reaction to any of the penicillins is a **contraindication**.

Side effects include *Clostridium difficile*-associated diarrhea (CDAD), thrombophlebitis, hypersensitivity reactions including rash, erythema multiforme and Stevens–Johnson syndrome, interstitial nephritis, hepatitis, nausea, vomiting, diarrhea, stomatitis, black or hairy tongue, hyperactivity and seizures, anemia, thrombocytopenia, neutropenia, andeosinophilia.

 DRUG INTERACTIONS/FOOD INTERACTIONS

Chloramphenicol, macrolides, sulfonamides, and tetracyclines may interfere with the bactericidal effects of penicillins.

When oxacillin and warfarin are used concomitantly, the prothrombin time should be closely monitored. High urine concentrations of oxacillin may result in false-positive reactions when testing for the presence of glucose in urine using *Clinitest®*. It is recommended that glucose tests based on enzymatic glucose oxidase reactions (such as *Clinistix®*) be used.

 DOSING

The usual IV or IM dosage for adults is 250–500 mg every 4–6 hours.

For severe infections, 1 g every 4–6 hours is recommended.

 SPECIAL POPULATIONS

RENAL IMPAIRMENT: No dose adjustment is necessary.

HEPATIC DYSFUNCTION: No dose adjustment is necessary.

Combined renal and hepatic insufficiency: Measurement of oxacillin serum levels should be performed and dosage adjusted accordingly.

Antibiotics Manual: A Guide to Commonly Used Antimicrobials, Second Edition. David Schlossberg and Rafik Samuel.
© 2017 John Wiley & Sons Ltd. Published 2017 by John Wiley & Sons Ltd.

PEDIATRICS:

Infants and children < 40 kg: 50 mg/kg/day IM or IV in equally divided doses q 6 h for mild to moderate infections and 100 mg/kg/day IM or IV in equally divided doses q 4–6 h for severe infections.

Premature and neonates: 25 mg/kg/day IM or IV.

 THE ART OF ANTIMICROBIAL THERAPY

Clinical Pearls

1. Oxacillin does not need to be dose adjusted for renal dysfunction.
2. Oxacillin should be used with caution in patients with both renal and hepatic insufficiency.

BASIC CHARACTERISTICS

Class: Salicylic acid.

Mechanisms of Action: Inhibition of metabolism of *para*-aminobenzoic acid in mycobacteria.

Mechanisms of Resistance: Incompletely understood.

Metabolic Route: Acetylated in the liver and excreted in the urine.

 FDA-APPROVED INDICATIONS

Treatment of active tuberculosis in combination with other antimycobacterials.

 SIDE EFFECTS/TOXICITY

Nausea, vomiting, diarrhea, hepatotoxicity, coagulopathy, hypothyroidism, hypersensitivity, rash, leucopenia, thrombocytopenia, optic neuritis, and crystalluria.

 DRUG INTERACTIONS/FOOD INTERACTIONS

Drug should be sprinkled over apple sauce or yogurt or mixed with acidic juices, e.g., tomato, apple, or orange. The granules should not be chewed.

Decreases levels of digoxin, warfarin, and orally administered B12.

 DOSING

PAS is packaged as granules, which are 4 grams/packet. The usual dose is 8–12 grams/day divided 2–3 times/day.

 SPECIAL POPULATIONS

RENAL IMPAIRMENT: No dose adjustment, but use with caution. It is recommended that PAS be avoided in severe renal failure, but some authorities suggest its cautious use in this situation, if benefit outweighs risk.

HEPATIC DYSFUNCTION: No dose adjustment, but use with caution.

PEDIATRICS: 200–300 mg/kg/day divided 2–4 times daily

 THE ART OF ANTIMICROBIAL THERAPY

Clinical Pearls

1. PAS should never be used alone in the treatment of active tuberculosis.
2. PAS should be refrigerated.
3. PAS should be taken with acidic food to minimize GI discomfort.
4. Shells of the PAS granules may be seen in stool.

Antibiotics Manual: A Guide to Commonly Used Antimicrobials, Second Edition. David Schlossberg and Rafik Samuel.
© 2017 John Wiley & Sons Ltd. Published 2017 by John Wiley & Sons Ltd.

5. Patients should drink plenty of fluids to limit crystalluria.

6. Monitor TSH and LFTs while patients are on PAS.

7. Patients tolerate PAS best if the dosage is gradually escalated, e.g., beginning with 2 grams bid for a few days, then 2 grams AM and 4 grams hs for a few days, and then 4 grams bid.

8. Hypothyroidism is more common when PAS is coadministered with ethionamide.

BASIC CHARACTERISTICS

Class: Pegylated interferon.

Mechanism of Action:

After binding to the cell-surface receptor, production of several interferon-stimulated gene products lead to antiviral, antipro-liferative, and immunomodulatory effects, regulation of cell surface major histocompatibility antigen (HLA class I and class II) expression, and regulation of cytokine expression.

Mechanism of Resistance: Unknown.

Metabolic Route: Peginterferon alfa-2a is metabolized into amino acids.

 FDA-APPROVED INDICATIONS

Peginterferon alfa-2a, as part of a combination regimen with other hepatitis C virus antiviral drugs, is indicated for the treatment of adults with chronic hepatitis C with compensated liver disease. Peginterferon alfa-2a monotherapy is only indicated for the treatment of patients with chronic hepatitis C with compensated liver disease if there are **contraindications** or significant intolerance to other HCV antiviral drugs.

Peginterferon alfa-2a is indicated for the treatment of adult patients with HBeAg positive and HBeAg negative chronic hepatitis B who have compensated liver disease and evidence of viral replication and liver inflammation.

 SIDE EFFECTS/TOXICITY

> **WARNING:** Alpha interferons, including peginterferon alfa-2a, may cause or aggravate fatal or life-threatening neuropsychiatric, autoimmune, ischemic, and infectious disorders. Patients should be monitored closely with periodic clinical and laboratory evaluations. Therapy should be withdrawn in patients with persistently severe or worsening signs or symptoms of these conditions. In many, but not all, cases, these disorders resolve after stopping peginterferon alfa-2a therapy.

Peginterferon alfa-2a is **contraindicated** in patients with known hypersensitivity to alpha interferons or to any component of the product, decompensated hepatic disease (cirrhosis with Child Pugh* >6), autoimmune hepatitis, neonates and infants.

*See Helpful Formulas, Equations, and Definitions for Child Pugh scoring.

Adverse events

General: fever, hypersensitivity.

Neuropsychiatric disorders: depression, suicide, psychosis, aggressive behavior, nervousness, anxiety, emotional lability, abnormal thinking, agitation, apathy, and relapse of drug addiction.

Infections

Bone marrow suppression

Cardiovascular disorders, including hypertension, tachycardia, palpitation, tachyarrhythmias, supraventricular arrhythmias, chest pain, and myocardial infarction.

Hypersensitivity

Endocrine disorders: hyperthyroidism, hypothyroidism, hyperglycemia, diabetes mellitus, and elevated serum triglycerides.

Autoimmune disorders: autoimmune thrombocytopenia, idiopathic thrombocytopenic purpura, psoriasis, SLE, thyroiditis, and rheumatoid arthritis.

Pulmonary: pneumonia and interstitial pneumonitis.

Gastrointestinal disorders: hemorrhagic/ischemic, ulcerative colitis, pancreatitis, and hepatic decompensation.

Ophthalmologic disorders: decrease or loss of vision, macular edema, retinal artery or vein thrombosis, retinal hemorrhages, cotton wool spots, optic neuritis, and papilledema.

Cerebrovascular disorders: ischemic and hemorrhagic cerebrovascular events.

 DRUG INTERACTIONS/FOOD INTERACTIONS

Theophylline serum levels should be monitored.

Patients should be monitored for signs and symptoms of methadone toxicity.

 DOSING

Chronic hepatitis C: 180 µg (1.0 mL vial or 0.5 mL prefilled syringe) once weekly by subcutaneous administration in the abdomen or thigh. Indications are as follows:

Patient Population	Medication	Duration
In combination with simeprevir and ribavirin:		
Genotype 1 or 4 without cirrhosis or with compensated cirrhosis	Simeprevir + Peg-IFN-alfa and RBV	12 weeks
	then	
	Peg-IFN-alfa and RBV	12 weeks
Genotype 1 or 4 prior nonresponders	Simeprevir + Peg-IFN-alfa and RBV	12 weeks
without cirrhosis or	**then**	
with compensated cirrhosis	Peg-IFN-alfa and RBV	36 weeks
In combination with sofosbuvir and ribavirin:		
Genotype 1 or 4	Sofosbuvir + ribavirin + Peg-IFN-alfa	12 weeks
In combination with Ribavirin only:		
Genotype 1 or 4	Peg-IFN-alfa and RBV	48 weeks
Genotype 2 or 3	Peg-IFN-alfa and RBV	24 weeks
Any Genotype, HIV coinfected	Peg-IFN-alfa and RBV	48 weeks

Chronic hepatitis B: 180 µg (1.0 mL vial or 0.5 mL prefilled syringe) once weekly for 48 weeks by subcutaneous administration in the abdomen or thigh.

SPECIAL POPULATIONS

RENAL IMPAIRMENT: End-stage renal disease requiring hemodialysis: 135 µg once weekly.

HEPATIC DYSFUNCTION: Peginterferon alpha-2a should not be administered to those with decompensated liver disease (see cirrhosis with Child Pugh >6) and LFTs should be monitored closely.

In chronic hepatitis C patients with ALT increases above baseline values, reduce the peginterferon alpha-2a dose to 135 µg; therapy can be resumed after ALT flares subside.

In chronic hepatitis B patients with elevations in ALT (>5 × ULN), reduce the dose of peginterferon alpha-2a to 135 µg or temporarily discontinue treatment. Therapy can be resumed after ALT flares subside. If flares are severe and persistent (ALT >10 times above the upper limit of normal), consider discontinuing treatment.

PEDIATRICS: In children over the age of 5 years, peginterferon alpha-2a is administered as 180 mcg/1.73 m^2 × BSA subcutaneously once weekly, to a maximum dose of 180 mcg, and should be given in combination with ribavirin. The recommended treatment duration for pediatric patients with HCV genotype 2 or 3 is 24 weeks and for other HCV genotypes is 48 weeks.

 ## THE ART OF ANTIMICROBIAL THERAPY

Clinical Pearls

1. Before initiating peginterferon alpha-2a, evaluate for psychiatric issues including depression.
2. Monitor CBC during therapy. Discontinue in patients who develop severe decreases in neutrophil (<0.5 × 109/L) or platelet counts (<50 × 109/L).
3. Hepatic function should be closely monitored, and interferon treatment should be immediately discontinued if symptoms of hepatic decompensation, such as jaundice, ascites, coagulopathy, or decreased serum albumin, are observed.
4. All patients should receive an eye examination at baseline. Patients with preexisting ophthalmologic disorders (e.g., diabetic or hypertensive retinopathy) should receive periodic ophthalmologic exams during interferon alpha treatment. Any patient who develops ocular symptoms should receive a prompt and complete eye examination.
5. Peginterferon alpha-2a is not recommended in transplant recipients.
6. Many options with better tolerability exist to treat chronic hepatitis B and hepatitis C. Please review the most updated guidelines for current recommendations.

■ PEGINTRON (Peginterferon alpha-2b)

 BASIC CHARACTERISTICS

Class: Alpha interferon.

Mechanism of Action: After binding to the cell-surface receptor, production of several interferon-stimulated gene products lead to antiviral, antiproliferative, and immunomodulatory effects, regulation of cell surface major histocompatibility antigen (HLA class I and class II) expression, and regulation of cytokine expression.

Mechanism of Resistance: Unknown.

Metabolic Route: Peginterferon alfa-2b is metabolized into amino acids.

 FDA-APPROVED INDICATIONS

Peginterferon alfa-2b, as part of a combination regimen, is indicated for the treatment of chronic hepatitis C in patients with compensated liver disease.

Peginterferon alfa-2b monotherapy should only be used in the treatment of chronic hepatitis C in patients with compensated liver disease if there are **contraindications** to or significant intolerance of ribavirin and is indicated for use only in previously untreated adult patients.

 SIDE EFFECTS/TOXICITY

> **WARNING:** Alpha interferons, including peginterferon alfa-2b, may cause or aggravate fatal or life-threatening neuropsychiatric, autoimmune, ischemic, and infectious disorders. Patients should be monitored closely with periodic clinical and laboratory evaluations. Patients with persistently severe or worsening signs or symptoms of these conditions should be withdrawn from therapy. In many, but not all cases, these disorders resolve after stopping peginterferon alfa-2b therapy.

Use with ribavirin: Ribavirin may cause birth defects and death of the unborn child. Extreme care must be taken to avoid pregnancy in female patients and in female partners of male patients. Ribavirin causes hemolytic anemia. The anemia associated with ribavirin therapy may result in a worsening of cardiac disease. Peginterferon alfa-2b is **contraindicated** in patients with known hypersensitivity to alpha interferons or to any component of the product, decompensated hepatic disease (cirrhosis with Child Pugh* >6), autoimmune hepatitis, neonates and infants.

*See Helpful Formulas, Equations, and Definitions for Child Pugh scoring.

Adverse events

General: fever, hypersensitivity.

Neuropsychiatric disorders: depression, suicide, psychosis, aggressive behavior, nervousness, anxiety, emotional lability, abnormal thinking, agitation, apathy, and relapse of drug addiction.

Infections

Bone marrow suppression

Cardiovascular disorders, including hypertension, tachycardia, palpitation, tachyarrhythmias, supraventricular arrhythmias, chest pain, and myocardial infarction.

Antibiotics Manual: A Guide to Commonly Used Antimicrobials, Second Edition. David Schlossberg and Rafik Samuel.
© 2017 John Wiley & Sons Ltd. Published 2017 by John Wiley & Sons Ltd.

Hypersensitivity

Endocrine disorders: hyperthyroidism, hypothyroidism, hyperglycemia, diabetes mellitus, and elevated serum triglycerides.

Autoimmune disorders: autoimmune thrombocytopenia, idiopathic thrombocytopenic purpura, psoriasis, SLE, thyroiditis, and rheumatoid arthritis.

Pulmonary: Pneumonia and interstitial pneumonitis.

Gastrointestinal disorders: hemorrhagic/ischemic, ulcerative colitis, pancreatitis, and hepatic decompensation.

Ophthalmologic disorders: decrease or loss of vision, macular edema, retinal artery or vein thrombosis, retinal hemorrhages, cotton wool spots, optic neuritis, and papilledema.

Cerebrovascular disorders: ischemic and hemorrhagic cerebrovascular events.

 DRUG INTERACTIONS/FOOD INTERACTIONS

Patients on methadone should be monitored for the signs and symptoms of methadone toxicity.

Theophyline serum levels should be monitored.

 DOSING

1.5 mcg/kg/week subcutaneously in combination with 800 to 1400 mg of ribavirin orally based on patient body weight. The treatment duration for patients with genotype 1 is 48 weeks. Patients with genotypes 2 and 3 should be treated for 24 weeks. If using peginterferon alpha-2b monotherapy, the dose is 1 mcg/kg/week for 48 weeks.

 SPECIAL POPULATIONS

RENAL IMPAIRMENT: Creatinine clearance 30–50 mL/min: dose reduction of 25 %.

Creatinine clearance 10–29 mL/min, or hemodialysis: dose reduction 50 %.

HEPATIC DYSFUNCTION: Peginterferon alpha-2b should not be administered to those with decompensated liver disease (see cirrhosis with Child Pugh >6). LFTs should be monitored closely.

PEDIATRICS: For children over the age of 3 years, the recommended dose is 60 mcg/m²/week subcutaneously.

 THE ART OF ANTIMICROBIAL THERAPY

Clinical Pearls

1. Before initiating peginterferon alpha-2b, evaluate for psychiatric issues including depression.
2. Monitor CBC during therapy. Discontinue in patients who develop severe decreases in neutrophil ($<0.5 \times 109/L$) or platelet counts ($<50 \times 109/L$).
3. Hepatic function should be closely monitored, and interferon treatment should be immediately discontinued if symptoms of hepatic decompensation, such as jaundice, ascites, coagulopathy, or decreased serum albumin, are observed.
4. All patients should receive an eye examination at baseline. Patients with preexisting ophthalmologic disorders (e.g., diabetic or hypertensive retinopathy) should receive periodic ophthalmologic exams during interferon alpha treatment. Any patient who develops ocular symptoms should receive a prompt and complete eye examination.
5. Many options with better tolerability exist to treat hepatitis C. Please review the most updated guidelines for current recommendations.

PENTOSTAM (Stibogluconate)

 BASIC CHARACTERISTICS

Class: Organometallic pentavalent antimonial.
Mechanism of Action: Inhibits DNA topoisomerase, glycolytic enzymes, and fatty acid oxidation.
Metabolic Route: Eliminated rapidly, mainly via the urine.
Used for: Active against all *Leishmania* spp. Used for visceral, cutaneous, and mucosal forms.

 SIDE EFFECTS/TOXICITY

Hepatitis, arthralgias, myalgias, thrombophlebitis, headache, anorexia, abdominal pain, nausea, vomiting, pancreatitis, metallic taste, pruritus, arrhythmias and prolongation of QT interval, elevated serum amylase thrombocytopenia, and leukopenia.

 DRUG INTERACTIONS/FOOD INTERACTIONS

No interactions are known, but drugs that may impair renal function or prolong the QT interval should be used with caution.

 DOSING

The recommended daily dose by is 20 mg/kg/day; however, bid or tid doses of 10 mg/kg have been used. It is given by slow intravenous infusion; IM administration is painful and PO absorption is inadequate.

Cutaneous leishmaniasis is treated for 20 days.

Visceral leishmaniasis is treated for 28–30 days.

Mucocutaneous leishmaniasis is treated for 28 days.

 SPECIAL POPULATIONS

RENAL IMPAIRMENT: An alternative drug such as liposomal amphotericin B should be used in patients with renal failure.

HEPATIC DYSFUNCTION: No dose adjustment is necessary.

PEDIATRICS: The dose of 20 mg/kg with an upper daily dose limit of 850 mg/day.

THE ART OF ANTIMICROBIAL THERAPY

Clinical Pearls

1. Antimonials are more toxic in HIV infected patients.
2. Children tolerate antimonials better than adults.
3. Alcohol should be avoided during therapy
4. EKG should be monitored and treatment interrupted for significant QTc prolongation.
5. Available from the CDC Drug Service, 404-639-3670. Evenings, weekends, and holidays: 770-488-7100; FAX 404-639-3717.

Antibiotics Manual: A Guide to Commonly Used Antimicrobials, Second Edition. David Schlossberg and Rafik Samuel.
© 2017 John Wiley & Sons Ltd. Published 2017 by John Wiley & Sons Ltd.

BASIC CHARACTERISTICS

Class: Ureodopenicillin.

Mechanism of Action: Binds penicillin-binding protein, disrupting cell wall synthesis.

Mechanisms of Resistance:

1. The PBP can be altered, with reduced affinity.
2. Production of a beta-lactamase, resulting in hydrolysis of the beta-lactam ring.
3. Decreased ability of the antibiotic to reach the PBP when bacteria decrease porin production, resulting in a decrease of the drug concentration within the cell.

Metabolic Route: Piperacillin is excreted by both biliary and renal routes.

 FDA-APPROVED INDICATIONS

Piperacillin is indicated in the treatment of infections due to susceptible (only beta-lactamase negative) strains of microorganisms in the conditions listed below:

Intra-abdominal infections

Urinary tract infections

Gynecologic infections

Septicemia

Lower respiratory tract infections

Skin and skin structure infections

Bone and joint infections

Uncomplicated gonococcal urethritis

Prophylaxis for surgery

 SIDE EFFECTS/TOXICITY

Contraindicated in patients with a history of allergic reactions to any of the penicillins, cephalosporins, or β-lactamase inhibitors.

Side effects include *Clostridium difficile*-associated diarrhea (CDAD), hypersensitivity reactions including anaphylaxis, rash including erythema multiforme and Stevens–Johnson syndrome, mucocutaneous candidiasis, nausea, vomiting, diarrhea, constipation, black hairy tongue, headache, arrhythmias, hyperactivity and seizures, confusion, hepatitis, renal dysfunction, crystalluria, anemia, thrombocytopenia, eosinophilia, leukopenia, and abnormalities of coagulation.

 DRUG INTERACTIONS/FOOD INTERACTIONS

Concurrent use of piperacillin and probenecid may result in increased and prolonged blood levels of piperacillin. Neuromuscular blockade produced by any of the nondepolarizing muscle relaxants could be prolonged in the presence of piperacillin. The clearance of methotrexate may be reduced.

Antibiotics Manual: A Guide to Commonly Used Antimicrobials, Second Edition. David Schlossberg and Rafik Samuel.
© 2017 John Wiley & Sons Ltd. Published 2017 by John Wiley & Sons Ltd.

Chloramphenicol, macrolides, sulfonamides, and tetracyclines may interfere with the bactericidal effects of penicillins.

High urine concentrations of piperacillin may result in false-positive reactions when testing for the presence of glucose in urine using *Clinitest®*. It is recommended that glucose tests based on enzymatic glucose oxidase reactions (such as *Clinistix®*) be used.

 ## DOSING

Piperacillin may be administered intramuscularly or intravenously.

Infection	Dose (maximum dose for serious infection: 24 g/day)
Sepsis	12–18 g IV daily divided every 4–6 h
Nosocomial pneumonia	12–18 g IV daily divided every 4–6 h
Intra-abdominal infections	12–18 g IV daily divided every 4–6 h
Gynecologic infections	12–18 g IV daily divided every 4–6 h
Skin and skin structure infections	12–18 g IV daily divided every 4–6 h
Complicated urinary tract infections	8–16 g IV daily divided every 6–8 h
Uncomplicated urinary tract infections	6–8 g IM or IV daily divided every 6–12 h
Uncomplicated gonococcal infections	2 g IM with 1 g of probenecid 30 min earlier
Prophylaxis for surgery	2 g 20–30 minutes prior to anesthesia

 ## SPECIAL POPULATIONS

RENAL IMPAIRMENT:

Creatine clearance, mL/min	Uncomplicated UTI	Complicated UTI	Serious infections
20–40	6–8 g IM or IV divided q 6–12 hours	3 g q 8 hours	4 g q 8 hours
<20	3 g every 12 hours	3 g q12 hours	4 g q 12 hours
Hemodialysis	Maximum daily dose is 2 g q 8 hours and 1 g after dialysis		
CAPD	Maximum daily dose is 2 g q 8 hours and 2 g after dialysis		
CRRT	3 grams every 8 hours		

HEPATIC DYSFUNCTION: No dose adjustment is necessary.

RENAL AND HEPATIC FAILURE: Should measure levels.

PEDIATRICS: Dosages in pediatric patients under 12 years of age have not been studied in adequate and well-controlled clinical trials.

 ## THE ART OF ANTIMICROBIAL THERAPY

Clinical Pearls

1. Piperacillin needs to be dose adjusted for renal dysfunction.
2. Piperacillin is a monosodium salt containing 1.85 meq of Na^+ per g (42.5 mg of Na^+ per g). This should be considered when treating patients requiring restricted salt intake.

3. Neuromuscular blockade produced by any of the non-depolarizing muscle relaxants could be prolonged in the presence of piperacillin.

4. As with other semisynthetic penicillins, piperacillin therapy has been associated with an increased incidence of fever and rash in cystic fibrosis patients.

5. When treating *Pseudomonas* infections, the piperacillin dose should be 24 g/day in 4 divided doses.

■ POLYMYXIN B INJECTION (Polymyxin B Sulfate)

 ## BASIC CHARACTERISTICS

Class: Polypeptide.
Mechanism of Action: Increases permeability of bacterial cell membrane leading to death of the cell.
Metabolic Route: Primarily excreted by the kidneys.

 ## FDA-APPROVED INDICATIONS

1. Acute infections caused by susceptible strains of *Pseudomonas aeruginosa* (urinary tract, meninges, and bloodstream).
2. It may be indicated in the following serious infections, if susceptible, when less toxic drugs cannot be used:
   H. influenzae meningitis, *E. coli* UTI, *Aerobacter aerogenes* bacteremia, and *Klebsiella pneumoniae* bacteremia.

 ## SIDE EFFECTS/TOXICITY

> **WARNING:** IM and/or intrathecal administration should be given only to hospitalized patients, so as to provide constant supervision by a physician. Carefully determine renal function; reduce dosage in patients with renal damage and nitrogen retention. Patients with nephrotoxicity due to polymyxin B usually show albuminuria, cellular casts, and azotemia; diminishing urine output and a rising BUN are indications for discontinuing therapy. Neurotoxic reactions may be manifested by irritability, weakness, drowsiness, ataxia, perioral paresthesia, numbness of the extremities, and blurring of vision. These are usually associated with high serum levels found in patients with renal impairment and/or nephrotoxicity. Avoid concurrent or sequential use of other neurotoxic and/or nephrotoxic drugs, particularly bacitracin, streptomycin, neomycin, kanamycin, gentamicin, tobramycin, amikacin, cephaloridine, paromomycin, viomycin, and colistin. Neurotoxicity of polymyxin B can result in respiratory paralysis from neuromuscular blockade, especially when the drug is given soon after anesthesia and/or muscle relaxants. Safety in human pregnancy has not been established.

Nephrotoxicity, neurotoxicity.

 ## DRUG INTERACTIONS/FOOD INTERACTIONS

Avoid concurrent use of a curariform muscle relaxant and other neurotoxic drugs (ether, tubocurarine, succinylcholine, gallamine, decamethonium, and sodium citrate), which may precipitate respiratory depression.

 ## DOSING (1 MG = 10 000 UNITS)

IV: 15 000–25 000 U/kg/day; may be divided q 12 h.
IM: 25 000–30 000 U/kg/day; may divide and give at either 4 or 6-hour intervals.
Intrathecal: 50 000 U q d for 3 to 4 days, then 50 000 U once qod for at least 2 weeks, after cerebrospinal fluid cultures are negative and sugar content has returned to normal.

Antibiotics Manual: A Guide to Commonly Used Antimicrobials, Second Edition. David Schlossberg and Rafik Samuel.
© 2017 John Wiley & Sons Ltd. Published 2017 by John Wiley & Sons Ltd.

SPECIAL POPULATIONS

RENAL IMPAIRMENT:

IV: Adults and children: Reduce from 15 000 U/kg downward.

IM: Adults and children: Reduce dose.

Hemodialysis, peritoneal dialysis: Adults: IM: 250 000 units every 24 hours; no supplemental dose necessary.

HEPATIC DYSFUNCTION: Probably no dose adjustment necessary.

PEDIATRICS:

1. **IV**:
   a. **Infants**:
      Maximum: 40 000 U/kg/day.
   b. **Children**:
      Usual: 15 000–25 000 U/kg/day divided q 12 h.
      Maximum: 25 000 U/kg/day.
2. **IM**:
   a. **Infants**:
      Maximum: 40 000 U/kg/day.
      Doses as high as 45 000 U/kg/day have been used in limited clinical studies in treating prematures and newborn infants for sepsis caused by *Pseudomonas aeruginosa*.
   b. **Children**:
      Usual: 25 000–30 000 U/kg/day; may divide and give at either 4 or 6 hour intervals.
3. **Intrathecal**:
   a. **<2 years**:
      Usual: 20 000 U q d for 3–4 days or 25 000 U qod. Continue with a dose of 25 000 U qod for at least 2 weeks after cerebrospinal fluid cultures are negative and sugar content has returned to normal.
   b. **>2 years**:
      Usual: 50 000 U q d for 3–4 days, then 50 000 U once qod for at least 2 weeks after cerebrospinal fluid cultures are negative and sugar content has returned to normal.

 THE ART OF ANTIMICROBIAL THERAPY

Clinical Pearls

1. Many gram-negative bacilli are resistant, including *Proteus, Serratia, Providentia, Burkholderia, Moraxella, Vibrio, Morganella, Helocobacter*, and *Edwardsiella*.
2. Monitor for nephrotoxicity, neurotoxicity, CDAD, superinfection, respiratory paralysis, and other adverse reactions.
3. Monitor urine output and BUN. Frequently monitor renal function and blood levels of the drug during parenteral therapy.
4. Administer only by intrathecal route in meningeal infections.

PREZCOBIX (Darunavir + Cobicistat)

 BASIC CHARACTERISTICS

Class: Protease inhibitor + CYP3A inhibitor.

Mechanism of Action: Darunavir reversibly binds the active site of the enzyme protease. Inhibition of protease prevents cleavage of the *gag* and *gag-pol* polyprotein, resulting in the production of immature, noninfectious virus.

Cobicistat is a mechanism-based CYP3A inhibitor.

Mechanism of Resistance: Development of mutations on the enzyme protease causes a conformational change that prevents darunavir from binding the active site, allowing protease activity to continue. There are many protease mutations identified for darunavir, of which 5 are required to inhibit its activity.

Metabolic Route: Both darunavir and cobicistat are metabolized in the liver and excreted in the feces.

 FDA-APPROVED INDICATIONS

In combination with other antiretroviral agents for the treatment of human immunodeficiency virus (HIV-1) infection in treatment-naïve and treatment-experienced adults with no darunavir resistance-associated substitutions.

 SIDE EFFECTS/TOXICITY

Darunavir is associated with new-onset diabetes mellitus, exacerbation of preexisting diabetes mellitus, hyperglycemia, increased bleeding, including spontaneous skin hematomas and hemarthrosis, in patients with hemophilia types A and B, redistribution/accumulation of body fat including central obesity, dorsocervical fat enlargement (buffalo hump), peripheral wasting, facial wasting, breast enlargement, "cushingoid appearance", immune reconstitution syndrome, hepatitis, rash, QTc prolongation, torsades de pointes, abdominal pain, headache, anorexia, dyspepsia, epigastric pain, hepatitis, mouth ulceration, pancreatitis, vomiting, anemia, leucopenia, thrombocytopenia, increases in alkaline phosphatase, amylase, creatine phosphokinase, lactic dehydrogenase, SGOT, SGPT, and gamma glutamyl transpeptidase; hyperlipemia, hyperuricemia, hyperglycemia, hypoglycemia, and dehydration.

Cobicistat decreases estimated creatinine clearance due to inhibition of tubular secretion of creatinine without affecting actual renal glomerular function. Renal impairment, including cases of acute renal failure and Fanconi syndrome when used with tenofovir DF. Other side effects reported include jaundice, rash, scleral icterus, nausea, diarrhea and headache.

In less than 2 %: abdominal pain, vomiting, fatigue, rhabdomyolysis, depression, abnormal dreams, insomnia, nephropathy, and nephrolithiasis.

 DRUG INTERACTIONS/FOOD INTERACTIONS

Darunavir/cobicistat should be taken with a meal.

Drugs that **should not be coadministered** with darunavir/cobicistat include amiodarone, quinidine, rifampin, ergot derivatives, St John's wort, HMG-CoA reductase inhibitors, simvastatin or lovastatin, pimozide, benzodiazepines, voriconazole, phenobarbital, phenytoin, carbamazepine, Prezista, ritonavir, lopinavir, saquinavir, nevirapine, efavirenz, fosamprenavir, tipranavir, etravirine, indinavir, alfuzosin, dronedarone, rivaroxaban, irinotecan, cisapride, avanafil, or sildenafil.

Antibiotics Manual: A Guide to Commonly Used Antimicrobials, Second Edition. David Schlossberg and Rafik Samuel.
© 2017 John Wiley & Sons Ltd. Published 2017 by John Wiley & Sons Ltd.

Darunavir and cobicistat are inhibitors of the CYP3A enzyme; coadministration of darunavir and drugs primarily metabolized by CYP3A may result in increased plasma concentrations of the other drug that could increase or prolong its therapeutic and adverse effects.

Darunavir is metabolized by CYP3A; coadministration of darunavir and drugs that induce CYP3A may decrease darunavir plasma concentrations and reduce its therapeutic effect. Coadministration of darunavir and drugs that inhibit CYP3A may increase darunavir plasma concentrations. Because of these metabolic effects, potential drug interactions that may require dosage change or clinical/laboratory monitoring are listed below:

Medication	Adjustment or action
Itraconzole	Do not exceed 200 mg of itraconazole
Ketoconazole	Do not exceed 200 mg of ketoconazole
Clarithromycin	Reduce clarithromycin dose in renal impairment
Rifabutin	Decrease rifabutin to 150/qod
Contraceptives	Use alternative or additional method
Atorvastatin	Use lowest possible dose with close monitoring
Pravastatin	Use lowest possible dose with close monitoring
Methadone	Monitor; may require higher methadone dose
Sildenafil	25 mg every 48 hours
Tadalafil	5 mg, no more than 10 mg in 72 hours
Vardenafil	2.5 mg in 24 hours
Paroxetine, sertraline	Monitor for antidepressant response
Tenofovir	Monitor for tenofovir toxicity
Maraviroc	Maraviroc dose should be 150 mg bid
Cyclosporine, tacrolimus, sirolimus	Monitor levels of immunosuppressants
Colchicine	Not recommended in renal or hepatic impairment
Bosentan	Bosentan dose 62.5 mg daily or qod

 ## DOSING

Darunavir/cobicistat is supplied in a fixed dose combination of darunavir 800 mg + cobicistat 150 mg.
The recommended dose is 1 pill daily.

 ## SPECIAL POPULATIONS

RENAL IMPAIRMENT: There is no adjustment needed.

HEPATIC DYSFUNCTION: No dose adjustment is required in patients with mild or moderate hepatic impairment. Darunavir/cobicistat is not recommended for use in patients with severe hepatic impairment.

PEDIATRICS: Not recommended under 18 years of age.

THE ART OF ANTIMICROBIAL THERAPY

Clinical Pearls

1. Darunavir/cobicistat should always be used in combination with other antiretrovirals.

2. Darunavir/cobicistat should be taken with food to increase absorption.

3. Darunavir has a sulfa moiety; use caution when using it in patients with sulfa allergies.

4. When assessing for resistance to darunavir, a phenotype assay may be helpful.

5. Whenever initiating darunavir, make sure to review all medications the patient is receiving, to minimize drug interactions.

6. Do not administer with agents containing the same components: Cobicistat, darunavir, Evotaz, Stribild, or Genvoya.

7. Do not administer with ritonavir.

8. When used with rifabutin, monitor for rifabutin-associated adverse reactions including neutropenia and uveitis.

Also available with Cobicistat as Prezcobix.

 ## BASIC CHARACTERISTICS

Class: Protease inhibitor.

Mechanism of Action: Darunavir reversibly binds the active site of the enzyme protease. Inhibition of protease prevents cleavage of the *gag* and *gag-pol* polyprotein, resulting in the production of immature, noninfectious virus.

Mechanism of Resistance: Development of mutations on the enzyme protease causes a conformational change that prevents darunavir from binding the active site, allowing protease activity to continue. There are many protease mutations identified for darunavir, of which 5 are required to inhibit its activity.

Metabolic Route: Darunavir is metabolized in the liver and excreted in the feces.

 ## FDA-APPROVED INDICATIONS

Treatment of HIV-1 in combinations with other antiretroviral agents.

 ## SIDE EFFECTS/TOXICITY

New-onset diabetes mellitus, exacerbation of preexisting diabetes mellitus, hyperglycemia, increased bleeding, including spontaneous skin hematomas and hemarthrosis, in patients with hemophilia types A and B, redistribution/accumulation of body fat including central obesity, dorsocervical fat enlargement (buffalo hump), peripheral wasting, facial wasting, breast enlargement, "cushingoid appearance", immune reconstitution syndrome, hepatitis, rash, QTc prolongation, torsades de pointes, abdominal pain, headache, anorexia, dyspepsia, epigastric pain, hepatitis, mouth ulceration, pancreatitis, vomiting, anemia, leucopenia, thrombocytopenia, increases in alkaline phosphatase, amylase, creatine phosphokinase, lactic dehydrogenase, SGOT, SGPT, gamma glutamyl transpeptidase, hyperlipemia, hyperuricemia, hyperglycemia, hypoglycemia, and dehydration.

 ## DRUG INTERACTIONS/FOOD INTERACTIONS

Darunavir should be taken with a meal.

Drugs that **should not be coadministered** with darunavir include colchicine, alfuzosin, dronaderone, ranolazine, lurasidone, cisapride, rifampin, rifapentine, ergot derivatives, St John's wort, simvastatin, lovastatin, pimozide, midazolam, triazolam, apixaban, rivaroxaban, voriconazole, simepravir, salmeterol, budesonide, fluticasone, lopinavir, saquinavir, or prezcobix.

Darunavir is an inhibitor of the CYP3A enzyme; coadministration of darunavir and drugs primarily metabolized by CYP3A may result in increased plasma concentrations of the other drug that could increase or prolong its therapeutic and adverse effects.

Darunavir is metabolized by CYP3A; coadministration of darunavir and drugs that induce CYP3A may decrease darunavir plasma concentrations and reduce its therapeutic effect. Coadministration of darunavir and drugs that inhibit CYP3A may

Antibiotics Manual: A Guide to Commonly Used Antimicrobials, Second Edition. David Schlossberg and Rafik Samuel.
© 2017 John Wiley & Sons Ltd. Published 2017 by John Wiley & Sons Ltd.

increase darunavir plasma concentrations. Because of these metabolic affects, potential drug interactions that may require dosage change or clinical/laboratory monitoring are listed below:

Medication	Adjustment or action
Itraconzole	Do not exceed 200 mg of itraconazole
Ketoconazole	Do not exceed 200 mg of ketoconazole
Clarithromycin	Reduce clarithromycin dose in renal impairment
Rifabutin	Decrease rifabutin to 150/qod
Contraceptives	Use alternative or additional method
Atorvastatin	Use lowest possible dose with close monitoring
Pravastatin	Use lowest possible dose with close monitoring
Methadone	Monitor; may require higher methadone dose
Sildenafil	25 mg every 48 hours
Tadalafil	5 mg, no more than 10 mg in 72 hours
Vardenafil	2.5 mg in 24 hours
Paroxetine, sertraline	Monitor for antidepressant response
Tenofovir	Monitor for tenofovir toxicity
Maraviroc	Maraviroc dose should be 150 mg bid
Cyclosporine, tacrolimus, sirolimus	Monitor levels of immunosuppressants
Quetiapine	Administer one-sixth of the quetiapine dose
Bosentan	Bosentan dose is 62.5 mg daily

 DOSING

Darunavir is supplied in 75 mg, 150 mg, 600 mg, and 800 mg tablets. It is also formulated in a liquid that contains 100 mg/mL. Darunavir **must** be taken with ritonavir to achieve adequate levels. The recommended dose of darunavir in adults with no darunavir resistance is 800 mg taken with ritonavir 100 mg once daily and with food. The type of food does not affect exposure to darunavir.

For those with documented resistance to darunavir, the recommended dose is 600 mg taken with ritonavir 100 mg twice daily and with food.

 SPECIAL POPULATIONS

RENAL IMPAIRMENT: There is no adjustment needed.

HEPATIC DYSFUNCTION: No dose adjustment is required in patients with mild or moderate hepatic impairment. Darunavir is not recommended for use in patients with severe hepatic impairment.

PEDIATRICS: Darunavir is approved for pediatric patients 3 years of age and older who weigh at least 10 kg.

For those who have no resistance to darunavir:

Body weight	Dose
10 kg to <11 kg	DRV 350 mg + RTV 64 mg once daily
11 kg to <12 kg	DRV 385 mg + RTV 64 mg once daily
12 kg to <13 kg	DRV 420 mg + RTV 80 mg once daily
13 kg to <14 kg	DRV 455 mg + RTV 80 mg once daily
14 kg to <15 kg	DRV 490 mg + RTV 96 mg once daily
15 kg to <30 kg	DRV 600 mg + RTV 100 mg once daily
30 kg to <40 kg	DRV 675 mg + RTV 100 mg once daily
40 kg and over	DRV 800 mg + RTV 100 mg once daily

For those who have resistance to darunavir:

Body weight	Dose
10 kg to <11 kg	DRV 200 mg + RTV 32 mg twice daily
11 kg to <12 kg	DRV 220 mg + RTV 32 mg twice daily
12 kg to < 13 kg	DRV 240 mg + RTV 40 mg twice daily
13 kg to <14 kg	DRV 260 mg + RTV 40 mg twice daily
14 kg to <15 kg	DRV 280 mg + RTV 48 mg twice daily
15 kg to <30 kg	DRV 375 mg + RTV 48 mg twice daily
30 kg to <40 kg	DRV 450 mg + RTV 600 mg twice daily
40 kg and over	DRV 600 mg + RTV 100 mg twice daily

 THE ART OF ANTIMICROBIAL THERAPY

Clinical Pearls

1. Darunavir should always be used in combination with other antiretrovirals.
2. Darunavir must be administered with ritonavir or cobicistat to achieve adequate levels when given once daily.
3. Do not use with cobicistat in the 600 mg twice daily dose; use only with ritonavir.
4. Darunavir should not be used with prezcobix.
5. Darunavir should be taken with food to increase absorption.
6. Darunavir has a sulfa moiety; use caution when using it in patients with sulfa allergies.
7. When assessing for resistance to darunavir, a phenotype assay may be helpful.
8. Whenever initiating darunavir, make sure to review all medications the patient is receiving, to minimize drug interactions.

■ PRIFTIN (Rifapentine)

BASIC CHARACTERISTICS

Class: Rifamycin.

Mechanisms of Action: Rifapentine inhibits DNA-dependent RNA polymerase activity in susceptible cells.

Mechanisms of Resistance: Resistance occurs as single-step mutations of the DNA-dependent RNA polymerase.

Metabolic Route: Rifapentine is rapidly eliminated in the bile and undergoes progressive deacetylation and is eliminated. However, up to 30 % of a dose is excreted in the urine, half of it as unchanged drug.

FDA-APPROVED INDICATIONS

Rifapentine is indicated in the treatment of pulmonary tuberculosis and for latent TB infection in combination with isoniazid.

SIDE EFFECTS/TOXICITY

Rifapentine is **contraindicated** in patients with a history of hypersensitivity to any of the rifamycins.

It is assumed that rifapentine's toxicity will resemble that of rifampin.

Adverse events: anaphylaxis, liver dysfunction, reddish coloration of the urine, sweat, sputum, and tears, "flu syndrome" (fever, chills, and malaise), rash, flushing, epigastric distress, anorexia, nausea, vomiting, flatulence, *Clostridium difficile*-associated diarrhea, disseminated intravascular coagulation, visual disturbances, confusion, renal insufficiency, elevations in serum uric acid, thrombocytopenia, leukopenia, hemolytic anemia, enhanced metabolism of endogenous substrates including adrenal hormones, thyroid hormones, and vitamin D.

DRUG INTERACTIONS/FOOD INTERACTIONS

Absorption of rifapentine is reduced when the drug is ingested with food, but absorption is usually adequate, and ingestion with food reduces GI intolerance.

It is assumed that rifapentine's drug interactions resemble those of rifampin.

Rifampin is known to induce certain cytochrome P-450 enzymes, and rifapentine shows 85 % of the enzyme induction of rifampin. Administration of rifapentine with drugs that undergo biotransformation through these metabolic pathways may accelerate elimination and decrease the therapeutic effect of these coadministered drugs, many of which require monitoring and possible adjustment during and following coadministration with rifampin. The list of drugs so affected includes the following drugs/classes:

anticonvulsants, antiarrhythmics, oral anticoagulants, antifungals, barbiturates, beta-blockers, calcium channel blockers, chloramphenicol, clarithromycin, corticosteroids, cyclosporine, cardiac glycoside preparations, clofibrate, hormonal contraceptives (patients should be advised to use nonhormonal methods of birth control during rifampin therapy), dapsone, diazepam, doxycycline, enalapril, fluoroquinolones, haloperidol, oral hypoglycemic agents, levothyroxine, methadone, narcotic analgesics, nortriptyline, progestins, quinine, tacrolimus, sulfapyridine, theophylline, tricyclic antidepressants, protease inhibitors, nonnucleoside reverse transcriptase inhibitors, CCR5 inhibitors, and zidovudine.

Rifampin levels may increase when coadministered with atovaquone, probenecid, and cotrimoxazole, and may decrease when given with ketoconazole and antacids (give rifampin at least 1 hour before the ingestion of antacids).

When rifampin is given concomitantly with either halothane or isoniazid, the potential for hepatotoxicity is increased, and concomitant use of rifampin and halothane should be avoided.

Antibiotics Manual: A Guide to Commonly Used Antimicrobials, Second Edition. David Schlossberg and Rafik Samuel.
© 2017 John Wiley & Sons Ltd. Published 2017 by John Wiley & Sons Ltd.

Drug/aboratory interactions

Cross-reactivity and false-positive urine screening tests for opiates have been reported in patients receiving rifampin.

Therapeutic levels of rifampin have been shown to inhibit standard microbiological assays for serum folate and vitamin B12.

 ## DOSING

Rifapentine is supplied as 150 mg tablets. Dose is 10 mg/kg, with a maximum dose of 600 mg.

 ## SPECIAL POPULATIONS

RENAL IMPAIRMENT: Not studied in patients with renal insufficiency.

HEPATIC DYSFUNCTION: Patients with impaired liver function should be given rifapentine only in cases of necessity and then with caution and monitoring of liver function.

PEDIATRICS: Not studied in children under 12 years of age.

For children over 12 years of age: 600 mg for those who weigh >45 kg, 450 mg for those <45 kg.

 ## THE ART OF ANTIMICROBIAL THERAPY

Clinical Pearls

1. Rifapentine is used in the continuation phase of therapy for tuberculosis (after the first two months), and is used ONLY for selected patients: those who are HIV-negative, have noncavitary pulmonary tuberculosis, and whose sputum smears are negative after two months of therapy.

2. Rifapentine is given once weekly, with INH, by DOT.

3. If the culture at two months is positive, the continuation phase of weekly INH and rifapentine should be extended to 7 months instead of 4 months. When used for treatment of latent TB, rifapentine is given with INH weekly for 12 weeks.

4. Liver function tests and symptoms of gastrointestinal intolerance should be monitored in all patients receiving rifapentine.

5. Rifapentine is a potent inducer of the p450 cytochrome system and coadministered medications may require discontinuation or monitoring for possible dosage adjustment.

6. Rifapentine should never be given alone, either for treatment of active tuberculous infection or for latent infection.

■ PRIMAQUINE (Primaquine Phosphate)

 BASIC CHARACTERISTICS

Class: Antimalarial agent.

Mechanism of Action: Primaquine phosphate is an 8-amino-quinoline compound that eliminates tissue (exoerythrocytic) infection. Thereby, it prevents the development of the blood (erythrocytic) forms of the parasite that are responsible for relapses in vivax malaria.

Primaquine phosphate is also active against gametocytes of *Plasmodium falciparum*.

 FDA-APPROVED INDICATIONS

Primaquine phosphate is indicated for the radical cure (prevention of relapse) of vivax malaria.

Also Used for: Radical cure of *P. ovale* and for prophylaxis of chloroquine-resistant *P. falciparum*.

 SIDE EFFECTS/TOXICITY

Hemolytic reactions: leukopenia, hemolytic anemia, methemoglobinemia; may occur in individuals with glucose-6-phosphate dehydrogenase (G-6-PD) or nicotinamide adenine dinucleotide (NADH) deficiency or history of favism. Other **toxicities** include nausea, vomiting, epigastric distress, and abdominal cramps.

 DRUG INTERACTIONS/FOOD INTERACTIONS

Insufficient data to make recommendations. Taking with food may minimize gastrointestinal toxicity.

 DOSING

Primaquine phosphate is supplied in tablets of 26.3 mg (=15 mg base).
Dose is 30 mg base/d PO × 14 d.

 SPECIAL POPULATIONS

RENAL IMPAIRMENT: There is no adjustment needed.

HEPATIC DYSFUNCTION: There is no adjustment needed.

PEDIATRICS: 0.5 mg/kg/d PO × 14 d.

 THE ART OF ANTIMICROBIAL THERAPY

Clinical Pearls

1. Primaquine is used in combination with chloroquine to eradicate the liver (nonerythrocytic) phase of *Plasmodium vivax* and *P. ovale*.
2. Patients should be screened for G6PD deficiency before administering primaquine.
3. CBC should be monitored during therapy.

Antibiotics Manual: A Guide to Commonly Used Antimicrobials, Second Edition. David Schlossberg and Rafik Samuel.
© 2017 John Wiley & Sons Ltd. Published 2017 by John Wiley & Sons Ltd.

BASIC CHARACTERISTICS

Class: Carbapenem.

Mechanism of Action: Binds penicillin-binding protein, disrupting cell wall synthesis.

Mechanisms of Resistance:

1. The PBP can be altered, with reduced affinity.
2. Production of a beta-lactamase, resulting in hydrolysis of the beta-lactam ring.
3. Decreased ability of the antibiotic to reach the PBP when bacteria decrease porin production, resulting in a decrease of the drug concentration within the cell.
4. Increased expression of efflux pump components.

Metabolic Route: Imipenem is metabolized in the kidneys by dehydropeptidase I, resulting in relatively low levels. Cilastatin sodium, an inhibitor of this enzyme, prevents renal metabolism; approximately 70 % of both imipenem and cilastatin are recovered in the urine.

 FDA-APPROVED INDICATIONS

Treatment of serious infections caused by susceptible strains of microorganisms in the conditions listed below:

1. **Lower respiratory tract infections**
2. **Urinary tract infections** (complicated and uncomplicated)
3. **Intra-abdominal infections**
4. **Gynecologic infections**
5. **Bacterial septicemia**
6. **Bone and joint infections**
7. **Skin and skin structure infections**
8. **Endocarditis**
9. **Polymicrobic infections**

 SIDE EFFECTS/TOXICITY

Imipenem is **contraindicated** in patients with known hypersensitivity to any component of this product or to other drugs in the same class or in patients who have demonstrated anaphylactic reactions to β-lactams. Before initiating therapy with imipenem, careful inquiries should be made concerning previous hypersensitivity reactions to penicillins, cephalosporins, other beta-lactams, and other allergens, because of the slightly increased possibility of hypersensitivity.

Seizures, phlebitis, fever, anaphylaxis, rash including Stevens–Johnson syndrome, erythema multiforme and toxic epidermal necrolysis, angioedema, hypotension, encephalopathy, hearing loss, diarrhea, *Clostridium difficile*-associated diarrhea and pseudomembranous colitis, oral candidiasis, glossitis, anorexia, nausea, vomiting, stomach cramps, hepatitis, renal impairment, genital pruritis, dyspnea, polyarthralgia, pyuria, hematuria, prolonged prothrombin time, pancytopenia, positive Coombs' test, decreased serum sodium, and increased potassium and chloride.

Antibiotics Manual: A Guide to Commonly Used Antimicrobials, Second Edition. David Schlossberg and Rafik Samuel.
© 2017 John Wiley & Sons Ltd. Published 2017 by John Wiley & Sons Ltd.

DRUG INTERACTIONS/FOOD INTERACTIONS

Ganciclovir should not be used with imipenem unless the potential benefits outweigh the risks.

Imipenem may reduce serum valproic acid concentrations; levels should be monitored.

It is not recommended that probenecid be given with imipenem.

 DOSING

Intravenous dosage schedule for adults with normal renal function and body weight ≥70 kg:

Type of infection	Susceptible	Moderately susceptible
Mild	250 mg q 6 hours	500 mg q 6 h
Moderate	500 mg q 8 or 6 hours	500 mg q 6 h or 1 g q 8 h
Severe	500 mg q 6 hours	1 g q 8 or 6 h
Uncomplicated UTI	250 mg q 6 hours	250 mg q 6 h
Complicated UTI	500 mg q 6 hours	500 mg q 6 h

 SPECIAL POPULATIONS

RENAL IMPAIRMENT:

Creatinine clearance, mL/min	Dose
50–80	500 mg q 6 hours
10–50	500 mg q 8 hours
<10	250 mg q 12 hours
<5	Avoid
After hemodialysis or peritoneal dialysis	250 mg
CRRT	500 mg q 8 hours

HEPATIC DYSFUNCTION: No dose adjustment is necessary.

PEDIATRICS:

<1 week of age	25 mg/kg every 12 hours
1–4 weeks of age	25 mg/kg every 8 hours
4 weeks–3 months of age	25 mg/kg every 6 hours
3 months to <3 years of age	25 mg/kg/dose q 6 hours
3–12 years of age	15 mg/kg/dose q 6 hours

Imipenem is not recommended in pediatric patients <30 kg with impaired renal function.

THE ART OF ANTIMICROBIAL THERAPY

Clinical Pearls

1. Imipenem must be dose-adjusted for renal dysfunction.
2. Cross allergy with penicillins is <10%.
3. Imipenem is not indicated in patients with meningitis because safety and efficacy have not been established and seizure potential is increased in the presence of CNS inflammation.
4. Imipenem is active against many organisms carrying extended spectrum beta-lactamases.

PROLOPRIM (Trimethoprim)

 BASIC CHARACTERISTICS

Class: Antimetabolite.

Mechanism of Action: Trimethoprim blocks the production of tetrahydrofolic acid from dihydrofolic acid by binding to and reversibly inhibiting the required enzyme, dihydrofolate reductase.

Mechanisms of Resistance: Plasmid-mediated alterations in dihydrofolate reductase and changes in cell permeability.

Metabolic Route: Ten to twenty percent of trimethoprim is metabolized in the liver; the remainder is excreted unchanged in the urine.

 FDA-APPROVED INDICATIONS

Treatment of initial episodes of uncomplicated urinary tract infections due to susceptible organisms.

Also Used for: Trimethoprim can be combined with dapsone for the treatment of PCP.

 SIDE EFFECTS/TOXICITY

Contraindicated in individuals hypersensitive to trimethoprim and in those with documented megaloblastic anemia due to folate deficiency.

Side effects include serious hypersensitivity reactions with anaphylaxis, exfoliative dermatitis, erythema multiforme, Stevens–Johnson syndrome, toxic epidermal necrolysis (Lyell syndrome), pruritus, phototoxicity, epigastric distress, nausea, vomiting, glossitis, aseptic meningitis, thrombocytopenia, leukopenia, neutropenia, megaloblastic anemia, methemoglobinemia, hyperkalemia, hyponatremia, increases in BUN, serum creatinine, serum transaminase, and bilirubin.

 DRUG INTERACTIONS/FOOD INTERACTIONS

Trimethoprim can be administered with or without food.

Trimethoprim increases phenytoin half-life.

Trimethoprim can interfere with a serum methotrexate assay and with the Jaffé alkaline picrate reaction assay for creatinine, resulting in overestimations of about 10 % in the range of normal values.

 DOSING

Trimethoprim is administered in 100 mg and 200 mg tablets.

The usual dosage is 100 mg every 12 hours or 200 mg every 24 hours, each for 10 days.

Antibiotics Manual: A Guide to Commonly Used Antimicrobials, Second Edition. David Schlossberg and Rafik Samuel.
© 2017 John Wiley & Sons Ltd. Published 2017 by John Wiley & Sons Ltd.

SPECIAL POPULATIONS

RENAL IMPAIRMENT:

Creatinine clearance, mL/min	Dose
10–50	Usual dose every 18 hours
<10	Usual dose every 24 hours
Hemodialysis	Usual dose after dialysis only
CAPD	Usual dose every 24 hours
CRRT	No data

HEPATIC DYSFUNCTION: Use with caution.

PEDIATRICS: Safety and effectiveness in pediatric patients below the age of 2 months have not been established. The effectiveness of trimethoprim as a single agent has not been established in pediatric patients under 12 years of age.

 THE ART OF ANTIMICROBIAL THERAPY

Clinical Pearls

1. Complete blood counts should be obtained if any of these signs are noted in a patient receiving trimethoprim and the drug discontinued if a significant reduction in the count of any formed blood element is found.
2. Trimethoprim should not be given to patients with documented megaloblastic anemia due to folate deficiency.
3. It may be beneficial to measure levels of concomitantly administered phenytoin.

PYRAZINAMIDE

 ## BASIC CHARACTERISTICS

Class: Pyrazine analog of nicotinamide.
Mechanisms of Action: Unknown.
Mechanisms of Resistance: Point mutations in the pyrazinamidase gene.
Metabolic Route: Hydrolyzed in the liver and excreted in the urine.

 ## FDA-APPROVED INDICATIONS

Treatment of active tuberculosis in combination with other antimycobacterials.

 ## SIDE EFFECTS/TOXICITY

Pyrazinamide inhibits renal excretion of urates, leading to hyperuricemia or gout; more commonly, it produces nongouty polyarthralgias. Also seen: fever, hypersensitivity, anorexia, nausea, vomiting, diarrhea, hepatitis, cutaneous flushing, porphyria, dysuria, thrombocytopenia, and sideroblastic anemia.

 ## DRUG INTERACTIONS/FOOD INTERACTIONS

Interferes with Ketostix and Acetest, producing a brown color.
Food impairs absorption slightly, but this is of minimal clinical significance and improves G-I tolerance.

 ## DOSING

15–30 mg/kg orally once daily, with a maximum of 2 grams per day.
Twice-weekly dose: 40–55 kg: 2000 mg; 56–75 kg: 3000 mg; 76–90 kg: 4000 mg (maximum).
Thrice-weekly dose: 40–55 kg: 1500 mg; 56–75 kg: 2500 mg; 76–90 kg: 3000 mg (maximum).

 ## SPECIAL POPULATIONS

RENAL IMPAIRMENT: 25–35 mg/kg, 3 times/week (not daily).

HEPATIC DYSFUNCTION: No dose adjustment, but use with caution.

PEDIATRICS: It is administered orally 15–30 mg/kg once daily, with a maximum of 2 grams per day. Twice-weekly dose: 50 mg/kg, maximum 4 grams.

THE ART OF ANTIMICROBIAL THERAPY

Clinical Pearls

1. Pyrazinamide should never be used alone in the treatment of active tuberculosis.
2. The regimen of pyrazinamide plus rifampin for treatment of latent TB is no longer indicated, due to hepatotoxicity.

Antibiotics Manual: A Guide to Commonly Used Antimicrobials, Second Edition. David Schlossberg and Rafik Samuel.
© 2017 John Wiley & Sons Ltd. Published 2017 by John Wiley & Sons Ltd.

3. Patients with acute gout should not receive pyrazinamide.

4. Pyrazinamide should be used with caution in patients with liver disease and avoided if possible in patients with severe liver damage.

5. Hepatic and hematologic function should be monitored at least monthly in all patients.

6. The dosage of pyrazinamide should not be divided; it is given as a single daily dose.

QUINIDINE

 BASIC CHARACTERISTICS

Class: Antimalarial agent and class 1a antiarrhythmic.

Mechanism of Action: Quinidine acts primarily as an intraerythrocytic schizonticide, with little effect upon sporozoites or upon pre-erythrocytic parasites. Quinidine is gametocidal to *Plasmodium vivax* and *P. malariae*, but not to *P. falciparum*.

Metabolic Route: Most quinidine is metabolized by the liver's cytochrome p450 system.

 FDA-APPROVED INDICATIONS

Approved for treatment of various arrhythmias.

Also Used for: Parenteral treatment of severe malaria (all *Plasmodium* species) and life-threatening *Plasmodium falciparum* malaria.

 SIDE EFFECTS/TOXICITY

> **WARNING:** Increased mortality in patients who take quinidine to treat or prevent arrhythmias.

Quinidine is **contraindicated**:

1. In patients who are known to be allergic to it or who have developed thrombocytopenic purpura during prior therapy with quinidine or quinine.
2. In the absence of a functioning artificial pacemaker, quinidine is also **contraindicated** in any patient whose cardiac rhythm is dependent upon a junctional or idioventricular pacemaker, including patients in complete atrioventricular block.
3. In those with myasthenia gravis and others who might be adversely affected by an anticholinergic agent.

Other **toxicity** includes: fever, angioedema rash, **cinchonism** (a syndrome that may also include tinnitus, reversible high-frequency hearing loss, deafness, vertigo, blurred vision, diplopia, photophobia, headache, confusion, and delirium), prolongation of QTc interval leading to torsades de pointes, other ventricular arrhythmias, paradoxical increase in ventricular rate in atrial flutter/fibrillation, bradycardia in patients with sick sinus syndrome, hepatotoxicity, bronchospasm, pneumonitis, lymphadenopathy, uveitis, visual disturbances, the sicca syndrome, arthralgia, myalgia, vasculitis, a lupus-like syndrome, psychosis, seizures, and ataxia, elevation in serum levels of skeletal–muscle enzymes, hemolytic anemia, thrombocytopenic purpura, and agranulocytosis.

DRUG INTERACTIONS/FOOD INTERACTIONS

Quinidine levels may be **increased** by drugs that alkalinize the urine (carbonic anhydrase inhibitors, sodium bicarbonate, thiazide diuretics), amiodarone or cimetidine, ketaconazole, and diltiazem.

Quinidine levels may be **decreased** by nifedipine, phenobarbital, phenytoin, rifampin, and verapamil.

Quinidine may result in **increased levels** or potentiated effects of digoxin warfarin, drugs metabolized by cytochrome P450IID6 (e.g., phenothiazines, polycyclic antidepressants, codeine, hydrocodone), procainamide, verapamil haloperidol and calcium channel blockers, and depolarizing neuromuscular blocking agents.

Antibiotics Manual: A Guide to Commonly Used Antimicrobials, Second Edition. David Schlossberg and Rafik Samuel.
© 2017 John Wiley & Sons Ltd. Published 2017 by John Wiley & Sons Ltd.

DOSING

10 mg/kg IV loading dose (maximum 600 mg) in normal saline over 1–2 hours, followed by continuous hours, followed by continuous infusion of 0.02 mg/kg/min until PO therapy can be started.

 SPECIAL POPULATIONS

RENAL IMPAIRMENT: Quinidine levels may increase, so dose reduction is recommended.

HEPATIC DYSFUNCTION: Quinidine levels may increase, so dose reduction is recommended.

PEDIATRICS: for treatment: Same dose as adults.

 THE ART OF ANTIMICROBIAL THERAPY

Clinical Pearls

1. Overly rapid infusion of quinidine may cause peripheral vascular collapse and severe hypotension.
2. Patients should be monitored for the adverse events listed above, particularly blood pressure, serum glucose, and EKG (e.g., for QTc prolongation).
3. Quinidine has many drug–drug interactions, which affect the levels of coadministered drugs as well as the levels of quinidine.

QUININE

Quinine sulfate is available as Qualaquin for PO administration; quinine can also be administered intravenously or intramuscularly.

 BASIC CHARACTERISTICS

Class: Antimalarial agent.

Mechanism of Action: Quinine inhibits nucleic acid synthesis, protein synthesis, and glycolysis in *Plasmodium falciparum* and can bind with hemazoin in parasitized erythrocytes.

Metabolic Route: Quinine is metabolized by the liver and excreted partially in the urine.

 FDA-APPROVED INDICATIONS

PO quinine sulfate is indicated only for treatment of uncomplicated *Plasmodium falciparum* malaria.

Also Used for: *P. vivax* malaria and babesiosis.

⚜ SIDE EFFECTS/TOXICITY

Quinine is **contraindicated** in patients with a prolonged QT interval, G-6-PD deficiency, myasthenia gravis, optic neuritis, or known hypersensitivity to quinine, mefloquine, or quinidine.

Side effects: "Cinchonism" occurs to some degree in almost all patients taking quinine. Symptoms include headache, vasodilation and sweating, nausea, tinnitus, hearing impairment, vertigo or dizziness, blurred vision, and disturbance in color perception. More severe symptoms of cinchonism are vomiting, diarrhea, abdominal pain, deafness, blindness, and disturbances in cardiac rhythm or conduction. Most symptoms of cinchonism are reversible and resolve with discontinuation of quinine.

Other side effects include:

General: fever, chills, sweating, flushing, asthenia, lupus-like syndrome, and hypersensitivity reactions.

Hematologic: agranulocytosis, hypoprothrombinemia, thrombocytopenia, disseminated intravascular coagulation, hemolytic anemia, hemolytic uremic syndrome, thrombotic thrombocytopenic purpura, coagulopathy, and lupus anticoagulant.

Neuropsychiatric: headache, diplopia, confusion, seizures, coma, tremors, ataxia, acute dystonic reaction, aphasia, and suicide.

Dermatologic: rashes, pruritus, erythema multiforme, Stevens–Johnson syndrome, toxic epidermal necrolysis, photosensitivity reactions, acral necrosis, and cutaneous vasculitis.

Cardiovascular: chest pain, vasodilatation, hypotension, postural hypotension, tachycardia, bradycardia, palpitations, syncope, atrioventricular block, atrial fibrillation, irregular rhythm, unifocal premature ventricular contractions, nodal escape beats, U waves, QT prolongation, ventricular fibrillation, ventricular tachycardia, torsades de pointes, and cardiac arrest.

Gastrointestinal: nausea, vomiting, diarrhea, abdominal pain, gastric irritation, and esophagitis.

Miscellaneous: hepatitis, asthma, dyspnea, pulmonary edema, hypoglycemia, myalgias and muscle weakness, hemoglobinuria, renal failure, acute interstitial nephritis, visual disturbances, optic neuritis, blindness, vertigo, tinnitus, hearing impairment, and deafness.

Antibiotics Manual: A Guide to Commonly Used Antimicrobials, Second Edition. David Schlossberg and Rafik Samuel.
© 2017 John Wiley & Sons Ltd. Published 2017 by John Wiley & Sons Ltd.

DRUG INTERACTIONS/FOOD INTERACTIONS

Quinine should be taken with food to minimize GI discomfort.

The concomitant administration of the following should be **avoided**: antacids, rifampin, troleandomycin, erythromycin, astemizole, cisapride, terfenadine, halofantrine, pimozide, mefloquine, and quinidine.

Concomitant administration of the following may result in changes in the level of quinine and/or the coadministered drug, and monitoring is recommended:

Aminophylline: aminophylline levels decreased.

Carbamazepine: decreased levels of quinine, increased levels of carbamazepine.

CYP2D6 substrates: e.g., desipramine, flecainide, debrisoquine, dextromethorphan, metoprolol, or paroxetine-increased level of the CYP2D6 substrate.

Digoxin: increased levels of digoxin.

Histamine H2-receptor blockers: increased levels of quinine.

HMG-CoA reductase (statins): levels of statins increased.

Ketoconazole: increased levels of quinine.

Neuromuscular blocking agents, succinylcholine and tubocurarine: levels of neuromuscular blocking agents increased.

Phenobarbital: decreased levels of quinine, increased levels of phenobarbital.

Phenytoin: decreased levels of quinine.

Tetracycline: increased levels of quinine.

Theophylline: theophylline levels decreased.

Warfarin: increased levels of warfarin.

Quinine may produce an elevated value for urinary 17-ketogenic steroids when the Zimmerman method is used.

 DOSING

For treatment of uncomplicated *P. falciparum* or *P. vivax* malaria in adults, dosage of PO quinine sulfate is 648 mg PO (two capsules) q 8 h for 3–7 days.

For severe illness, quinine is given intravenously (not FDA approved), as follows:

Loading dose of 20 mg/kg in 5 % dextrose over 4 hours, followed by 10 mg/kg over 2–4 hours q 8 h (maximum 1800 mg/d until PO therapy can be started.

Babesiosis: 648 mg PO tid or qid × 7–10 d.

 SPECIAL POPULATIONS

RENAL IMPAIRMENT: In patients with acute uncomplicated malaria and severe chronic renal failure, the following modified dosage regimen is recommended: one loading dose of 648 mg followed 12 hours later by maintenance doses of 324 mg every 12 hours.

The effects of mild and moderate renal impairment on the pharmacokinetics and safety of quinine sulfate are not known.

HEPATIC DYSFUNCTION: Patients with mild to moderate hepatic impairment (Child Pugh A and Child Pugh B, respectively) should be monitored closely for adverse reactions; dosage reduction is not warranted.

The effects of severe hepatic impairment (Child Pugh C) on the safety and pharmacokinetics of quinine sulfate are not known.

PEDIATRICS:

Malaria: 30 mg/kg/d PO in 3 doses × 3 **or** 7 d 11.

Babesiosis: 24 mg/kg/d (maximum 600 mg/dose) PO in 3 doses × 7–10 d.

IV dosage: same as for adults.

 THE ART OF ANTIMICROBIAL THERAPY

Clinical Pearls

1. Quinine is not approved for patients with severe or complicated *P. falciparum* malaria or the prophylaxis of malaria.
2. Quinine is not recommended for the treatment of leg cramps.
3. Serologic testing for quinine-specific antibody may be useful for identifying the specific cause of thrombocytopenia in individual cases.
4. Continuous EKG, blood pressure, and glucose monitoring are recommended.
5. IV quinine is not available in the United States. It may be available through a compounding pharmacy: Call the National Association of Compounding Pharmacies (800-687-7850) or Professional Compounding Centers of America (800-331-2498, www.pccarx.com).

BASIC CHARACTERISTICS

Class: Neuraminidase inhibitor.

Mechanism of Action: Inhibitor of influenza virus neuraminidase.

Mechanisms of Resistance: Amino acid substitutions in the viral neuraminidase or hemagglutinin proteins.

Metabolic Route: Cleared by renal excretion and can be cleared by hemodialysis.

 ## FDA-APPROVED INDICATIONS

Acute uncomplicated influenza in patients 18 years and older who have been symptomatic for no more than 2 days.

 ## SIDE EFFECTS/TOXICITY

Diarrhea, serious skin reactions, hallucinations, delirium, abnormal behavior, hepatitis, hyperglycemia, elevated CPK, constipation, insomnia, hypertension, and neutropenia.

 ## DRUG INTERACTIONS/FOOD INTERACTIONS

Not known.

 ## DOSING

Administer within 2 days of onset of symptoms of influenza. The recommended dose in adult patients 18 years of age or older with acute uncomplicated influenza is a single 600 mg dose, administered via intravenous infusion for 15 to 30 minutes.

 ## SPECIAL POPULATIONS

RENAL IMPAIRMENT:

Creatinine clearance, mL/min	Dose, mg
>50	600
30–49	200
10–29	100

HD: give adjusted dose after dialysis.

If hemodialysed, give after hemodialysis on hemodialysis days.

HEPATIC DYSFUNCTION: No adjustment is necessary.

PEDIATRICS: Safety and effectiveness in pediatric patients younger than 18 years has not been established.

Antibiotics Manual: A Guide to Commonly Used Antimicrobials, Second Edition. David Schlossberg and Rafik Samuel.
© 2017 John Wiley & Sons Ltd. Published 2017 by John Wiley & Sons Ltd.

THE ART OF ANTIMICROBIAL THERAPY

Clinical Pearls

1. Inactivated influenza vaccine can be administered at any time relative to use of peramivir.

2. Avoid use of LAIV within 2 weeks before or 48 hours after administration of peramivir unless medically indicated.

3. Peramivir is only indicated for uncomplicated influenza.

BASIC CHARACTERISTICS

Class: Neuraminidase inhibitor.

Mechanism of Action: Zanamivir is an inhibitor of influenza virus neuraminidase affecting release of viral particles.

Mechanism of Resistance: Mutations in the viral neuraminidase or viral hemagglutinin (or both).

Metabolic Route: Up to 17 % of the inhaled compound is absorbed systemically. It is excreted unchanged in the urine.

 FDA-APPROVED INDICATIONS

Treatment of uncomplicated influenza A and B virus in adults and pediatric patients 7 years of age and older who have been symptomatic for no more than 2 days.

Prophylaxis of influenza in adults and pediatric patients 5 years of age and older.

 SIDE EFFECTS/TOXICITY

Zanamivir is not recommended for treatment or prophylaxis of influenza in individuals with underlying airways disease (such as asthma or chronic obstructive pulmonary disease). Serious cases of bronchospasm, including fatalities, have been reported in patients with and without underlying airways disease. Zanamivir should be discontinued in any patient who develops bronchospasm or decline in respiratory function.

Zanamivir should not be used in patients with allergies to milk products.

Other adverse reactions include allergic-like reactions, including oropharyngeal edema, serious skin rashes, and anaphylaxis, delirium, seizures and abnormal behavior, arrhythmias, syncope, seizures, rash, sinusitis, dizziness, fever, chills, and arthralgias.

 DRUG INTERACTIONS/FOOD INTERACTIONS

Live attenuated influenza vaccine (LAIV) should not be administered within 2 weeks before or 48 hours after administration of zanamivir.

 DOSING

Administration to the respiratory tract by oral inhalation only, using the DISKHALER device provided. The recommended dose of zanamivir for treatment of influenza in adults and pediatric patients 7 years of age and older is 10 mg twice daily (approximately 12 hours apart) for 5 days.

The recommended dose of zanamivir for prophylaxis of influenza in adults and pediatric patients 5 years of age and older in a household setting is 10 mg once daily for 10 days.

The recommended dose of zanamivir for prophylaxis of influenza in adults and adolescents in a community setting is 10 mg once daily for 28 days.

Antibiotics Manual: A Guide to Commonly Used Antimicrobials, Second Edition. David Schlossberg and Rafik Samuel.
© 2017 John Wiley & Sons Ltd. Published 2017 by John Wiley & Sons Ltd.

SPECIAL POPULATIONS

RENAL IMPAIRMENT: No dose adjustment is recommended.

HEPATIC DYSFUNCTION: Zanamivir has not been studied in those with hepatic impairment.

PEDIATRICS: Used for treatment in children 7 years and older and prophylaxis for children 5 years and older. The dose is the same as for adults.

 THE ART OF ANTIMICROBIAL THERAPY

Clinical Pearls
1. Zanamivir has activity against both influenza A and B.
2. Zanamivir is active against avian H5N1 and novel H1N1 influenza.
3. Resistance in zanamivir leads to resistance in oseltamivir; however, zanamivir remains active against novel H1N1 in the presence of oseltamivir resistance.
4. Do not administer zanamivir at the same time as the live influenza vaccine.
5. Zanamivir is not recommended for treatment or prophylaxis of influenza in patients with underlying airways disease.
6. Zanamivir has not been proven effective for prophylaxis in nursing home residents.

Also available combined with lamivudine as Combivir and with both lamivudine and abacavir as Trizivir.

 BASIC CHARACTERISTICS

Class: Nucleoside reverse transcriptase inhibitor (NRTI) with activity against HIV.

Mechanism of Action: Converted by cellular enzymes to its active drug zidovudine triphosphate, an analog of thymidine triphosphate. The zidovudine triphosphate competes with the naturally occurring nucleotide for incorporation in newly forming HIV DNA. Since zidovudine triphosphate does not have a terminal hydroxyl group, it halts transcription and replication of the virus.

Mechanism of Resistance: Changes in the structure of HIV reverse transcriptase leads to pyrophosphorolysis of the nucleoside analog that allows transcription of DNA to continue. Resistance mutations include the "TAMS": 41L, 67N, 70R, 210W, 215F, and 219E.

Metabolic Route: Zidovudine is primarily eliminated by hepatic metabolism. The major metabolite of zidovudine is 3′-azido-3′-deoxy-5′-O-β-D-glucopyranuronosylthymidine.

 FDA-APPROVED INDICATIONS

Treatment of HIV infection, in combination with other antiretrovirals.

 SIDE EFFECTS/TOXICITY

> **WARNING:** Zidovudine is associated with **hematologic toxicity** including neutropenia and severe anemia particularly in patients with advanced HIV.
>
> Prolonged use of zidovudine has been associated with symptomatic **myopathy**.
>
> **Lactic acidosis and severe hepatomegaly with steatosis**, including fatal cases, have been reported with the use of nucleoside analogs alone or in combination, including zidovudine.

Other side effects: Immune reconstitution inflammatory syndrome, fat redistribution including central obesity and dorsocervical fat enlargement, peripheral wasting, facial wasting, breast enlargement, fever, cough, headache, malaise, nausea, anorexia, and vomiting.

 DRUG INTERACTIONS/FOOD INTERACTIONS

Zidovudine can be taken with or without food and is unaffected by pH.

Zidovudine should not be used with stavudine since they are both thymidine analogs and may be antagonistic.

Zidovudine should not be administered with ribavirin or doxorubicin.

 DOSING

Zidovudine is administered in 100 and 300 mg tablets, via intravenous injection or in a pale strawberry flavored liquid, which contains 50 mg/cc. The recommended adult dose is 300 mg twice daily.

Antibiotics Manual: A Guide to Commonly Used Antimicrobials, Second Edition. David Schlossberg and Rafik Samuel.
© 2017 John Wiley & Sons Ltd. Published 2017 by John Wiley & Sons Ltd.

SPECIAL POPULATIONS

RENAL IMPAIRMENT: In patients on dialysis, the recommended dose is 100 mg every 8 hours.

HEPATIC DYSFUNCTION: No dose adjustment necessary.

PEDIATRICS: The approved dose is 160 mg/m^2 every 8 hours (480 mg/m^2/day up to a maximum of 200 mg every 8 hours).

 THE ART OF ANTIMICROBIAL THERAPY

Clinical Pearls

1. Zidovudine should be used in combination with other antiretroviral agents.
2. Zidovudine is present in three different medications: Retrovir, Trizivir, and Combivir.
3. Unlike other NRTIs, pharmacokinetic studies do not support once daily dosing.

Also available with cobicistat as Evotaz.

 BASIC CHARACTERISTICS

Class: Protease inhibitor.

Mechanism of Action: Atazanavir reversibly binds the active site of the enzyme protease. Inhibition of protease prevents cleavage of the *gag* and *gag-pol* polyprotein, resulting in the production of immature, noninfectious virus.

Mechanism of Resistance: Development of mutations on the enzyme protease causes a conformational change that prevents atazanavir from binding the active site, allowing protease activity to continue. The most frequent resistance mutations include I50L.

Metabolic Route: Atazanavir is mostly excreted in the feces.

 FDA-APPROVED INDICATIONS

Treatment of HIV-1 in combinations with other antiretroviral agents.

 SIDE EFFECTS/TOXICITY

New-onset diabetes mellitus, exacerbation of preexisting diabetes mellitus, hyperglycemia, increased bleeding, including spontaneous skin hematomas and hemarthrosis, in patients with hemophilia types A and B, redistribution/accumulation of body fat including central obesity, dorsocervical fat enlargement (buffalo hump), peripheral wasting, facial wasting, breast enlargement, "cushingoid appearance", immune reconstitution syndrome, rash, nephrolithiasis, prolongation of PR interval, QTc prolongation, torsades de pointes, abdominal pain, headache, anorexia, dyspepsia, epigastric pain, hepatitis, mouth ulceration, pancreatitis, vomiting, anemia, leucopenia, thrombocytopenia, increases in alkaline phosphatase, amylase, creatine phosphokinase, lactic dehydrogenase, SGOT, SGPT, indirect bilirubin, gamma glutamyl transpeptidase, hyperlipemia, hyperuricemia, hyperglycemia, hypoglycemia, and dehydration.

 DRUG INTERACTIONS/FOOD INTERACTIONS

Atazanavir should be taken with a meal, even when given with ritonavir.

Drugs that should not be coadministered with atazanavir include alfuzosin, rifampin, irinotecan, lurasidone, pimozide, midazolam, triazolam, ergot derivatives, cisapride, simvastatin, lovastatin, indinavir, nevirapine, salmeterol, fluticasone, colchicine in renal or hepatic impairment, or Evotaz.

Atazanavir is an inhibitor of the CYP3A enzyme and UGT1A1; coadministration of atazanavir and drugs primarily metabolized by CYP3A or UGT1A1 may result in increased plasma concentrations of the other drug, which could increase or prolong its therapeutic and adverse effects.

Atazanavir is metabolized by CYP3A; coadministration of atazanavir and drugs that induce CYP3A may decrease atazanavir plasma concentrations and reduce its therapeutic effect. Coadministration of atazanavir and drugs that inhibit CYP3A may increase atazanavir plasma concentrations. Because of these metabolic affects, potential drug interactions that may require dosage change or clinical/laboratory monitoring are listed below:

Antibiotics Manual: A Guide to Commonly Used Antimicrobials, Second Edition. David Schlossberg and Rafik Samuel.
© 2017 John Wiley & Sons Ltd. Published 2017 by John Wiley & Sons Ltd.

Medication	Adjustment or action
Itraconazole	Monitor for toxicity
Voriconazole	Monitor for toxicity
Rifabutin	Decrease rifabutin to 150/qod or 3 × week
Contraceptives	Use lowest effective dose
Atorvastatin	Use lowest possible dose with close monitoring
Phenobarbital, phenytoin or carbamazepine	Monitor anticonvulsant level; consider alternative
Sildenafil	25 mg every 48 hours
Tadalafil	5 mg, no more than 10 mg in 72 hours
Vardenafil	2.5 mg in 24 hours
Diltiazem	ECG monitoring recommended
H2 receptors	Not recommended with unboosted atazanavir.
	Dose should not exceed 40 mg bid equivalent of famotidine if ritonavir with boosted atazanavir is used
PPI	Not recommended with unboosted atazanavir.
	Dose should not exceed 20 mg equivalent of omeprazole and should be given 12 hours before ritonavir with boosted atazanavir
Antacids	Administer 2 hours apart
Didanosine	Administer separately from atazanavir
Tenofovir	Not recommended with unboosted atazanavir
Efavirenz	Not recommended with unboosted atazanavir
Maraviroc	Maraviroc dose is 150 mg bid
Quetiapine	Administer one-sixth of the quetiapine dose
Bosentan	Bosentan dose is 62.5 mg daily

 ## DOSING

Atazanavir is available in 150, 200, and 300 mg capsules.

It is also available in an oral powder with 50 mg per packet.

For treatment-naive patients, the recommended dosage is atazanavir 300 mg with ritonavir 100 mg once daily (all as a single dose with food).

For treatment-naive patients who are unable to tolerate ritonavir, the recommended dosage is atazanavir 400 mg (without ritonavir) once daily taken with food.

For treatment-experienced patients, the recommended dose is atazanavir 300 mg with ritonavir 100 mg once daily (all as a single dose with food).

 ## SPECIAL POPULATIONS

RENAL IMPAIRMENT: For patients with renal impairment, including those with severe renal impairment who are not managed with hemodialysis, no dose adjustment is required.

Treatment-naive patients with end-stage renal disease managed with hemodialysis should receive atazanavir 300 mg with ritonavir 100 mg. Atazanavir should not be administered to HIV-treatment-experienced patients with end-stage renal disease managed with hemodialysis.

HEPATIC DYSFUNCTION: Atazanavir should be used with caution in patients with mild-to-moderate hepatic impairment. For patients with Child Pugh* class B who have not experienced prior virologic failure, a dose reduction to 300 mg once daily should be considered. Atazanavir should not be used in patients with Child Pugh class C. Atazanavir/ritonavir has not been studied in subjects with hepatic impairment and is not recommended.

PEDIATRICS: The recommended daily dosage of atazanavir with ritonavir in patients at least 3 months of age and at least 5 kg:

Weight	Atazanavir	Ritonavir
5 kg to <15 kg	200 mg (powder)	80 mg
15 kg to <25 kg	250 mg (powder)	80 mg
15 kg to <20 kg	150 mg capsule	100 mg
20 kg to <40	200 mg capsule	100 mg
40 kg and over	300 mg capsule	100 mg

For treatment-naive patients at least 13 years of age and at least 40 kg, who are unable to tolerate ritonavir, the recommended dose is atazanavir 400 mg (without ritonavir) once daily with food.

 ## THE ART OF ANTIMICROBIAL THERAPY

Clinical Pearls

1. Atazanavir should always be used in combination with other antiretrovirals.
2. Atazanavir should be taken with food to increase absorption.
3. Atazanavir should be boosted with ritonavir or cobicistat when combined with tenofovir.
4. When atazanavir is boosted with ritonavir, the 2 medications should be administered at the same time.
5. Avoid PPI or H2 blockers if atazanavir is given unboosted.
6. Whenever initiating atazanavir, make sure to review all medications the patient is receiving to minimize drug interactions.
7. Atazanavir causes an increase in indirect bilirubin by inhibiting glucuronidation.
8. Atazanavir causes nephrolithiasis; patients should be advised to drink adequate water.
9. Rash is not infrequent on atazanavir even though it does not contain a sulfa moiety.
10. Atazanavir dose should be increased to 400 mg with 100 mg of ritonavir if given with tenofovir during the second or third trimesters.

* See Helpful Formulas, Equations, and Definitions for definitions.

Also available combined with INH as Rifamate and combined with INH plus pyrazinamide as Rifater.

 BASIC CHARACTERISTICS

Class: Rifamycin.

Mechanisms of Action: Rifampin inhibits DNA-dependent RNA polymerase activity in susceptible cells.

Mechanisms of Resistance: Resistance occurs as single-step mutations of the DNA-dependent RNA polymerase.

Metabolic Route: Rapidly eliminated in the bile and undergoes progressive deacetylation and is eliminated. However, up to 30% of a dose is excreted in the urine, with about half of this being unchanged drug.

 FDA-APPROVED INDICATIONS

Treatment of all forms of tuberculosis.

Treatment of asymptomatic carriers of *Neisseria meningitidis* to eliminate meningococci from the nasopharynx.

Also Used for:

Treatment of latent tuberculosis (LTBI).

Combination therapy for *Staphylococcus aureus* infections.

Combination therapy for prosthetic valve endocarditis due to coagulase negative staphylococci.

Other foreign body infections in combination with tetracyclines and fluoroquinolones.

 SIDE EFFECTS/TOXICITY

Rifampin is **contraindicated** in patients with a history of hypersensitivity to any of the rifamycins.

Adverse events: anaphylaxis, liver dysfunction, reddish coloration of the urine, sweat, sputum, and tears, "flu syndrome" (fever, chills, and malaise), rash, flushing, epigastric distress, anorexia, nausea, vomiting, flatulence, *Clostridium difficile*-associated diarrhea, disseminated intravascular coagulation, visual disturbances, adrenal insufficiency, confusion, renal insufficiency, elevations in serum uric acid, thrombocytopenia, leukopenia, and hemolytic anemia.

 DRUG INTERACTIONS/FOOD INTERACTIONS

Absorption of rifampin is reduced when the drug is ingested with food, but absorption is usually adequate, and ingestion with food reduces GI intolerance.

Rifampin is known to induce certain cytochrome P-450 enzymes. Administration of rifampin with drugs that undergo biotransformation through these metabolic pathways may accelerate elimination and decrease the therapeutic effect of these coadministered drugs, many of which require monitoring and possible adjustment during and following coadministration with rifampin.

The list of drugs so affected includes the following drugs/classes: anticonvulsants, antiarrhythmics, oral anticoagulants, antifungals, barbiturates, beta-blockers, calcium channel blockers, chloramphenicol, clarithromycin, corticosteroids, cyclosporine, cardiac glycoside preparations, clofibrate, hormonal contraceptives (patients should be advised to use nonhormonal methods of birth control during rifampin therapy), dapsone, diazepam, doxycycline, enalapril, fluoroquinolones, haloperidol,

Antibiotics Manual: A Guide to Commonly Used Antimicrobials, Second Edition. David Schlossberg and Rafik Samuel.
© 2017 John Wiley & Sons Ltd. Published 2017 by John Wiley & Sons Ltd.

oral hypoglycemic agents, levothyroxine, methadone, narcotic analgesics, nortriptyline, progestins, quinine, tacrolimus, sulfapyridine, theophylline, tricyclic antidepressants, protease inhibitors, nonnucleoside reverse transcriptase inhibitors, CCR5 inhibitors and zidovudine.

Rifampin levels may increase when coadministered with atovaquone, probenecid, and cotrimoxazole, and may decrease when given with ketoconazole and antacids (give rifampin at least 1 hour before the ingestion of antacids).

When rifampin is given concomitantly with either halothane or isoniazid, the potential for hepatotoxicity is increased and concomitant use of rifampin and halothane should be avoided.

Drug/laboratory interactions

Cross-reactivity and false-positive urine screening tests for opiates have been reported in patients receiving rifampin.

Therapeutic levels of rifampin have been shown to inhibit standard microbiological assays for serum folate and vitamin B12.

Anti-retroviral therapy interacts significantly with rifampin. The following caveats apply;

Rifampin	
Usual dose	Efavirenz (Sustiva, Atripla): usual dose
	Nevirapine: usual dose
	Maraviroc: 600 bid
	Raltegravir: 800 bid
	Dolutegravir (Triumeq): 50 bid if no INSTI mutations
Contraindicated	Complera, Descovy
Contraindicated	Genvoya, Stribild
Contraindicated	Prezcobix
Contraindicated	Descovy

DOSING

Rifampin is supplied as 150 mg and 300 mg tablets. It can also be administered intravenously.

Tuberculosis: 10 mg/kg, in a single daily administration up to 600 mg/day, oral or IV. The same dosage can be given twice or thrice weekly.

Meningococcal carriers: 600 mg rifampin administered twice daily for two days.

SPECIAL POPULATIONS

RENAL IMPAIRMENT: No dose adjustment is necessary.

HEPATIC DYSFUNCTION: Patients with impaired liver function should be given rifampin only in cases of necessity and then with caution and monitoring of liver function.

PEDIATRICS: Tuberculosis: 10–20 mg/kg, not to exceed 600 mg/day, oral or IV.

Meningococcal carriers 1 month of age or older: 10 mg/kg (not to exceed 600 mg per dose) every 12 hours for two days. Those under 1 month of age: 5 mg/kg every 12 hours for two days.

THE ART OF ANTIMICROBIAL THERAPY

Clinical Pearls

1. Rifampin should never be used alone in the treatment of active tuberculosis, since resistance may develop.

2. Liver function tests, symptoms of gastrointestinal intolerance and CBC should be monitored at least monthly in all patients receiving rifampin.

3. Rifampin is a potent inducer of the p450 cytochrome system and coadministered medications may require discontinuation or monitoring for possible dosage adjustment.

4. Rifampin penetrates foreign material well and can be used as synergy with tetracyclines and fluoroquinolones for foreign body infections (off-label use).

5. Some of the hypersensitivity-related toxicity seen with rifampin, e.g., flu-like illness and thrombocytopenia, may be more frequent with intermittent administration.

BASIC CHARACTERISTICS

Class: Rifampin—rifamycin;

Isoniazid—isonicotinic acid hydrazide.

Mechanisms of Action: Rifampin inhibits DNA-dependent RNA polymerase activity in susceptible cells.

Isoniazid inhibits the synthesis of mycolic acid, a constituent of the cell wall and inhibits catalase-peroxidase.

Mechanisms of Resistance: Resistance to rifampin occurs as single-step mutations of the DNA-dependent RNA polymerase.

Resistance to isoniazid occurs as point mutations in the catalase-peroxidase gene and the regulatory genes involved in mycolic acid synthesis.

Metabolic Route: Rifampin is rapidly eliminated in the bile and undergoes progressive deacetylation and is eliminated. However, up to 30 % of a dose is excreted in the urine, with about half of this being unchanged drug.

Isoniazid is metabolized by acetylation and dehydrazination. The rate of acetylation is genetically determined.

 FDA-APPROVED INDICATIONS

Pulmonary tuberculosis in which organisms are susceptible and when the patient has been titrated on the individual components and it has therefore been established that this fixed dosage is therapeutically effective.

 SIDE EFFECTS/TOXICITY

> **WARNING:** Severe and sometimes fatal hepatitis associated with isoniazid therapy may occur and may develop even after many months of treatment.

Rifamate is **contraindicated** in patients with a history of hypersensitivity to any of the rifamycins or isoniazid.

Adverse events: anaphylaxis, liver dysfunction, reddish coloration of the urine, sweat, sputum, and tears, "flu syndrome" (fever, chills, and malaise), rash, flushing, epigastric distress, anorexia, nausea, vomiting, flatulence, *Clostridium difficile*-associated diarrhea, disseminated intravascular coagulation, visual disturbances, adrenal insufficiency, confusion, renal insufficiency, elevations in serum uric acid, thrombocytopenia, leukopenia, hemolytic anemia, peripheral neuropathy, hypersensitivity, fever, skin eruptions, vasculitis, a systemic lupus erythematosus-like syndrome, nausea, vomiting, epigastric distress, seizures, encephalopathy, metabolic acidosis, optic neuritis, arthralgias, agranulocytosis, hemolytic or sideroblastic anemia, and thrombocytopenia.

Foods rich in histamine (e.g., cheese, wine, tuna) or tyramine (e.g., cured meats, soybeans, aged cheese) may produce flushing and headache due to the INH component.

Rifamate can enhance the metabolism of endogenous substrates including adrenal hormones, thyroid hormones, and vitamin D.

 DRUG INTERACTIONS/FOOD INTERACTIONS

Absorption of Rifamate is reduced when the drug is ingested with food, but absorption is usually adequate, and ingestion with food reduces GI intolerance.

Antibiotics Manual: A Guide to Commonly Used Antimicrobials, Second Edition. David Schlossberg and Rafik Samuel.
© 2017 John Wiley & Sons Ltd. Published 2017 by John Wiley & Sons Ltd.

INH inhibits the metabolism of many drugs, potentially increasing their serum levels; patients on anticoagulants, anticonvulsants, benzodiazepines, haloperidol, theophylline and cycloserine should be monitored for toxic effects; levels of carbamazepine, phenytoin, and valproate should be measured.

Rifamate is known to induce certain cytochrome P-450 enzymes. Administration of rifampin with drugs that undergo biotransformation through these metabolic pathways may accelerate elimination and decrease the therapeutic effect of these coadministered drugs, many of which require monitoring and possible adjustment during and following coadministration with rifampin.

The list of drugs so affected includes the following drugs/classes: anticonvulsants, antiarrhythmics, oral anticoagulants, antifungals, barbiturates, beta-blockers, calcium channel blockers, chloramphenicol, clarithromycin, corticosteroids, cyclosporine, cardiac glycoside preparations, clofibrate, hormonal contraceptives (patients should be advised to use nonhormonal methods of birth control during rifampin therapy), dapsone, diazepam, doxycycline, enalapril, fluoroquinolones, haloperidol, oral hypoglycemic agents, levothyroxine, methadone, narcotic analgesics, nortriptyline, progestins, quinine, tacrolimus, sulfapyridine, theophylline, tricyclic antidepressants, protease inhibitors, nonnucleoside reverse transcriptase inhibitors, CCR5 inhibitors, and zidovudine.

Rifamate levels may increase when coadministered with atovaquone, probenecid, and cotrimoxazole, and may decrease when given with ketoconazole and antacids (give Rifamate at least 1 hour before the ingestion of antacids).

When Rifamate is given concomitantly with halothane, the potential for hepatotoxicity is increased, and concomitant use of Rifamate and halothane should be avoided.

Acetaminophen and alcohol should be avoided, as they may increase hepatotoxicity, as should disulfiram, enflurane, stavudine, and vincristine.

Drug/laboratory interactions

Cross-reactivity and false-positive urine screening tests for opiates have been reported in patients receiving Rifamate.

Therapeutic levels of Rifamate have been shown to inhibit standard microbiological assays for serum folate and vitamin B12.

Significant interactions with antiretroviral medications:

Rifamate	
Usual dose	Efavirenz (Sustiva, Atripla): usual dose
	Nevirapine: usual dose
	Saquinavir: 400/ritonavir 400 bid
	Kaletra: 4 tablets bid
	Maraviroc: 600 bid
	Raltegravir: 800 bid (elvitegravir: **no**)
	Dolutegravir (Triumeq): 50 bid if no INSTI mutations; if mutations: RFB
Contraindicated	Complera, Descovy
Contraindicated	Stribild, Genvoya
Contraindicated	Prezcobix

 DOSING

Rifamate contains 300 mg of rifampin and 150 mg of isoniazid. Treatment should contain two Rifamate capsules once daily; for intermittent therapy, dosage is two capsules of Rifamate plus two 300-mg tablets of INH given twice weekly by DOT. Tolerance of Rifamate is improved if taken with food.

SPECIAL POPULATIONS

RENAL IMPAIRMENT: No dose adjustment is necessary.

HEPATIC DYSFUNCTION: Patients with impaired liver function should be given Rifamate only in cases of necessity and then with caution and monitoring of liver function.

PEDIATRICS: Not recommended for children or adolescents under the age of 15 (re-check prior to publication).

 THE ART OF ANTIMICROBIAL THERAPY

Clinical Pearls

1. When possible, Rifamate should be used for tuberculosis after the individual components have been started and have been shown to be tolerated.

2. Rifamate is helpful when DOT is not possible, as it minimizes inadvertent monotherapy and subsequent risk of acquired drug resistance.

3. Fixed-dose combinations like Rifamate may decrease the patient's pill burden.

4. Liver function tests and symptoms of gastrointestinal intolerance should be monitored in all patients receiving Rifamate.

5. Rifampin is a potent inducer of the p450 cytochrome system and coadministered medications may require discontinuation or monitoring for possible dosage adjustment.

6. Pyroxidine (25 mg/day) should be given to prevent B6 deficiency in those patients at risk for peripheral neuropathy, i.e., nutritional deficiency, diabetes, HIV infection, renal failure, alcoholism, pregnancy, and breastfeeding mothers.

7. Soft contact lenses may be permanently stained.

■ RIFATER (Rifampin + Isoniazid + Pyrazinamide)

 BASIC CHARACTERISTICS

Class: Rifampin—rifamycin;

    Isoniazid—isonicotinic acid hydrazide;

    Pyrazinamide—pyrazine analog of nicotinamide.

Mechanisms of Action: Rifampin inhibits DNA-dependent RNA polymerase activity in susceptible cells.

Isoniazid inhibits the synthesis of mycolic acid, a constituent of the cell wall and inhibits catalase-peroxidase.

Pyrazinamide: unknown.

Mechanisms of Resistance: Resistance to rifampin occurs as single-step mutations of the DNA-dependent RNA polymerase.

Resistance to isoniazid occurs as point mutations in the catalase-peroxidase gene and the regulatory genes involved in mycolic acid synthesis.

Resistance to pyrazinamide occurs as point mutations in the pyrazinamidase gene.

Metabolic Route: Rifampin is rapidly eliminated in the bile and undergoes progressive deacetylation and is eliminated. However, up to 30 % of a dose is excreted in the urine, with about half of this being unchanged drug.

Isoniazid is metabolized by acetylation and dehydrazination. The rate of acetylation is genetically determined.

Pyrazinamide is hydrolyzed in the liver and excreted in the urine.

 FDA-APPROVED INDICATIONS

Rifater is indicated in the initial phase of the short-course treatment of pulmonary tuberculosis. During this phase, which should last 2 months, Rifater should be administered on a daily, continuous basis.

 SIDE EFFECTS/TOXICITY

> **WARNING:** Severe and sometimes fatal hepatitis associated with isoniazid therapy may occur and may develop even after many months of treatment.

Rifater is **contraindicated** in patients with a history of hypersensitivity to any of the rifamycins or isoniazid.

Adverse events include peripheral neuropathy, hypersensitivity, fever, vasculitis, a systemic lupus erythematosus-like syndrome, seizures, encephalopathy, metabolic acidosis, optic neuritis, arthralgias, agranulocytosis, hemolytic or sideroblastic anemia, and thrombocytopenia.

Rifater inhibits renal excretion of urates, leading to hyperuricemea or gout; more commonly, it produces nongouty polyarthralgias. Also seen: anorexia, nausea, vomiting, diarrhea, flatulence, hepatitis, cutaneous flushing, porphyria, dysuria, reddish coloration of the urine, sweat, sputum, and tears, "flu syndrome" (fever, chills and malaise), rash, *Clostridium difficile*-associated diarrhea, disseminated intravascular coagulation, confusion, and renal insufficiency. Rifampin can enhance the metabolism of endogenous substrates including adrenal hormones, thyroid hormones, and vitamin D.

Antibiotics Manual: A Guide to Commonly Used Antimicrobials, Second Edition. David Schlossberg and Rafik Samuel.
© 2017 John Wiley & Sons Ltd. Published 2017 by John Wiley & Sons Ltd.

DRUG INTERACTIONS/FOOD INTERACTIONS

Absorption of Rifater is reduced when the drug is ingested with food, but absorption is usually adequate and ingestion with food reduces GI intolerance.

Foods rich in histamine (e.g., cheese, wine, tuna) or tyramine (e.g., cured meats, soybeans, aged cheese) may produce flushing and headache. Antacids may impair absorption and should be separated from INH ingestion by 2 hours.

INH inhibits the metabolism of many drugs, potentially increasing their serum levels; patients on anticoagulants, anticonvulsants, benzodiazepines, haloperidol, theophylline and cycloserine should be monitored for toxic effects; levels of carbamazepine, phenytoin, and valproate should be measured. Acetaminophen and alcohol should be avoided, as they may increase hepatotoxicity, as should disulfiram, enflurane, stavudine, and vincristine.

Rifampin is known to induce certain cytochrome P-450 enzymes. Administration of Rifater with drugs that undergo biotransformation through these metabolic pathways may accelerate elimination and decrease the therapeutic effect of these coadministered drugs, many of which require monitoring and possible adjustment during and following coadministration with Rifater.

The list of drugs so affected includes the following drugs/classes: anticonvulsants, antiarrhythmics, oral anticoagulants, antifungals, barbiturates, beta-blockers, calcium channel blockers, chloramphenicol, clarithromycin, corticosteroids, cyclosporine, cardiac glycoside preparations, clofibrate, hormonal contraceptives (patients should be advised to use nonhormonal methods of birth control during Rifater therapy), dapsone, diazepam, doxycycline, enalapril, fluoroquinolones, haloperidol, oral hypoglycemic agents, levothyroxine, methadone, narcotic analgesics, nortriptyline, progestins, quinine, tacrolimus, sulfapyridine, theophylline, tricyclic antidepressants, protease inhibitors, nonnucleoside reverse transcriptase inhibitors, CCR5 inhibitors, and zidovudine.

Rifampin levels may increase when coadministered with atovaquone, probenecid, and cotrimoxazole, and may decrease when given with ketoconazole and antacids (give Rifater at least 1 hour before the ingestion of antacids).

When Rifater is given concomitantly with halothane, the potential for hepatotoxicity is increased and concomitant use of Rifater and halothane should be avoided.

Drug/laboratory interactions

Cross-reactivity and false-positive urine screening tests for opiates have been reported in patients receiving rifampin.

Therapeutic levels of Rifater have been shown to inhibit standard microbiological assays for serum folate and vitamin B12.

Rifater may interfere with Ketostix and Acetest, producing a brown color.

Anti-retroviral therapy interacts significantly with rifampin. The following caveats apply:

Rifater	
Usual dose	Efavirenz (Sustiva, Atripla): usual dose
	Nevirapine: usual dose
	Maraviroc: 600 bid
	Raltegravir: 800 bid
	Dolutegravir (Triumeq): 50 bid if no INSTI mutations
Contraindicated	Complera, Descovy
Contraindicated	Stribild, Genvoya
Contraindicated	Prezcobix

DOSING

Rifater contains 120 mg rifampin, 50 mg isoniazid, and 300 mg pyrazinamide. Treatment is weight based as follows:

Patients weighing ≤44 kg	4 tablets daily
Patients weighing between 45–54 kg	5 tablets daily
Patients weighing ≥55 kg	6 tablets daily

To obtain an adequate dose of PZA in persons heavier than 90 kg, additional PZA tablets must be given.

 SPECIAL POPULATIONS

RENAL IMPAIRMENT: Rifater should not be used, because of the potential need to adjust PZA dosage.

HEPATIC DYSFUNCTION: Patients with impaired liver function should be given rifater only in cases of necessity and then with caution and monitoring of liver function.

PEDIATRICS: The ratio of the drugs in Rifater may not be appropriate in pediatric patients under the age of 15 (e.g., higher mg/kg doses of isoniazid are usually given in pediatric patients than in adults).

 THE ART OF ANTIMICROBIAL THERAPY

Clinical Pearls

1. Rifater should be used for the induction phase of tuberculosis therapy.
2. Liver function tests and symptoms of gastrointestinal intolerance should be monitored in all patients receiving Rifater.
3. Rifampin is a potent inducer of the p450 cytochrome system, and coadministered medications may require discontinuation or monitoring for possible dosage adjustment.
4. Pyroxidine (25 mg/day) should be given to prevent INH-related B6 deficiency in those at risk for peripheral neuropathy, i.e., nutritional deficiency, diabetes, HIV infection, renal failure, alcoholism, pregnancy, and breastfeeding mothers.
5. Patients with acute gout should not receive any medication containing pyrazinamide.
6. Fixed-dose combinations like Rifater minimize inadvertent monotherapy and the subsequent risk of acquired drug resistance. They should be used when possible if therapy cannot be given via DOT.
7. Soft contact lenses may be permanently stained.

BASIC CHARACTERISTICS

Class: Third generation cephalosporin.

Mechanism of Action: Binds penicillin-binding protein, disrupting cell wall synthesis.

Mechanisms of Resistance:

1. The PBP can be altered, with reduced affinity.
2. Production of a beta-lactamase, resulting in hydrolysis of the beta-lactam ring.
3. Decreased ability of the antibiotic to reach the PBP when bacteria decrease porin production, resulting in a decrease of the drug concentration within the cell.

Metabolic Route: Approximately 33 % is excreted in the urine, 67 % in the feces.

 FDA-APPROVED INDICATIONS

Treatment of the following syndromes when caused by susceptible organisms:

Lower respiratory tract infections

Acute bacterial otitis media

Skin and skin structure infections

Urinary tract infections

Uncomplicated gonorrhea

Pelvic inflammatory diseases

Bacterial septicemia

Bone and joint infections

Intra-abdominal infections

Meningitis

It is also indicated for surgical prophylaxis for certain patients when administered preoperatively.

 SIDE EFFECTS/TOXICITY

Ceftriaxone is **contraindicated** in patients with cephalosporin allergy and in neonates who are hyperbilirubinemic or who require **calcium-containing IV solutions**.

Ceftriaxone should be used with caution if hypersensitivity exists to penicillin.

Toxicity includes inflammation at the site of injection, fever, anaphylaxis, rash including Stevens–Johnson syndrome, erythema multiforme and toxic epidermal necrolysis, angioedema, flushing, serum-sickness-like reactions, encephalopathy, seizures, myoclonus, diarrhea, *Clostridium difficile*-associated diarrhea and pseudomembranous colitis, oral candidiasis, anorexia, nausea, vomiting, stomach cramps, flatulence, hepatitis, renal impairment, genital moniliasis, vaginitis, hemorrhage, prolonged prothrombin time, pancytopenia, hemolytic anemia, positive Coombs' test. Crystallization of ceftriaxone salt in the gallbladder may produce gallbladder sludge.

Antibiotics Manual: A Guide to Commonly Used Antimicrobials, Second Edition. David Schlossberg and Rafik Samuel.
© 2017 John Wiley & Sons Ltd. Published 2017 by John Wiley & Sons Ltd.

DRUG INTERACTIONS/FOOD INTERACTIONS

Ceftriaxone and intravenous calcium-containing products should not be mixed or coadministered to any patient, even via different sites. Cephalosporins may cause false-positive urine glucose determinations when using cupric sulfate solution (Benedict's solution, *Clinitest®*). Tests utilizing glucose oxidase (*Tes-Tape®*, *Clinistix®*) are not affected by cephalosporins.

 ## DOSING

Ceftriaxone is given intravenously in doses of 1–2 grams daily depending on the type and severity of infection. The total dose may be given once a day or divided equally and given twice a day.

Meningitis: up to 4 grams twice daily.

Gonorrhea: 250 mg intramuscularly – single dose.

Surgical prophylaxis: 1 gram 30–60 minutes given preoperatively.

 ## SPECIAL POPULATIONS

RENAL IMPAIRMENT: No dose adjustment is necessary.

HEPATIC DYSFUNCTION: No dose adjustment is necessary; however, a dose of 2 grams daily should not be exceeded.

PEDIATRICS: **Skin and skin structure infections**: 50–75 mg/kg/day (given once a day or in equally divided doses twice a day); not to exceed a daily dose of 2 grams.

Acute bacterial otitis media: 50 mg/kg (not to exceed one gram) as a single IM dose.

Serious miscellaneous infections other than meningitis: 50–75 mg/kg/day; not to exceed 2 grams, in divided doses q 12 h.

Meningitis: initial dose of 100 mg/kg (not to exceed 4 grams), followed by a total daily dose of 100 mg/kg (not to exceed 4 grams), administered once daily or in equally divided doses q 12 h.

Neonates with hyperbilirubinemia should not receive ceftriaxone.

 ## THE ART OF ANTIMICROBIAL THERAPY

Clinical Pearls

1. Ceftriaxone is not dose adjusted for renal dysfunction.
2. Cross allergy with penicillins is <10 % and can be used in life-threatening infections (e.g., meningitis) with caution if the allergy is not severe.
3. Crystallization of ceftriaxone in the gallbladder can occur.
4. Coadministration of ceftriaxone and intravenous calcium products should be avoided.
5. Neonates with hyperbilirubinemia should not receive ceftriaxone.

BASIC CHARACTERISTICS

Class: Macrolide.

Mechanism of Action: Binds to the 50 S subunit of bacterial ribosomes, resulting in blockage of the transpeptidation or translocation reactions.

Mechanisms of Resistance: Unknown.

Metabolic Route: Metabolized in the liver and excreted in the bile.

Used for: Prevention of congenital toxoplasmosis.

 SIDE EFFECTS/TOXICITY

Patients with hypersensitivity reactions to other macrolides may also have hypersensitivity to spiramycin.

Also seen: hypersensitivity reactions, anaphylaxis, urticaria, pruritus, rash, nausea, vomiting, diarrhea, abdominal pain, esophagitis, hepatitis, pseudomembranous colitis, QT prolongation, ventricular arrhythmias, neuromuscular blockade, paraesthesias, and thrombocytopenia.

 DRUG INTERACTIONS/FOOD INTERACTIONS

Spiramycin may be taken with or without food

Decreases carbidopa absorption and levodopa concentrations. Increased risk of ventricular arrhythmias when used with astemizole, cisapride, and terfenadine. Risk of dystonia when used with fluphenazine.

 DOSING

Spiramycin is administered as tablets, capsules, intravenously, or by rectal suppositories.

Toxoplasmosis in pregnancy: 3 grams per day, divided into three or four doses.

 SPECIAL POPULATIONS

RENAL IMPAIRMENT: No dose adjustment is necessary.

HEPATIC DYSFUNCTION: Biliary obstruction or hepatic function impairment may decrease the elimination of spiramycin.

 THE ART OF ANTIMICROBIAL THERAPY

Clinical Pearls

1. Spiramycin is not commercially available. However, it can be obtained from Aventis through IND from the FDA (301-796-1600) following confirmation of the diagnosis by a recognized laboratory (i.e., Palo Alto Medical Foundation, Toxoplasmosis Laboratory, 650-853-4828). It may also be available through a compounding pharmacy. Call National

Antibiotics Manual: A Guide to Commonly Used Antimicrobials, Second Edition. David Schlossberg and Rafik Samuel.
© 2017 John Wiley & Sons Ltd. Published 2017 by John Wiley & Sons Ltd.

Association of Compounding Pharmacies (800-687-7850) or the Professional Compounding Centers of America (800-331-2498, www.pccarx.com).

2. For prevention of congenital toxoplasmosis, women who develop toxoplasmosis during the first trimester of pregnancy should be treated with spiramycin (3–4 g/d). After the first trimester, if there is no documented transmission to the fetus, spiramycin can be continued until delivery. If fetal transmission is documented, therapy with pyrimethamine and sulfadiazine should be started, but only after the first trimester because of pyrimethamine's teratogenicity.

BASIC CHARACTERISTICS

Class: CCR5 coreceptor antagonist.

Mechanism of Action: Maraviroc is an antagonist of the interaction between human CCR5 and HIV-1 gp120. Blocking this interaction prevents CCR5-tropic HIV-1 entry into cells.

Maraviroc is not active against all HIV viruses, only those that use CCR5 solely as the co-receptor for entry.

Mechanism of Resistance: Two amino acid residue substitutions in the V3-loop region of the HIV-1 envelope glycoprotein gp160, A316T, and I323V lead to resistance to maraviroc.

Metabolic Route: Maraviroc is principally metabolized by the cytochrome P450 system.

FDA-APPROVED INDICATIONS

Treatment of HIV-1 in combinations with other antiretroviral agents for adult patients infected with only CCR5-tropic HIV-1.

SIDE EFFECTS/TOXICITY

> **WARNING: Hepatotoxicity** has been reported with maraviroc use. Severe rash or evidence of a **systemic allergic reaction** (e.g., pruritic rash, eosinophilia, or elevated IgE) prior to the development of hepatotoxicity may occur. Patients with signs or symptoms of hepatitis or allergic reaction following use of maraviroc should be evaluated immediately.

Other side effects include: hypersensitivity fever, rash, eosinophilia, hepatotoxicity, upper respiratory tract infection, cough, dizziness, diarrhea, edema, sleep disorders, symptomatic postural hypotension, immune reconstitution syndrome.

Maraviroc antagonizes the CCR5 coreceptor located on some immune cells, and therefore could potentially increase the risk of developing infections. Patients should be monitored closely for evidence of infections while receiving maraviroc.

Due to maraviroc's mechanism of action it could affect immune surveillance and increase the risk of malignancy. Use with caution in patients at increased risk for cardiovascular events.

DRUG INTERACTIONS/FOOD INTERACTIONS

Maraviroc can be taken with or without food.

St John's wort should not be taken with maraviroc.

Since maraviroc is metabolized by CYP3A, coadministration of maraviroc and drugs that induce CYP3A may decrease maraviroc plasma concentrations and reduce its therapeutic effect. Coadministration of maraviroc and drugs that inhibit CYP3A may increase maraviroc plasma concentrations. Because of these metabolic effects, potential drug interactions that may require dosage change or clinical/laboratory monitoring are listed below:

Medication	*Adjustment or action*
Itraconazole and ketoconazole	Decrease maraviroc to 150 mg bid
Voriconazole	Monitor for toxicities
Clarithromycin	Decrease maraviroc to 150 mg bid

Antibiotics Manual: A Guide to Commonly Used Antimicrobials, Second Edition. David Schlossberg and Rafik Samuel.
© 2017 John Wiley & Sons Ltd. Published 2017 by John Wiley & Sons Ltd.

Medication	Adjustment or action
Rifampin	Increase maraviroc to 600 mg bid
Rifabutin	If used with CYP3A inhibitor, decrease maraviroc to 150 mg bid
	If used with CYP3A inducer, regular dose
Phenobarbital, phenytoin, or carbamazepine	Increase maraviroc to 600 mg bid
All PIs except tipranavir	Decrease maraviroc to 150 mg bid
Efavirenz	Increase maraviroc to 600 mg bid
Tipranavir/ritonavir, nevirapine, all NRTIs, and enfurvirtide	Maraviroc dose, 300 mg bid

DOSING

Maraviroc is supplied in 25 mg, 75 mg, 150 mg and 300 mg tablets. It is also supplied as an oral solution that contains 20 mg per mL. The normal dose is 300 mg given twice daily.

SPECIAL POPULATIONS

RENAL IMPAIRMENT: Maraviroc should not be used in patients with creatinine clearance <30 mL/min when given potent CYP3A 4 inhibitors or inducers.

HEPATIC DYSFUNCTION: Maraviroc should be used with caution in those with hepatic impairment.

PEDIATRICS: Can be given to children over 2 years of age that weigh at least 10 kg as follows:

10 kg to <20 kg	20 kg to <30 kg	30 kg to <40 kg	≥40 kg
With potent inhibitors of p450:			
50 mg twice daily	75 mg twice daily	100 mg twice daily	150 mg twice daily
With no interactions:			
No recommendation	No recommendation	300 mg twice daily	300 mg twice daily
With potent inducers of p450:			
Not recommended			

THE ART OF ANTIMICROBIAL THERAPY

Clinical Pearls

1. Maraviroc should always be used in combination with other antiretrovirals.
2. A tropism test must be done to see if the patient has a virus that uses only the CCR5 receptor, to ensure that maraviroc's use is appropriate.
3. If the virus uses the CXCR4 coreceptor or is dual tropic, maraviroc should not be used.
4. Whenever initiating maraviroc, make sure to review all medications the patient is receiving to minimize drug interactions.

BASIC CHARACTERISTICS

Class: Analog of D-alanine.

Mechanisms of Action: Cycloserine inhibits cell-wall synthesis in gram-positive and gram-negative bacteria and in *Mycobacterium tuberculosis*.

Mechanisms of Resistance: Incompletely understood.

Metabolic Route: About 2/3 is excreted in the urine and the other 1/3 is metabolized to unknown substances.

 FDA-APPROVED INDICATIONS

Treatment of active pulmonary and extrapulmonary tuberculosis when the causative organisms are susceptible to this drug and when treatment with the primary medications has proved inadequate.

Treatment of urinary tract infections caused by susceptible strains of gram-positive and gram-negative bacteria, but should be considered only when conventional therapy has failed

 SIDE EFFECTS/TOXICITY

Contraindicated in patients with hypersensitivity to cycloserine, epilepsy, depression, severe anxiety, psychosis, or excessive use of alcohol.

CNS toxicity, including inability to concentrate and lethargy, headache, tremor, vertigo, paresis, dysarthria, seizure, depression, psychosis, and suicidal ideation, peripheral neuropathy, allergic dermatitis, lichenoid eruptions, Stevens–Johnson syndrome, elevated serum transaminases, congestive heart failure, vitamin B12 and/or folic acid deficiency, megaloblastic anemia, and sideroblastic anemia.

 DRUG INTERACTIONS/FOOD INTERACTIONS

Absorption modestly decreased by food; avoid large fatty meals.

Concurrent administration of ethionamide has been reported to potentiate neurotoxic side effects.

Alcohol and cycloserine are incompatible because alcohol increases the risk of epileptic episodes.

Concurrent administration of isoniazid may result in increased incidence of CNS effects, such as dizziness or drowsiness.

 DOSING

10–15 mg/kg/day usually: 250 mg PO twice a day; can increase to 250 mg.

PO 3 times a day or 250 mg AM and 500 mg hs if peak levels are kept below 35 mcg/mL.

 SPECIAL POPULATIONS

RENAL IMPAIRMENT: The manufacturer contraindicates its use in severe renal insufficiency; if it must be used, for patients with CC <30 mL/h or on hemodialysis give 250 mg once daily or 500 mg/dose 3 times/week; monitor levels.

Antibiotics Manual: A Guide to Commonly Used Antimicrobials, Second Edition. David Schlossberg and Rafik Samuel.
© 2017 John Wiley & Sons Ltd. Published 2017 by John Wiley & Sons Ltd.

HEPATIC DYSFUNCTION: No adjustment necessary.

PEDIATRICS: Safety and effectiveness in pediatric patients have not been established. If it must be used: 10–20 mg/kg/day divided every 12 hours (daily maximum 1 gram).

 ## THE ART OF ANTIMICROBIAL THERAPY

Clinical Pearls

1. Cycloserine should never be used alone in the treatment of active tuberculosis.
2. Cycloserine should only be used if resistance to first line antimycobacterial agents is noted.
3. Cycloserine may cause increased neurotoxic side effects when administered with ethionamide.
4. Even though cycloserine has activity against usual bacteria, it is not routinely used to treat nonmycobacterial infection.
5. Alcohol should not be consumed while on cycloserine.
6. Neuropsychiatric side effects usually occur at serum levels >35 mcg/mL; serum levels of cycloserine should be monitored, with a goal of peak levels (2 hours after a dose) of 20–35 mcg/mL.
7. Hematologic, renal, and hepatic functions should be monitored.
8. Some patients tolerate cycloserine best if treatment is begun with a small dose that is gradually increased over a few days to a week (ramping).
9. All patients should receive vitamin B6 while taking cycloserine. Adults need 100–300 mg (or 50 mg per 250 mg of cycloserine) and children should receive a dose proportionate to their weight.

BASIC CHARACTERISTICS

Class: Diarylquinoline.

Mechanism of Action: Inhibits mycobacterial ATP (adenosine 5'-triphosphate) synthase, by binding to subunit c of the enzyme that is essential for the generation of energy in *M. tuberculosis*.

Mechanisms of Resistance: Modification of the *atpE* target gene and/or upregulation of the MmpS5-MmpL5 efflux pump.

Metabolic Route: Primarily eliminated in feces.

 FDA-APPROVED INDICATIONS

Indicated as part of combination therapy in the treatment of adults (18 years and older) with pulmonary multidrug resistant tuberculosis (MDR-TB).

 SIDE EFFECTS/TOXICITY

> **WARNING:**
> 1. Increased mortality.
> 2. QT Prolongation.

Use with drugs that prolong the QT interval may cause additive QT prolongation. Monitor ECGs. Other **toxicity** includes increased mortality and hepatotoxicity.

 DRUG INTERACTIONS/FOOD INTERACTIONS

Bedaquiline exposure may be reduced during coadministration with inducers of CYP3A4 and increased during coadministration with inhibitors of CYP3A4.

Concomitant administration of bedaquiline and efavirenz, or other moderate CYP3A inducers, should be avoided.

Use bedaquiline with caution when coadministered with lopinavir/ritonavir and only if the benefit outweighs the risk.

Should be taken with food.

 DOSING

The recommended dosage of bedaquiline is 400 mg orally once daily for the first two weeks, followed by 200 mg orally three times per week (with at least 48 hours between doses) for 22 weeks (total duration of 24 weeks).

The bedaquiline tablet should be swallowed whole with water and taken with food.

 SPECIAL POPULATIONS

RENAL IMPAIRMENT: In severe renal impairment or end-stage renal disease requiring hemodialysis or peritoneal dialysis, bedaquiline should be used with caution.

Antibiotics Manual: A Guide to Commonly Used Antimicrobials, Second Edition. David Schlossberg and Rafik Samuel.
© 2017 John Wiley & Sons Ltd. Published 2017 by John Wiley & Sons Ltd.

HEPATIC DYSFUNCTION: Bedaquiline should be used with caution in patients with severe hepatic dysfunction and only when the benefits outweigh the risks.

PEDIATRICS: Safety and effectiveness in pediatric patients has not been established.

 ## THE ART OF ANTIMICROBIAL THERAPY

Clinical Pearls

1. Do not use bedaquiline for the treatment of latent tuberculosis, drug-sensitive tuberculosis, extrapulmonary tuberculosis, or infections caused by nontuberculous mycobacteria.

2. The safety and efficacy of bedaquiline in the treatment of HIV infected patients with MDR-TB have not been established as clinical data are limited.

3. Administer bedaquiline by directly observed therapy (DOT).

4. *M. tuberculosis* isolates resistant to bedaquiline via mutations in the Rv0678 gene that lead to upregulation of the MmpS5-MmpL5 efflux pump are less susceptible to clofazimine.

5. Prior to and during treatment, obtain and monitor the following: ECG, serum potassium, calcium, and magnesium concentrations, liver enzymes.

6. Only use bedaquiline in combination with at least 3 other drugs to which the patient's MDR-TB isolate has been shown to be susceptible *in vitro*. If *in vitro* testing results are unavailable, bedaquiline treatment may be initiated in combination with at least 4 other drugs to which the patient's MDR-TB isolate is likely to be susceptible.

7. Discontinue bedaquiline if there is evidence of serious ventricular arrhythmia or QTc interval is greater than 500 ms.

BASIC CHARACTERISTICS

Class: Oxazolidinone.

Mechanism of Action: The antibacterial activity of tedizolid is mediated by binding to the 50S subunit of the bacterial ribosome, resulting in inhibition of protein synthesis.

Mechanism of Resistance: Organisms resistant to oxazolidinones via mutations in chromosomal genes encoding 23S rRNA or ribosomal proteins (L3 and L4) are generally cross-resistant to tedizolid.

Metabolic Route: Primarily excreted in feces.

 FDA-APPROVED INDICATIONS

Acute bacterial skin and skin structure infections (ABSSSI) caused by susceptible *Staphylococcus aureus* (including MRSA) and streptococci.

 SIDE EFFECTS/TOXICITY

Toxicity includes nausea, **headache**, **diarrhea**, **vomiting**, and **dizziness**, anemia, palpitations, tachycardia, asthenopia, blurred vision, visual impairment, vitreous floaters, infusion-related reactions, drug hypersensitivity, *Clostridium difficile* colitis, oral candidiasis, vulvovaginal mycotic infection, elevated hepatic transaminases, decreased white blood cell count, hypoesthesia, paresthesia, VII nerve paralysis, peripheral neuropathy, optic neuropathy, insomnia, pruritus, urticaria, dermatitis, flushing, hypertension, and myelosuppression.

 DRUG INTERACTIONS/FOOD INTERACTIONS

Tedizolid is a reversible inhibitor of monoamine oxidase (MAO) *in vitro*. The interaction with MAO inhibitors could not be evaluated in Phase 2 and 3 trials, as subjects taking such medications were excluded from the trials.

Tedizolid can be administered with or without food.

 DOSING

200 mg administered once daily orally or as an intravenous (IV) infusion over 1 hour.

 SPECIAL POPULATIONS

RENAL IMPAIRMENT: No dosage adjustment is necessary.

HEPATIC DYSFUNCTION: No dose adjustment is necessary.

PEDIATRICS: Safety and effectiveness in pediatric patients below the age of 18 have not been established.

Antibiotics Manual: A Guide to Commonly Used Antimicrobials, Second Edition. David Schlossberg and Rafik Samuel.
© 2017 John Wiley & Sons Ltd. Published 2017 by John Wiley & Sons Ltd.

THE ART OF ANTIMICROBIAL THERAPY

Clinical Pearls

1. The safety and efficacy of tedizolid in patients with neutropenia (neutrophil counts <1000 cells/mm^3) have not been adequately evaluated.

2. Tedizolid has activity against enterococci.

3. Tedizolid is not a good choice for bacteremia.

BASIC CHARACTERISTICS

Class: Nucleotide reverse transcriptase inhibitor for hepatitis C NS5B polymerase.

Mechanism of Action: Sofosbuvir undergoes intracellular metabolism to form the pharmacologically active uridine analog triphosphate, which can be incorporated into HCV RNA by the NS5B polymerase and acts as a chain terminator.

Mechanism of Resistance: The substitution S282T can lead to decreased incorporation of the uridine analog triphosphate, allowing replication of the virus to continue.

Metabolic Route:

Metabolized in the liver to its active form. It is predominantly excreted in the urine.

 FDA-APPROVED INDICATIONS

Sofosbuvir is indicated for the treatment of genotype 1, 2, 3, or 4 chronic hepatitis C virus (HCV) infection as a component of a combination antiviral treatment regimen.

 SIDE EFFECTS/TOXICITY

Patients taking beta-blockers, or those with underlying cardiac comorbidities and/or advanced liver disease, may be at increased risk for symptomatic bradycardia with coadministration of sofosbuvir and amiodarone.

Other side effects include: fatigue, headache, nausea, insomnia, pruritus, anemia, asthenia, rash, chills, influenza-like illness, pyrexia, and diarrhea.

Lab abnormalities including elevated bilirubin and creatinine kinase have been reported.

 DRUG INTERACTIONS/FOOD INTERACTIONS

Sofosbuvir may be taken without regard to food.

When sofosbuvir is used in combination with ribavirin or peginterferon alfa/ribavirin, the contraindications applicable to those agents are applicable to combination therapies.

Do not coadminister sofosbuvir with Harvoni (ledipasvir/sofosbuvir), rifampin, rifabutin, rifapentine, St John's wort, amiodarone, carbamazepine, phenytoin, phenobarbital, oxcarbazepine, or tipranavir/ritonavir.

 DOSING

One 400 mg tablet, taken orally, once daily with or without food.

Patient population	Medication	Duration
Genotype 1 or 4	Sofosbuvir + ribavirin + pegylated interferon	12 weeks
Genotype 2	Sofosbuvir + ribavirin	12 weeks
Genotype 3	Sofosbuvir + ribavirin	24 weeks

Antibiotics Manual: A Guide to Commonly Used Antimicrobials, Second Edition. David Schlossberg and Rafik Samuel.
© 2017 John Wiley & Sons Ltd. Published 2017 by John Wiley & Sons Ltd.

SPECIAL POPULATIONS

RENAL IMPAIRMENT: Do not use if creatinine clearance is <30 mL/ minute.

HEPATIC DYSFUNCTION: No dose adjustment necessary.

PEDIATRICS: Do not use in patients under 18 years of age.

 ## THE ART OF ANTIMICROBIAL THERAPY

Clinical Pearls

1. Sofosbuvir is active against HCV genotypes 1, 2, 3, and 4.

2. Sofosbuvir in combination with ribavirin for 24 weeks can be considered as a therapeutic option for patients with genotype 1 infection who are ineligible to receive an interferon-based regimen.

3. Administer sofosbuvir in combination with ribavirin for up to 48 weeks or until the time of liver transplantation, whichever occurs first, to prevent posttransplant HCV reinfection.

4. Although not in the sofosbuvir package insert, sofosbuvir + simeprevir for 12 weeks is approved for the treatment of HCV genotype 1. Refer to simeprevir.

5. Although not in the sofosbuvir package insert, sofosbuvir + daclatasvir for 12 weeks is approved for the treatment of HCV genotypes 1 and 3. Refer to daclatasvir.

6. Significant bradycardia has been reported if sofosbuvir is combined with amiodarone.

7. Do not administer sofosbuvir with Harvoni (ledipasvir/sofosbuvir).

8. Sofosbuvir can be used in HIV coinfected patients.

9. Review the most current hepatitis C treatment guidelines because they are changing rapidly: http://www.cdc.gov/hepatitis/HCV/index.htm.

BASIC CHARACTERISTICS

Class: Third generation cephalosporin.

Mechanism of Action: Binds penicillin-binding protein, disrupting cell wall synthesis.

Mechanisms of Resistance:

1. The PBP can be altered, with reduced affinity.
2. Production of a beta-lactamase, resulting in hydrolysis of the beta-lactam ring.
3. Decreased ability of the antibiotic to reach the PBP when bacteria decrease porin production, resulting in a decrease of the drug concentration within the cell.

Metabolic Route: Cefditoren is excreted unchanged in the urine.

 FDA-APPROVED INDICATIONS

Treatment of the following infections in adults and adolescents (12 years and older) when caused by susceptible organisms:

Acute bacterial exacerbation of chronic bronchitis

Community-acquired pneumonia

Pharyngitis/tonsillitis

Uncomplicated skin and skin-structure infections

 SIDE EFFECTS/TOXICITY

Cefditoren is **contraindicated** in patients with allergy to cephalosporins, in patients with carnitine deficiency, and patients with milk protein hypersensitivity (not lactose intolerance), since cefditoren contains sodium caseinate, a milk protein.

Cefditoren should be used with caution if hypersensitivity exists to penicillins.

Toxicity includes fever, anaphylaxis, rash including Stevens–Johnson syndrome, erythema multiforme and toxic epidermal necrolysis, angioedema, flushing, serum-sickness-like reactions, encephalopathy, seizures, abnormal dreams, diarrhea, *Clostridium difficile*-associated diarrhea and pseudomembranous colitis, oral candidiasis, anorexia, nausea, vomiting, stomach cramps, flatulence, hepatitis, renal impairment, arthralgia, genital moniliasis, vaginitis, hemorrhage, prolonged prothrombin time, pancytopenia, hemolytic anemia, and positive Coombs' test.

 DRUG INTERACTIONS/FOOD INTERACTIONS

Cefditoren should be taken with food.

Probenecid inhibits the renal excretion of cefditoren.

Antacids and H2-receptor antagonists may reduce the absorption of cefditoren.

Cephalosporins may cause false-positive urine glucose determinations when using cupric sulfate solution (Benedict's solution, *Clinitest*®). Tests utilizing glucose oxidase (*Tes-Tape*®, *Clinistix*®) are not affected by cephalosporins. False-positive reaction for ketones in the urine may occur with tests using nitroprusside, but not with those using nitroferricyanide.

Antibiotics Manual: A Guide to Commonly Used Antimicrobials, Second Edition. David Schlossberg and Rafik Samuel.
© 2017 John Wiley & Sons Ltd. Published 2017 by John Wiley & Sons Ltd.

DOSING

Cefditoren is supplied as 200 mg and 400 mg tablets.

Infection	Dosage	Duration
Community acquired pneumonia	400 mg q 12 h	14 days
Acute exacerbations of chronic bronchitis	400 mg q 12 h	10 days
Pharyngitis	200 mg q 12 h	10 days
Uncomplicated skin and skin structure	200 mg q 12 h	10 days

 ## SPECIAL POPULATIONS

RENAL IMPAIRMENT:

Creatinine clearance, mg/mL	Dose
30–49	200 mg q 12 h
<30	200 mg daily
Hemodialysis	200 mg daily and 200 mg after HD
CAPD	No data
CRRT	No data

HEPATIC DYSFUNCTION: No dose adjustment is necessary.

PEDIATRICS: Use of cefditoren pivoxil is not recommended for pediatric patients less than 12 years of age. Dosage in pediatric patients over 12 years of age should follow adult recommendations.

 ## THE ART OF ANTIMICROBIAL THERAPY

Clinical Pearls

1. Cefditoren must be adjusted for renal insufficiency.
2. Cross allergy with penicillins is <10 %.
3. It is not recommended that cefditoren be taken with antacids or H2 receptor antagonists.

BASIC CHARACTERISTICS

Class: Triazole.

Mechanism of Action: Inhibition of lanosterol 14-α-demethylase, which is involved in the synthesis of ergosterol, an essential component of fungal cell membranes.

Mechanisms of Resistance:

1. Point mutations in the gene (*ERG11*) encoding for the target enzyme lead to an altered target with decreased affinity for azoles.

2. Overexpression of *ERG11* results in the production of high concentrations of the target enzyme, creating the need for higher intracellular drug concentrations to inhibit all of the enzyme molecules in the cell.

3. Active efflux of itraconazole out of the cell through the activation of two types of multidrug efflux transporters.

Metabolic Route: Itraconazole is metabolized predominantly by the cytochrome P450 3A4 isoenzyme system, resulting in the formation of several metabolites, including hydroxyitraconazole, the major metabolite.

 FDA-APPROVED INDICATIONS

Itraconazole oral solution is indicated for treatment of oropharyngeal and esophageal candidiasis.

For the **immunocompromised** or **nonimmunocompromised** hosts, itraconazole capsules are indicated for the treatment of blastomycosis, nonmeningeal histoplasmosis, and aspergillosis in patients who are intolerant of or refractory to amphotericin B therapy.

In nonimmunocompromised patients, itraconazole capsules are indicated for onychomycosis due to dermatophytes (tinea unguium).

 SIDE EFFECTS/TOXICITY

WARNING: Congestive heart failure, cardiac effects and drug interactions

Itraconazole should not be administered for the treatment of onychomycosis in patients with evidence of ventricular dysfunction such as congestive heart failure (CHF) or a history of CHF. If signs or symptoms of congestive heart failure occur during administration of itraconazole, discontinue administration. When itraconazole was administered intravenously to dogs and healthy human volunteers, negative inotropic effects were seen.

Drug interactions

Coadministration of the following drugs are contraindicated with itraconazole: methadone, disopyramide, dofetilide, dronedarone, quinidine, ergot alkaloids (such as dihydroergotamine, ergometrine (ergonovine), ergotamine, methylergometrine (methylergonovine), irinotecan, lurasidone, oral midazolam, pimozide, triazolam, felodipine, nisoldipine, ivabradine, ranolazine, eplerenone, cisapride, lovastatin, simvastatin, ticagrelor, and, in subjects with varying degrees of renal or hepatic impairment, colchicine, fesoterodine, telithromycin, and solifenacin. Coadministration with itraconazole can cause elevated plasma concentrations of these drugs and may increase or prolong both the pharmacologic effects and/or adverse reactions to these drugs. For example, increased plasma concentrations of some of these drugs can lead to QT prolongation and ventricular tachyarrhythmias, including occurrences of torsades de pointes, a potentially fatal arrhythmia.

Antibiotics Manual: A Guide to Commonly Used Antimicrobials, Second Edition. David Schlossberg and Rafik Samuel.
© 2017 John Wiley & Sons Ltd. Published 2017 by John Wiley & Sons Ltd.

Other toxic effects include severe hepatotoxicity, neuropathy, transient or permanent hearing loss, fever, rash, rhinitis, pharyngitis, sinusitis, increased appetite, nausea, diarrhea, constipation dyspepsia, flatulence, abdominal pain, dizziness, cystitis, urinary tract infection, gastritis, gastroenteritis, headache, tremor, myalgia, and abnormal dreams.

 DRUG INTERACTIONS/ADMINISTRATION

Itraconazole capsules should be administered with a full meal and must be swallowed whole.

Itraconazole oral solution should be taken without food.

The absorption of itraconazole may be decreased with the concomitant administration of antacids or gastric acid secretion suppressors.

Itraconazole, a potent cytochrome P450 3A4 isoenzyme system (CYP3A4) inhibitor, may increase plasma concentrations of drugs metabolized by this pathway. In addition, drugs that enhance or inhibit CYP3A4 activity may decrease or elevate levels of itraconazole, respectively.

Itaconazole should not be coadministered with: methadone, disopyramide, dofetilide, dronedarone, quinidine, ergot alkaloids (such as dihydroergotamine, ergometrine (ergonovine), ergotamine, methylergometrine (methylergonovine)), irinotecan, lurasidone, oral midazolam, pimozide, triazolam, felodipine, nisoldipine, ivabradine, ranolazine, eplerenone, cisapride, lovastatin, simvastatin, tamsulosin, rifabutin, rifampin, apixaban, rivaroxaban, carbamazapine, axitinib, dabrafenib, dasatinib, ibrutinib, nilotinib, sunitinib, trabectedin, simepravir, aliskiren, sildenafil for the treatment of pulmonary hypertension, everolimus, temsirolimus, salmeterol, darifenacin, vardenafil, conivaptan, tolvaptan, ticagrelor, and, in subjects with varying degrees of renal or hepatic impairment, colchicine, fesoterodine, telithromycin, and solifenacin.

The following list includes significant drug interactions with itraconazole:

Benzodiazepines: alprazolam, diazepam levels increased. **Cyclosporine, tacrolimus, sirolimus**: levels elevated.

Dexamethasone: levels elevated.

Digoxin: digoxin levels increased.

Docetaxel: levels increased.

Disopyramide: levels increased.

Fentanyl: levels elevated.

H2-receptor antagonists: decrease itra levels.

HMG CoA-reductase inhibitors (statins): atorvastatin and cerivastatin may have elevated levels.

Isoniazid: decrease itraconazole levels.

Macrolides (clarithromycin, erythromycin): increase itra levels.

Oral hypoglycemics: levels elevated.

NNRTIs: decrease itraconazole levels.

Phenobarbitol: decrease itraconazole levels.

Phenytoin: decrease itraconazole levels.

Protease inhibitors (indinivir, ritonavir, saquinavir): levels elevated; also, itra levels elevated.

Proton pump inhibitors: decrease itra levels.

Trimetraxate: levels elevated.

Warfarin: levels elevated.

Vinca alkaloids: levels increased.

DOSING

Itraconazole is available as a 100 mg capsule and in a solution containing 10 mg of itraconazole per mL.

Blastomycosis and histoplasmosis

The recommended dose is 200 mg once daily. The dose can be increased in 100 mg increments to a maximum of 400 mg daily if no response is noted. Doses above 200 mg/day should be given in two divided doses.

Treatment of aspergillosis

The recommended oral dose is 200 mg to 400 mg daily. In life-threatening situations it is recommended that a loading dose of 200 mg three times daily be given for the first 3 days of treatment.

Treatment of onychomycosis

Toenails: 200 mg once daily for 12 consecutive weeks.

Fingernails only: 2 treatment regimen pulses, each consisting of 200 mg bid for 1 week. The pulses are separated by a 3-week period.

Treatment of oropharyngeal and esophageal candidiasis

The oral solution should be vigorously swished in the mouth (10 mL at a time) for several seconds and swallowed.

Oropharyngeal candidiasis: 200 mg daily for 1–2 weeks.

Esophageal candidiasis: 100 mg daily for 3 weeks or 2 weeks after symptoms resolve (whichever is longer).

 SPECIAL POPULATIONS

RENAL IMPAIRMENT: Use caution when administered in patients with renal impairment.

HEPATIC DYSFUNCTION: Caution should be used when used in patients with hepatic dysfunction. Liver function tests should be monitored. Use in patients with elevated liver function tests is strongly discouraged.

PEDIATRICS: The efficacy and safety of itraconazole have not been established in pediatric patients. If used, 100 mg/day of itraconazole capsules for systemic fungal infections can be used.

 THE ART OF ANTIMICROBIAL THERAPY

Clinical Pearls

1. Itraconazole requires a low pH for absorption. In achlorhydric patients, administration of a cola beverage increases absorption.
2. The capsules should be given with a full meal; the oral solution should be given without food.
3. Drug exposure is greater with the oral solution than with the capsules when the same dose of drug is given.
4. Only the oral solution has been demonstrated effective for oral and/or esophageal candidiasis.
5. Itraconazole is an inhibitor of cytochrome P450 and can enhance the activity of many commonly used drugs, e.g., oral hypoglycemics and anticoagulants.
6. The intravenous formulation of itraconazole is no longer being made.

◼ STREPTOMYCIN

 BASIC CHARACTERISTICS

Class: Aminoglycoside. **Mechanisms of Action:**

Binds the 30S subunit of the bacterial ribosome, which terminates protein synthesis.

Mechanism of Resistance:

1. Gram-negative bacteria inactivate aminoglycosides by acetylation.
2. Some bacteria alter the 30S ribosomal subunit, which prevents streptomycin's interference with protein synthesis.
3. Low-level resistance may result from inhibition of streptomycin uptake by the bacteria.

Metabolic Route: The drug is excreted unchanged in the urine.

 FDA-APPROVED INDICATIONS

1. *Mycobacterium tuberculosis*.
2. Infections due to *Yersinia pestis*, *Francisella tularensis*, *Brucella* spp., *Calymmatobacterium granulomatis*, *H. ducreyi*, *H. influenzae*, *K. pneumoniae* pneumonia, *E.coli*, *Proteus* spp., *A. aerogenes*, *K. pneumoniae*, and *Enterococcus faecalis* in urinary tract infections, and gram-negative bacillary bacteremia (concomitantly with another antibacterial agent).
3. Synergy with penicillin to treat endocardial infections with *Streptococcus* viridans and *Enterococcus faecalis*.

 SIDE EFFECTS/TOXICITY

> **WARNINGS:**
>
> **Ototoxicity**: vestibular toxicity and auditory ototoxicity, especially in patients with renal damage, those treated with higher doses, and those with prolonged treatment. Avoid use with potent diuretics such as ethacrynic acid because of additive ototoxicity.
>
> **Nephrotoxicity**: especially in patients with impaired renal function and those treated with higher doses or prolonged treatment. Avoid concurrent use with other nephrotoxic agents and potent diuretics, which can cause dehydration.
>
> **Neuromuscular blockade**: especially in those receiving anesthetics, neuromuscular blocking agents or massive transfusions.

Additional neurotoxicity includes optic nerve dysfunction, peripheral neuritis, arachnoiditis and encephalopathy. Other adverse effects include nausea, vomiting, rash, fever, pancytopenia, and hemolytic anemia.

 DRUG INTERACTIONS

Streptomycin should not be administered with other medications that are nephrotoxic or ototoxic.

Antibiotics Manual: A Guide to Commonly Used Antimicrobials, Second Edition. David Schlossberg and Rafik Samuel.
© 2017 John Wiley & Sons Ltd. Published 2017 by John Wiley & Sons Ltd.

DOSING

Intramuscular only

1. Tuberculosis: 15 mg/kg/day up to 1 gram; given daily at first, then 2–3 times/week after a period of daily administration. For patients >59 years of age, 10 mg/kg/dose (maximum 750 mg).

2. Tularemia: One to 2 g daily in divided doses for 7 to 14 days until the patient is afebrile for 5 to 7 days.

3. Plague: Two grams of streptomycin daily in two divided doses should be administered intramuscularly. A minimum of 10 days of therapy is recommended.

4. Bacterial endocarditis: *Streptococcal endocarditis*: 1 g bid for the first week and 500 mg bid for the second week. If the patient is over 60 years of age, the dosage should be 500 mg bid for the entire 2-week period in combination with penicillin.

   Enterococcal endocarditis: 1 g bid for 2 weeks and 500 mg bid for an additional 4 weeks in combination with penicillin.

 SPECIAL POPULATIONS

RENAL IMPAIRMENT: In patients with renal impairment, the usual dose is administered; however, the interval is increased as described in the table below. Levels should be measured.

Creatinine clearance, mL/min	Dose
>50	Usual dose
10–50	Increase interval to 3 × usual interval
<10	Increase interval to 4 × usual interval
Hemodialysis	Administer half the usual dose after dialysis
CRRT	Increase interval to 3 × usual interval

PEDIATRICS: 20–40 mg/kg/day up to 1 gram a day for tuberculosis as well as severe bacterial infections.

 THE ART OF ANTIMICROBIAL THERAPY

Clinical Pearls

1. Streptomycin is administered by intramuscular injection only.

2. When streptomycin must be given for prolonged periods of time, alkalinization of the urine may minimize or prevent renal damage.

3. Although streptomycin is recommended as the fourth agent for routine treatment of TB, ethambutol is usually used in its place.

4. If treating tuberculosis, never use streptomycin alone.

5. The peak concentration should be between 35 and 45 mcg/mL.

6. Streptomycin is considered a second line agent for the treatment of gram-negative bacillary bacteremia, meningitis, and pneumonia, brucellosis, granuloma inguinale, chancroid, and urinary tract infection.

7. Monitor renal function, hearing, and vestibular function during therapy.

BASIC CHARACTERISTICS

Class: Nucleotide reverse transcriptase inhibitor + nucleotide reverse transcriptase inhibitor + integrase inhibitor + CYP3A inhibitor.

Mechanism of Action: Tenofovir and emtricitabine are converted by cellular enzymes to their active drugs, tenofovir biphosphate (an analog of adenosine triphosphate) and emtricitabine triphosphate (an analog of cytosine triphosphate). These drugs compete with the naturally occurring nucleotides for incorporation in newly forming HIV DNA. Since they do not have a terminal hydroxyl group, they halt transcription and replication of the virus.

Elvitegravir is an HIV-1 integrase strand transfer inhibitor (INSTI). Inhibition of integrase prevents the integration of HIV-1 DNA into host genomic DNA, blocking propagation of the viral infection.

Cobicistat is a CYP3A inhibitor indicated to increase systemic exposure of elvitegravir.

Mechanism of Resistance: Changes in the structure of HIV reverse transcriptase leads to preferred incorporation of adenosine triphosphate and cytosine triphosphate with decreased incorporation of tenofovir biphosphate and emtricitabine triphosphate, which allows transcription of DNA to continue. Resistance mutations include K65R, M184V, and "TAMS": 41 L, 67 N, 70R, 210W, 215 F, and 219E.

Changes in the structure of HIV integrase prevents elvitegravir from binding to the active site of the enzyme and allowing integrase activity to continue. Resistance mutations that emerge in patients taking elvitegravir include T66A/I, E92G/Q, S147G, and Q148R.

Metabolic Route: Tenofovir and emtricitabine are excreted in the urine unchanged.

Elvitegravir undergoes primarily oxidative metabolism via CYP3A and is secondarily glucuronidated via UGT1A1/3 enzymes in the liver and excreted.

Metabolized by CYP3A and to a minor extent by CYP2D6 enzymes in the liver and excreted.

 FDA-APPROVED INDICATIONS

Stribild is indicated as a complete regimen for the treatment of HIV-1 infection in adult patients who have no antiretroviral treatment history or to replace the current antiretroviral regimen in those who are virologically suppressed on a stable antiretroviral regimen for at least 6 months with no history of treatment failure and no known substitutions associated with resistance to the individual components of Stribild.

 SIDE EFFECTS/TOXICITY

> **WARNING: Severe acute exacerbations of hepatitis** have been reported in hepatitis B-infected patients who have discontinued antihepatitis B therapy, including Stribild or any medications containing either tenofovir or emtricitabine. Hepatic function should be monitored closely with both clinical and laboratory follow-up for at least several months in patients who discontinue antihepatitis B therapy, including Stribild. If appropriate, resumption of antihepatitis B therapy may be warranted.
>
> **Lactic acidosis** and hepatomegaly with steatosis have been reported with nucleoside analogs, including tenofovir. If this syndrome occurs, the drug should be discontinued.

Antibiotics Manual: A Guide to Commonly Used Antimicrobials, Second Edition. David Schlossberg and Rafik Samuel.
© 2017 John Wiley & Sons Ltd. Published 2017 by John Wiley & Sons Ltd.

Other adverse events: Immune reconstitution inflammatory syndrome, fat redistribution including central obesity and dorso-cervical fat enlargement, peripheral wasting, facial wasting, breast enlargement, diarrhea, nausea, fatigue, headache, dizziness, depression, insomnia, abnormal dreams, rash, renal impairment, including acute renal failure and Fanconi syndrome, and decreased bone mineral density.

In less than 2 %: abdominal pain, dyspepsia, vomiting, suicidal ideation and suicide attempt, rhabdomyolysis, and nephrolithiasis.

Decreases estimated creatinine clearance due to inhibition of tubular secretion of creatinine without affecting actual renal glomerular function.

DRUG INTERACTIONS/FOOD INTERACTIONS

Stribild should be administered with food.

Stribild should not be given with didanosine because of decreased CD4 counts in patients maintained on this regimen. If didanosine is given with Stribild or any medication containing tenofovir, the didanosine should be decreased to 250 mg daily.

Elvitegravir and cobicistat are metabolized by CYP3A. Drugs that induce or inhibit CYP3A activity are expected to affect the clearance of elvitegravir and cobicistat.

Do not coadminister Stribild with efavirenz, nevirapine, indinavir, saquinavir, nelfinavir, phenobarbital, phenytoin, carbamazepine, oxcarbazepine, rifampin, rifabutin, rifapentine, dexamethasone, St John's wort, norgestimate/ethinyl estradiol, Kaletra, fosamprenavir, tipranavir, etravirine, alfuzosin, dronedarone, rivaroxaban, irinotecan, dihydroergotamine, ergotamine, methylergonovine, cisapride, lovastatin, simvastatin, pimozide, avanafil, sildenafil, triazolam, or midazolam.

Medication	Adjustment or action
Maraviroc	Maraviroc dose 150 bid
Antacid	Administer 2 hours apart
Colchicine	Not recommended in renal or hepatic impairment
Bosentan	Bosentan dose 62.5 mg daily or qod
Cyclosporine, tacrolimus	Monitor levels of the immunosuppressants
Sildenafil	25 mg every 48 hours
Tadalafil	No more than 10 mg in 72 hours
Vardenafil	No more than 2.5 mg in 24 hours

DOSING

Stiribild is a fixed formulation of tenofovir DF 300 mg + emtricitabine 200 mg + elvitegravir 150 mg + cobicistat 150 mg. The recommended adult dose is one tablet once daily.

SPECIAL POPULATIONS

RENAL IMPAIRMENT: Initiation of Stribild in patients with estimated creatinine clearance below 70 mL per minute is not recommended. Stribild should be discontinued if estimated creatinine clearance declines below 50 mL per minute during treatment.

HEPATIC DYSFUNCTION: Not recommended for use in patients with severe hepatic impairment.

PEDIATRICS: Not studied in patients under 18 years of age.

 THE ART OF ANTIMICROBIAL THERAPY

Clinical Pearls

1. Stribild should not be used with any medications that include its components including: Viread, Emtriva, Truvada, Descovy, Atripla, Genvoya, Complera, Odefsey, Vitekta, or Tybost.

2. Stribild is an integrase inhibitor and should not be used with Triumeq, Isentress, or Tivicay.

3. Stribild contains emtricitabine and should not be used with any medication containing lamivudine including: Epivir, Triumeq, Epzicom, Trizivir, or Combivir.

4. Stribild and didanosine combinations should be administered with caution.

5. Stribild should be given with food.

BASIC CHARACTERISTICS

Class: Avermectin antiparasitic.

Mechanism of Action: Ivermectin selectively binds to glutamate-gated chloride ion channels, which occur in invertebrate nerve and muscle cells. This leads to an increase in the permeability of the cell membrane to chloride ions with hyperpolarization of the nerve or muscle cell, resulting in paralysis and death of the parasite.

Metabolic Route: Metabolized by the liver and excreted in the feces.

 FDA-APPROVED INDICATIONS

The treatment of strongyloidiasis of the intestinal tract and onchocerciasis (river blindness).

Also Used for: Cutaneous larva migrans, scabies, body lice, trichostrongyliasis, ascariasis, and trichuriasis.

 SIDE EFFECTS/TOXICITY

Hypotension, dizziness, pruritus, worsening of bronchial asthma, toxic epidermal necrolysis, Stevens–Johnson syndrome, seizures, and hepatotoxicity. If patients with onchocerciasis are coinfected with Loa Loa and receive ivermectin, encephalopathy and other neurologic and ophthalmologic side effects are rarely seen.

Mazzotti reaction (fever, rash, adenopathy, arthralgia, etc.) may be seen in patients treated for onchocerciasis; though the Mazzotti reaction is not a direct toxic effect of ivermectin and probably results from antigenic products of the treated parasite, it may resemble drug toxicity and should be anticipated.

 DRUG INTERACTIONS/FOOD INTERACTIONS

Ivermectin should be taken on an empty stomach with a glass of water.

Increased INR when administered with warfarin.

 DOSING

Strongyloidiasis: A single oral dose of 200 mcg of ivermectin per kg of body weight.

Onchocerciasis: A single oral dose of 150 mcg of ivermectin per kg of body weight.

 SPECIAL POPULATIONS

RENAL IMPAIRMENT: There is no dose adjustment for renal insufficiency.

HEPATIC DYSFUNCTION: There is no dose adjustment for hepatic dysfunction.

PEDIATRICS: Not studied in children under 15 kg weight.

Antibiotics Manual: A Guide to Commonly Used Antimicrobials, Second Edition. David Schlossberg and Rafik Samuel.
© 2017 John Wiley & Sons Ltd. Published 2017 by John Wiley & Sons Ltd.

THE ART OF ANTIMICROBIAL THERAPY

Clinical Pearls

1. Although ivermectin is indicated only for the treatment of strongyloidiasis and onchocerciasis, it is also used for multiple additional parasitic infections, as listed above.

2. Although not approved for use in scabies, ivermectin has been found particularly helpful in Norwegian or crusted scabies, in view of the difficulty of penetrating the crusts with topical therapy alone.

3. When treating strongyloidiasis in HIV-infected patients, more than one course of therapy may be needed.

4. Follow-up stool examinations should be performed to verify eradication of infection.

5. Mazzotti reaction (see above) is a possible complication of therapy for onchocerciasis.

BASIC CHARACTERISTICS

Class: Sulfonamide.

Mechanism of Action: Sulfonamides competitively inhibit the incorporation of *para*-aminobenzoic acid into dihydropteroic acid.

Mechanisms of Resistance:

1. Overproduction of *para*-aminobenzoic acid.
2. Structural change in dihydropteroate synthesis.

Metabolic Route: Sulfadiazine is excreted in the urine.

 FDA-APPROVED INDICATIONS

Chancroid

Trachoma

Inclusion conjunctivitis

Nocardiosis

Urinary tract infections in the absence of obstructive uropathy or foreign bodies

Toxoplasmosis encephalitis as adjunctive therapy with pyrimethamine

Malaria due to chloroquine-resistant strains of *Plasmodium falciparum*, when used as adjunctive therapy

Prophylaxis of meningococcal meningitis for sulfa-sensitive group A strains

Meningococcal meningitis

Acute otitis media

Prophylaxis against recurrences of rheumatic fever, as an alternative to penicillin

H. influenzae **meningitis**, as adjunctive therapy with parenteral streptomycin.

 SIDE EFFECTS/TOXICITY

Contraindicated in patients with hypersensitivity to sulfonamides, infants less than 2 months of age (except as adjunctive therapy with pyrimethamine in the treatment of congenital toxoplasmosis), and in pregnancy at term and during the nursing period, because sulfonamides cross the placenta and are excreted in breast milk and may cause kernicterus.

Side effects include: hypersensitivity reactions including fever and rash (erythema multiforme (Stevens–Johnson syndrome), generalized skin eruptions, epidermal necrolysis, urticaria, serum sickness, pruritus, exfoliative dermatitis), nausea, emesis, abdominal pains, hepatitis, diarrhea, pancreatitis, stomatitis, renal failure, stone formation, headache, peripheral neuritis, depression, convulsions, ataxia, hallucinations, tinnitus, vertigo, goiter, diuresis, hypoglycemia aplastic anemia, thrombocytopenia, leukopenia, hemolytic anemia, purpura, hypoprothrombinemia, methemoglobinemia, hemolysis in individuals deficient in glucose-6-phosphate dehydrogenase.

Antibiotics Manual: A Guide to Commonly Used Antimicrobials, Second Edition. David Schlossberg and Rafik Samuel.
© 2017 John Wiley & Sons Ltd. Published 2017 by John Wiley & Sons Ltd.

DRUG INTERACTIONS/FOOD INTERACTIONS

Sulfadiazine can be taken with or without food.

Administration of a sulfonamide may increase the effect of oral anticoagulants, sulfonylurea hypoglycemic agents, thiazide diuretics, uricosuric agents, and methotrexate.

Agents such as indomethacin, probenecid, and salicylates may displace sulfonamides from plasma albumin and increase the concentrations of free drug in plasma.

 DOSING

Sulfadiazine is administered in 500 mg tablets.

Loading dose of 2–4 grams followed by 2 to 4 g, divided into 3 to 6 doses, every 24 hours.

 SPECIAL POPULATIONS

RENAL IMPAIRMENT: Use with caution.

HEPATIC DYSFUNCTION: Use with caution.

RENAL AND HEPATIC FAILURE: Should measure levels.

PEDIATRICS: Sulfadiazine is contraindicated in infants less than 2 months of age except as adjunctive therapy with pyrimethamine in the treatment of congenital toxoplasmosis.

For those over 2 months of age:

A loading dose of one-half the 24-hour dose followed by a maintenance dose of 150 mg/kg or 4 g/m^2, divided into 4 to 6 doses, every 24 hours, with a maximum of 6 g every 24 hours.

Rheumatic fever prophylaxis, under 30 kg, 500 mg every 24 hours; over 30 kg, 1 g every 24 hours.

 THE ART OF ANTIMICROBIAL THERAPY

Clinical Pearls

1. Complete blood counts and urinalyses with careful microscopic examinations should be done frequently in patients receiving sulfonamides.
2. Patients taking sulfadiazine should drink adequate amounts of water to decrease the likelihood of crystalluria and stone formation.
3. Systemic sulfonamides are contraindicated in infants under 2 months of age except as adjunctive therapy with pyrimethamine in the treatment of congenital toxoplasmosis.
4. The sulfonamides should **not** be used for the **treatment** of group A beta-hemolytic streptococcal infections; in an established infection, they will not eradicate the streptococcus.

BASIC CHARACTERISTICS

Class: Third generation cephalosporin.

Mechanism of Action: Binds penicillin-binding protein, disrupting cell wall synthesis.

Mechanisms of Resistance:

1. The PBP can be altered, with reduced affinity.

2. Production of a beta-lactamase, resulting in hydrolysis of the beta-lactam ring.

3. Decreased ability of the antibiotic to reach the PBP when bacteria decrease porin production, resulting in a decrease of the drug concentration within the cell.

Metabolic Route: Cefixime is excreted unchanged in the urine.

 FDA-APPROVED INDICATIONS

Treatment of the following infections when caused by susceptible organisms:

Uncomplicated urinary tract infections

Otitis media

Pharyngitis and tonsillitis

Acute exacerbations of chronic bronchitis

Uncomplicated gonorrhea

 SIDE EFFECTS/TOXICITY

Cefixime is **contraindicated** in patients with cephalosporin allergy and should be used with caution if hypersensitivity exists to penicillin.

Toxicity includes fever, anaphylaxis, rash including Stevens–Johnson syndrome, erythema multiforme and toxic epidermal necrolysis, angioedema, flushing, serum-sickness-like reactions, encephalopathy, seizures, diarrhea, *Clostridium difficile*-associated diarrhea and pseudomembranous colitis, oral candidiasis, anorexia, nausea, vomiting, stomach cramps, flatulence, hepatitis, renal impairment, genital moniliasis, vaginitis, hemorrhage, prolonged prothrombin time, pancytopenia, hemolytic anemia, and positive Coombs' test.

 DRUG INTERACTIONS/FOOD INTERACTIONS

Cefixime can be taken with or without food.

Increased levels of carbamazepine and prothrombin time may be seen when carbamazepine and warfarin are administered with cefixime.

Cephalosporins may cause false-positive urine glucose determinations when using cupric sulfate solution (Benedict's solution, *Clinitest*®). Tests utilizing glucose oxidase (*Tes-Tape*®, *Clinistix*®) are not affected by cephalosporins. A false-positive reaction for ketones in the urine may occur with tests using nitroprusside but not with those using nitroferricyanide.

Antibiotics Manual: A Guide to Commonly Used Antimicrobials, Second Edition. David Schlossberg and Rafik Samuel.
© 2017 John Wiley & Sons Ltd. Published 2017 by John Wiley & Sons Ltd.

DOSING

Cefixime is available as a 400 mg tablet and an oral suspension of 100 mg/5 mL.

The recommended dose of the suspension is 400 mg daily.

For the treatment of uncomplicated cervical/urethral gonococcal infections, a single oral dose of 400 mg is recommended.

 SPECIAL POPULATIONS

RENAL IMPAIRMENT:

Creatinine Clearance	Dose
21 and 60 mL/min or hemodialysis	300 mg daily
<20 mL/min or peritoneal dialysis	200 mg daily
CRRT	N/A

HEPATIC DYSFUNCTION: No dose adjustment is necessary.

PEDIATRICS: Safety and effectiveness of cefixime in children aged less than six months old have not been established.

The recommended dose is 8 mg/kg/day of the suspension. This may be administered as a single daily dose or may be given in two divided doses, as 4 mg/kg every 12 hours.

Children weighing more than 50 kg or older than 12 years should be treated with the recommended adult dose.

 THE ART OF ANTIMICROBIAL THERAPY

Clinical Pearls

1. Cefixime is dose adjusted for renal dysfunction.
2. Cross allergy with penicillins is <10 %.
3. Monitoring is essential when cefixime is coadministered with warfarin and carbamazepine.

Also available combined with tenofovir and emtricitabine as Atripla.

 ## BASIC CHARACTERISTICS

Class: Nonnucleoside reverse transcriptase inhibitor.

Mechanism of Action: Efavirenz inhibits reverse transcriptase activity by binding the enzyme.

Mechanism of Resistance: Changes in the structure of reverse transcriptase leads to the inability of efavirenz to bind the enzyme and allow transcription to continue. The most frequent resistance mutations include K103N and Y181C.

Metabolic Route: Metabolized by the cytochrome P450 system to hydroxylated metabolites with subsequent glucuronidation.

 ## FDA-APPROVED INDICATIONS

Treatment of HIV-1 in combinations with other antiretroviral agents.

 ## SIDE EFFECTS/TOXICITY

Serious psychiatric toxicity, including severe depression, suicidal ideation, nonfatal suicide attempts, aggressive behavior, paranoid reactions, manic reactions, insomnia, impaired concentration, somnolence, dizziness, abnormal dreams, and hallucinations.

Other adverse events include rash, elevated liver enzymes, convulsions, elevated cholesterol, fat redistribution, immune reconstitution syndrome, nausea and vomiting, headache, and fatigue.

 ## DRUG INTERACTIONS/FOOD INTERACTIONS

Efavirenz should be taken on an empty stomach at bedtime to decrease CNS side effects.

Efavirenz should not be administered concurrently with astemizole, bepridil, cisapride, midazolam, pimozide, triazolam, ergot derivatives, St John's wort, simepravir, atovaquone/proguanil, or etravirine.

Efavirenz causes hepatic enzyme induction of CYP3A4; coadministration of efavirenz with drugs primarily metabolized by 2C9, 2C19, and 3A4 isozymes may result in altered plasma concentrations of the coadministered drug. Drugs that induce CYP3A4 activity would be expected to increase the clearance of efavirenz, resulting in lowered plasma concentrations. Because of these metabolic activities, the following drug interactions warrant consideration of dosage adjustment and monitoring of clinical effects and serum levels of affected drugs:

Medication	Adjustment or action
Voriconazole	Increase voriconazole to 400 bid and decrease efavirenz to 300 daily
Clarithromycin	Consider alternative agent
Rifabutin	Increase rifabutin to 450–600/q d or 600 3 × week
Rifampin	Consider increasing efavirenz to 800/day
Contraceptives	Use alternative or additional method
Phenobarbitol, phenytoin, or carbamazepine	Monitor anticonvulsant level consider alternative

Antibiotics Manual: A Guide to Commonly Used Antimicrobials, Second Edition. David Schlossberg and Rafik Samuel.
© 2017 John Wiley & Sons Ltd. Published 2017 by John Wiley & Sons Ltd.

Medication	Adjustment or action
Methadone	Opiate withdrawal common; titrate methadone
Warfarin	Monitor INR closely
Fosamprenavir	fAPV 1400 + RTV 300 daily or usual BID dose
Darunavir	Monitor levels with normal dosing
Indinavir	IDV 800 bid + RTV 100 bid
Maraviroc	Increase maraviroc to 600 mg bid

 DOSING

Efavirenz is administered in 50 mg, 200 mg, and 600 mg tablets.

The recommended dosage of efavirenz is 600 mg orally, once daily, in combination with other antiretrovirals.

 SPECIAL POPULATIONS

RENAL IMPAIRMENT: There is no adjustment needed.

HEPATIC DYSFUNCTION: Not recommended in those with moderate to severe hepatic dysfunction.

PEDIATRICS: Should only be administered to children older than 3 years of age as follows:

Weight, kg	Dose, mg/day
3.5 to <5	100
5 to <7.5	150
7.5 to < 15	200
15 to <20	250
20 to <25	300
25 to <32.5	350
32.5 to <40	400
≥40	600

 THE ART OF ANTIMICROBIAL THERAPY

Clinical Pearls

1. Efavirenz should always be used in combination with other antiretrovirals.
2. Efavirenz should be dosed at bedtime to decrease the CNS adverse events.
3. If efavirenz is given without food, less is absorbed and side effects can be decreased.
4. Efavirenz has a very long half-life. If stopping antiretroviral regimen, to decrease resistance, the other medications should be continued for at least another 48 hours.
5. Women receiving efavirenz should use 2 methods of birth control.
6. Whenever initiating efavirenz, make sure to review all medications the patient is receiving, to limit drug interactions.

BASIC CHARACTERISTICS

Class: Neuraminidase inhibitor.

Mechanism of Action: Oseltamivir carboxylate is an inhibitor of influenza virus neuraminidase, affecting the release of viral particles.

Mechanism of Resistance: Mutations in the viral neuraminidase or viral hemagglutinin (or both).

Metabolic Route: Oseltamivir phosphate is an ethyl ester prodrug requiring ester hydrolysis for conversion to the active form, oseltamivir carboxylate. It is excreted unchanged in the urine.

 FDA-APPROVED INDICATIONS

Treatment of influenza A and B in patients two weeks and older.

Prophylaxis of influenza A and B in patients one year and older.

 SIDE EFFECTS/TOXICITY

Nausea, vomiting, bronchitis, insomnia, vertigo, rash including Stevens–Johnson syndrome, delirium, and seizure.

 DRUG INTERACTIONS/FOOD INTERACTIONS

Oseltamivir is well absorbed orally, with or without food.

Live attenuated influenza vaccine should not be given 2 weeks before or 2 days after taking oseltamivir.

 DOSING

Oseltamivir phosphate is available as 30 mg, 45 mg, or 75 mg capsules and as a powder for oral suspension, which when constituted with water as directed contains 6 mg/mL of oseltamivir base.

Dose for treatment in those 13 years and older is 75 mg twice daily for 5 days.

Dose for prophylaxis in those 13 years and older is 75 mg once daily for at least 10 days.

 SPECIAL POPULATIONS

RENAL IMPAIRMENT:

Creatinine clearance, mL/min	Treatment	Prophylaxis
>60–90	75 mg twice daily	75 mg once daily
>30–60	30 mg twice daily	30 mg once daily
>10–30	30 mg once daily	30 mg every other day
Hemodialysis	30 mg then 30 mg after alternate HD	30 mg then 30 mg after every HD
Peritoneal dialysis	Single 30 mg dose	30 mg dose weekly

Antibiotics Manual: A Guide to Commonly Used Antimicrobials, Second Edition. David Schlossberg and Rafik Samuel.
© 2017 John Wiley & Sons Ltd. Published 2017 by John Wiley & Sons Ltd.

HEPATIC DYSFUNCTION: No dose adjustment is recommended for patients with mild or moderate hepatic impairment. It should not be administered to those with severe hepatic impairment.

PEDIATRIC: Oseltamivir is indicated for treatment of influenza in pediatric patients 2 weeks and older. It is indicated for prophylaxis of influenza in pediatric patients 1 year and older.

Weight	Treatment	Prophylaxis
Patients 2 weeks to 1 year:		
Any weight	3 mg/kg twice daily	Not applicable
Patients over 1 year of age:		
≤15 kg	30 mg twice daily	30 mg once daily
>15 kg to 23 kg	45 mg twice daily	45 mg once daily
>23 kg to 40 kg	60 mg twice daily	60 mg once daily
>40 kg	75 mg twice daily	75 mg once daily

 THE ART OF ANTIMICROBIAL THERAPY

Clinical Pearls

1. Oseltamivir has activity against both influenza A and B.
2. Oseltamivir is active against avian H5N1 and novel H1N1 influenza.
3. An increased incidence of resistance to oseltamivir has been described.
4. Resistance to oseltamivir may not lead to resistance to zanamavir.
5. Delerium and abnormal behavior have been seen in pediatric patients.

BASIC CHARACTERISTICS

Class: Ombitasvir is a hepatitis C virus NS5A inhibitor.

Paritaprevir is a hepatitis C virus NS3/4A protease inhibitor.

Ritonavir is a CYP3A inhibitor.

Mechanism of Action: Ombitasvir is an inhibitor of HCV NS5A, which is essential for viral RNA replication and virion assembly.

Paritaprevir is an inhibitor of the HCV NS3/4A protease, which is necessary for the proteolytic cleavage of the HCV encoded polyprotein and is essential for viral replication.

Ritonavir is a CYP3A inhibitor that inhibits CYP3A mediated metabolism of paritaprevir.

Mechanism of Resistance: Ombitasvir activity is decreased by mutations on the NS5A protein: M28T/V, Q30E/R, L31V, H58D, and Y93C/H/L/N.

Paritaprevir activity is decreased by mutations on the protease enzyme: F43L, R155G/K/S, A156T, D168A/E/F/H/N/V/Y, and Q80K.

Metabolic Route: Ombitasvir is metabolized by amide hydrolysis.

Pariteprevir is metabolized by CYP 3A4.

Ritonavir is metabolized by the CYP 3A4.

 FDA-APPROVED INDICATIONS

Technivie is indicated in combination with ribavirin for the treatment of patients with genotype 4 chronic hepatitis C virus (HCV) infection without cirrhosis.

 SIDE EFFECTS/TOXICITY

Hepatic decompensation and hepatic failure, including liver transplantation or fatal outcomes, increased the risk of ALT and bilirubin elevations.

Other side effects include fatigue, nausea, pruritis, rash, insomnia, asthenia, and anemia.

 DRUG INTERACTIONS/FOOD INTERACTIONS

Ombitasvir and paritaprevir are inhibitors of UGT1A1 and ritonavir is an inhibitor of CYP3A4. Paritaprevir is an inhibitor of OATP1B1 and OATP1B3 and paritaprevir, and ritonavir is an inhibitor of BCRP. Coadministration of Technivie with drugs that are substrates of CYP3A, UGT1A1, BCRP, OATP1B1, or OATP1B3 may result in increased plasma concentrations of such drugs.

The **contraindications** to ribavirin also apply to this combination regimen. Refer to the ribavirin prescribing information for a list of **contraindications**.

Technivie should not be administered with alfuzosin, carbamazepine, phenobarbital, phenytoin, colchicine, rifampin, rifapentine, ergotamine, dihydroergotamine, methylergonovine, ethinyl estradiol, St John's wort, lovastatin, pravastatin, pimozide, efavirenz, sildenafil, triazolam, midazolam, voriconazole, fluticasone, atazanavir, Kaletra, rilpivirine, or salmeterol.

Antibiotics Manual: A Guide to Commonly Used Antimicrobials, Second Edition. David Schlossberg and Rafik Samuel.
© 2017 John Wiley & Sons Ltd. Published 2017 by John Wiley & Sons Ltd.

Dose adjustments needed are as follows:

Medication	Adjustment or action
Valsartan, losartan, candesartan	Lower the dose of the ARB
Digoxin	Decrease dose 30–50 % and monitor levels
Antiarrhythmics	Monitor levels
Ketoconazole	Maximum dose of ketoconazole should be 200 mg
Quetiapine	Decrease the dose of quetiapine to one-sixth
Calcium channel blockers	Decrease the calcium channel blocker by 50 %
Darunavir	Darunavir 800 mg must be taken at the same time as Technivie
Pravastatin	Maximum dose of pravastatin is 40 mg
Cyclosporine	Decrease cyclosporine to one-fifth the dose and monitor levels
Tacrolimus	Reduce dose to 0.5 mg every 7 days and monitor levels
Buprenorphine/naloxone	Monitor closely
Alprazolam	Monitor closely
Rifabutin	150 mg/d or 300 mg 3 ×/week and monitor

 DOSING

Technivie is ombitasvir 12.5 mg, paritaprevir 75 mg, ritonavir 50 mg fixed dose combination. The recommended oral dosage is two ombitasvir, paritaprevir, ritonavir tablets once daily (in the morning). Take Technivie with a meal without regard to fat or calorie content.

Patient population	Medication	Duration
Genotype 4 without cirrhosis	Technivie + ribavirin	12 weeks

 SPECIAL POPULATIONS

RENAL IMPAIRMENT: No dosage adjustment.

HEPATIC DYSFUNCTION: Not recommended for patients with moderate or severe hepatic impairment.

PEDIATRICS: Do not use in those under 18 years of age.

THE ART OF ANTIMICROBIAL THERAPY

Clinical Pearls
1. Technivie is only indicated for HCV genotype 4.
2. Monitor liver chemistry tests before and during Technivie therapy.
3. Technivie contains ritonavir, so all patients with HIV must be on treatment to prevent HIV resistance.
4. Review the most current hepatitis C treatment guidelines because they are changing rapidly: http://www.cdc.gov/hepatitis/HCV/index.htm.

BASIC CHARACTERISTICS

Class: Cephalosporin.

Mechanism of Action: Binds penicillin-binding protein, disrupting cell wall synthesis.

Mechanisms of Resistance:

1. The PBP can be altered, with reduced affinity.

2. Production of a beta-lactamase, resulting in hydrolysis of the beta-lactam ring.

3. Decreased ability of the antibiotic to reach the PBP when bacteria decrease porin production, resulting in a decrease of the drug concentration within the cell.

Metabolic Route: Primarily excreted by the kidneys.

 FDA-APPROVED INDICATIONS

Acute bacterial skin and skin structure infections (ABSSSI) caused by susceptible gram-positive (including MRSA) and gram-negative organisms.

Community-acquired bacterial pneumonia caused by susceptible organisms.

 SIDE EFFECTS/TOXICITY

Contraindicated in patients who have shown serious hypersensitivity to ceftaroline or other beta-lactam antibiotics. If other forms of hypersensitivity to beta-lactams exist, use with caution.

Toxicity includes *Clostridium difficile*-associated diarrhea (CDAD), direct Coombs' test, **diarrhea**, **nausea**, and **rash**, anemia, eosinophilia, neutropenia, thrombocytopenia, bradycardia, palpitations, abdominal pain, pyrexia, hepatitis, hypersensitivity, hyperglycemia, hyperkalemia, dizziness, convulsion, renal failure, and urticaria.

 DRUG INTERACTIONS/FOOD INTERACTIONS

There is minimal potential for drug–drug interactions between ceftaroline and CYP450 substrates, inhibitors, or inducers.

 DOSING

Type of infection	Dose	Duration
ABSSSI	600 mg q 12 h	5–14 days
CABP	600 mg q 12 h	5–7 days

Antibiotics Manual: A Guide to Commonly Used Antimicrobials, Second Edition. David Schlossberg and Rafik Samuel.
© 2017 John Wiley & Sons Ltd. Published 2017 by John Wiley & Sons Ltd.

SPECIAL POPULATIONS

RENAL IMPAIRMENT:

Creatinine clearance	Dose
>30 to <50	400 mg IV q 12 h
>15 to <30	300 mg IV q 12 h

End-stage renal disease, including HD 200 mg IV q 12 h

If hemodialysed, give after hemodialysis on hemodialysis days

HEPATIC DYSFUNCTION: No dose adjustment necessary.

PEDIATRICS: Safety and effectiveness in pediatric patients has not been established.

 THE ART OF ANTIMICROBIAL THERAPY

Clinical Pearls

1. Ceftaroline is not active against gram-negative bacteria producing extended spectrum beta-lactamases (ESBLs) or carbapenemases.

2. Ceftaroline is not active against *Pseudomonas*.

3. Ceftaroline is the only cephalosporin active against MRSA.

4. Although not FDA approved, ceftaroline has been used to treat MRSA bacteremia, but the dose should be increased to 600 mg every 8 hours.

BASIC CHARACTERISTICS

Class: Tetracycline.

Mechanism of Action: They reversibly bind the 30s ribosomal subunit, preventing the addition of new amino acids into the growing peptide chain.

Mechanisms of Resistance: Decreased entry into the cell or increased excretion of the drug. Rarely the tetracyclines are inactivated.

Metabolic Route: They are concentrated by the liver in the bile, and excreted in the urine and feces at high concentrations and in a biologically active form.

 FDA-APPROVED INDICATIONS

Tetracycline is indicated for the treatment of serious infections caused by susceptible strains of microorganisms in the conditions listed below:

Respiratory tract infections, skin and soft tissue infections, urinary tract infections, Rocky Mountain spotted fever, typhus group infections, Q fever, rickettsial pox, psittacosis infections caused by *Chlamydia trachomatis* such as uncomplicated urethral, endocervical, or rectal infections, inclusion conjunctivitis, trachoma and lymphogranuloma venereum, *Granuloma inguinale*, relapsing fever, bartonellosis, chancroid, tularemia, plague, cholera, brucellosis, infections due to *Campylobacter fetus*, amebiasis, acne, syphilis and yaws, Vincent's infection, infections caused by *Neisseria gonorrhoeae*, anthrax, listeriosis, actinomycosis, and infections due to *Clostridium* species.

 SIDE EFFECTS/TOXICITY

This drug is **contraindicated** in persons who have shown hypersensitivity to any of the tetracyclines.

Tetracyclines should not be used during pregnancy or up to the age of 8 years unless absolutely necessary and no reasonable alternative exists.

Side effects include hypersensitivity reactions, including rash, anaphylaxis, urticaria, angioneurotic edema, serum sickness, photosensitivity, pericarditis, and exacerbation of systemic lupus erythematosus, nausea, vomiting, diarrhea, glossitis, esophagitis, hepatotoxicity, pseudomembranous colitis, bulging fontanels in infants and benign intracranial hypertension in adults, vertigo, pseudotumor cerebri, tinnitus and decreased hearing, dose-related rise in BUN, hemolytic anemia, thrombocytopenia, neutropenia, and eosinophilia.

 DRUG INTERACTIONS/FOOD INTERACTIONS

Tetracycline hydrochloride tablets should be taken at least one hour before meals or 2 hours after meals.

1. Concurrent use of tetracycline may render oral contraceptives less effective.
2. Patients who are on anticoagulant therapy may require downward adjustment of their anticoagulant dosage.
3. It is advisable to avoid giving tetracycline-class drugs in conjunction with penicillin.
4. Absorption of oral tetracycline is impaired by antacids containing aluminum, calcium, or magnesium, and iron-containing preparations.

Antibiotics Manual: A Guide to Commonly Used Antimicrobials, Second Edition. David Schlossberg and Rafik Samuel.
© 2017 John Wiley & Sons Ltd. Published 2017 by John Wiley & Sons Ltd.

5. The concurrent use of tetracycline and methoxyflurane has resulted in fatal renal toxicity.

6. Pregnant women with renal disease may be more prone to develop tetracycline-associated liver failure.

 DOSING

Tetracycline is administered as 250 mg and 500 mg tablets. The **usual daily dose** is 500 mg bid or 250 mg qid. Higher doses such as 500 mg qid may be required for severe infections or for those infections that do not respond to the smaller doses. Therapy is usually continued for at least 24–48 hours after symptoms and fever have subsided.

Brucellosis: 500 mg qid × 3 weeks (in combination with other antibiotics).

Syphilis: 500 mg qid × 15 days for syphilis of less than one year's duration and × 30 days for syphilis of more than one year's duration.

Gonorrhea, chlamydial urogenital infection: 500 mg qid × 7 days.

 SPECIAL POPULATIONS

RENAL IMPAIRMENT:

Creatinine clearance, mL/min	Dose
10–50	Usual dose every 12–24 hours
<10	Usual dose once daily
Hemodialysis, CAPD, and CRRT	N/A

HEPATIC DYSFUNCTION: Data incomplete.

PEDIATRICS: **For children above eight years of age:** The usual daily dose is 10 to 20 mg/lb (25 to 50 mg/kg) body weight divided in four equal doses.

 THE ART OF ANTIMICROBIAL THERAPY

Clinical Pearls

1. To reduce the risk of esophageal irritation and ulceration, tetracycline should be taken with adequate amounts of fluid and should not be taken immediately before going to bed.

2. Tetracycline can cause fetal harm when administered to a pregnant woman.

3. The use of drugs of the tetracycline class during tooth development (last half of pregnancy, infancy, and childhood to the age of 8 years) may cause permanent discoloration of the teeth (yellow–gray–brown).

4. Tetracycline should not be administered with calcium or other cations.

BASIC CHARACTERISTICS

Class: Glycylcycline.

Mechanism of Action: Tigecycline inhibits protein translation in bacteria by binding to the 30S ribosomal subunit and blocking entry of amino-acyl tRNA molecules into the A site of the ribosome.

Mechanisms of Resistance: Tigecycline is not affected by the major tetracycline-resistance mechanism, ribosomal protection.

Tigecycline resistance in some bacteria is associated with multidrug-resistant efflux pumps.

Metabolic Route: 60 % in feces and the remainder in the urine.

 FDA-APPROVED INDICATIONS

Complicated skin and skin structure infections caused by susceptible organisms.

Complicated intra-abdominal infections caused by susceptible organisms.

Community-acquired bacterial pneumonia caused by susceptible organisms.

 SIDE EFFECTS/TOXICITY

> **WARNING: All-cause mortality**: An increase in all-cause mortality has been observed in a meta-analysis of Phase 3 and 4 clinical trials in tygecycline-treated patients versus a comparator. The cause of this mortality risk difference of 0.6 % (95 % CI 0.1, 1.2) has not been established. Tigecycline should be reserved for use in situations when alternative treatments are not suitable.

Contraindicated for use in patients who have known hypersensitivity to tigecycline.

Side effects include anaphylaxis/anaphylactoid reactions, liver dysfunction and liver failure, fetal harm when administered to a pregnant woman, permanent discoloration of teeth (yellow–gray–brown) if administered during tooth development (last half of pregnancy, infancy, and childhood to the age of 8 years), nausea, vomiting, diarrhea, abdominal pain, *Clostridium difficile*-associated diarrhea, headache, hypocalcemia, hypoglycemia, hyponatremia, and thrombocytopenia.

Tigecycline is structurally similar to tetracycline-class antibiotics and may have similar adverse effects seen with tetracyclines, including photosensitivity, pseudotumor cerebri, pancreatitis, and antianabolic action (which has led to increased BUN, azotemia, acidosis, and hyperphosphatemia).

 DRUG INTERACTIONS/FOOD INTERACTIONS

1. Prothrombin time should be monitored if tigecycline is administered with warfarin.
2. Concurrent use of antibacterial drugs with oral contraceptives may render oral contraceptives less effective.

 DOSING

The recommended dosage regimen is an initial dose of 100 mg IV, followed by 50 mg every 12 hours.

Antibiotics Manual: A Guide to Commonly Used Antimicrobials, Second Edition. David Schlossberg and Rafik Samuel.
© 2017 John Wiley & Sons Ltd. Published 2017 by John Wiley & Sons Ltd.

SPECIAL POPULATIONS

RENAL IMPAIRMENT: No dose adjustment is necessary.

HEPATIC DYSFUNCTION: In patients with severe hepatic impairment (Child Pugh* C), the initial dose of tigecycline should be 100 mg followed by a reduced maintenance dose of 25 mg every 12 hours. Patients with severe hepatic impairment (Child Pugh C) should be treated with caution and monitored for a treatment response.

PEDIATRICS: Safety and efficacy in patients under the age of 18 have not been established.

 ## THE ART OF ANTIMICROBIAL THERAPY

Clinical pearls

1. Tigecycline can cause fetal harm when administered to a pregnant woman.
2. The use of drugs of the tetracycline class during tooth development (last half of pregnancy, infancy, and childhood to the age of 8 years) may cause permanent discoloration of the teeth (yellow–gray–brown).
3. Tigecycline is not active against *Pseudomonas* spp.
4. Tigecycline is associated with poor outcomes in hospital-associated pneumonia.
5. Caution is urged in patients with known hypersensitivity to tetracyclines.
6. Tigecycline is not indicated for the treatment of diabetic foot infections. A clinical trial failed to demonstrate noninferiority of tigecycline for treatment of diabetic foot infections.
7. Tigecycline is not indicated for the treatment of hospital-acquired or ventilator-associated pneumonia. In a comparative clinical trial, greater mortality and decreased efficacy were reported in tigecycline-treated patients.

---

* See Helpful Formulas, Equations, and Definitions for definitions.

BASIC CHARACTERISTICS

Class: Carboxypenicillin.

Mechanism of Action: Binds penicillin-binding protein, disrupting cell wall synthesis.

Mechanisms of Resistance:

1. The PBP can be altered, with reduced affinity.
2. Production of a beta-lactamase, resulting in hydrolysis of the beta-lactam ring.
3. Decreased ability of the antibiotic to reach the PBP when bacteria decrease porin production, resulting in a decrease of the drug concentration within the cell.

Metabolic Route: The majority of ticarcillin and half of clavulanate are excreted unchanged in the urine.

 FDA-APPROVED INDICATIONS

Ticarcillin–clavulanate is indicated in the treatment of infections due to susceptible strains of microorganisms in the conditions listed below:

Septicemia (including bacteremia)

Lower respiratory infections

Bone and joint infections

Skin and skin structure infections

Urinary tract infections

Gynecologic infections

Intra-abdominal infections

 SIDE EFFECTS/TOXICITY

A history of allergic reaction to any of the penicillins is a **contraindication**.

Side effects include *Clostridium difficile*-associated diarrhea (CDAD), hypersensitivity reactions including anaphylaxis, rash including erythema multiforme and Stevens–Johnson syndrome, mucocutaneous candidiasis, nausea, vomiting, diarrhea, constipation, black hairy tongue, headache, arrhythmias, hyperactivity and seizures, confusion, hepatitis, renal dysfunction, anemia, thrombocytopenia, eosinophilia, leukopenia, hypernatremia, hypokalemia, abnormalities of coagulation.

 DRUG INTERACTIONS/FOOD INTERACTIONS

Concurrent use of ticarcillin/clavulanate and probenecid may result in increased and prolonged blood levels of ticarcillin/clavulanate.

High urine concentrations of ticarcillin may produce false-positive urine protein reactions.

False-positive Coombs' test.

Chloramphenicol, macrolides, sulfonamides, and tetracyclines may interfere with the bactericidal effects of penicillins.

Antibiotics Manual: A Guide to Commonly Used Antimicrobials, Second Edition. David Schlossberg and Rafik Samuel.
© 2017 John Wiley & Sons Ltd. Published 2017 by John Wiley & Sons Ltd.

High urine concentrations of ticarcillin may result in false-positive reactions when testing for the presence of glucose in urine using *Clinitest*®. It is recommended that glucose tests based on enzymatic glucose oxidase reactions (such as *Clinistix*®) be used.

 DOSING

The usual dosage for **systemic and urinary tract infections** is 3.1 grams every 4 to 6 hours.

For **gynecologic infections**, moderate infections, 200 mg/kg/day in divided doses every 6 hours, and for severe infections, 300 mg/kg/day in divided doses every 4 hours.

 SPECIAL POPULATIONS

RENAL IMPAIRMENT:

Creatinine clearance, mL/min	*Dosage*
30–60	2 g q 4 hours
10–30	2 g q 8 hours
<10	2 g q 12 hours
<10 with hepatic impairment	2 g q 24 hours
CAPD	3.1 g q 12 hours
Hemodialysis	2 g q 12 hours with 3.1 g after dialysis
CRRT	Unknown

HEPATIC DYSFUNCTION: No dose adjustment is necessary.

PEDIATRICS: There are insufficient data to support the use in pediatric patients under 3 months of age.

Pediatric patients ≥3 months and <60 kg, 50 mg/kg every 6 hours for mild–moderate infections and every 4 hours for severe infections.

For patients ≥60 kg use the adult dosing recommendations.

 THE ART OF ANTIMICROBIAL THERAPY

Clinical Pearls

1. Ticarcillin/clavulanate needs to be dose adjusted for renal dysfunction.
2. The theoretical sodium content is 4.51 meq (103.6 mg) per gram of ticarcillin/clavulanate. This should be considered when treating patients requiring restricted salt intake.
3. Treatment of pseudomonas may be more successful with the addition of an aminoglycoside.

BASIC CHARACTERISTICS

Class: Synthetic antiprotozoal.

Mechanism of Action: Synthetic antiprotozoal.

Metabolic Route: Mostly excreted unchanged in the urine.

 FDA-APPROVED INDICATIONS

Treatment of trichomoniasis, giardiasis, intestinal amebiasis, amebic liver abscess, and bacterial vaginosis.

 SIDE EFFECTS/TOXICITY

> **WARNINGS:** Carcinogenicity has been seen in mice and rats treated chronically with metronidazole, another nitroimidazole agent. Although such data have not been reported for tinidazole, the two drugs are structurally related and have similar biologic effects.

The use of tinidazole is **contraindicated** in patients with a previous history of hypersensitivity to tinidazole or other nitroimidazole derivatives, during first trimester of pregnancy and in nursing mothers.

Adverse events include: fever, hypersensitivity, angioedema, rash including Stevens–Johnson syndrome and erythema multiforme, seizures, coma, confusion, peripheral neuropathy, vertigo, ataxia, insomnia, depression, drowsiness, tongue discoloration, stomatitis, diarrhea, urticaria, pruritus, rash, flushing, sweating, dryness of mouth, thirst, salivation, darkened urine, palpitations, bronchospasm, *Candida* overgrowth, raised transaminase level, arthralgias, arthritis, myalgias, neutropenia, leucopenia, and thrombocytopenia.

 DRUG INTERACTIONS/FOOD INTERACTIONS

Tinidazole should be taken with food.

Do not administer tinidazole with alcoholic beverages, preparations containing ethanol or propylene glycol or disulfiram, fluorouracil, or cholestyramine.

Coadministered drugs may affect the level of tinidazole or of the coadministered drug, as follows, where monitoring is recommended:

Cimetidine: increased levels of tinidazole

Cyclosporine: increased effect of cyclosporin

Fosphenytoin: decreased levels of tinidazole

Ketoconazole: increased levels of tinidazole

Lithium: increased effect of lithium

Phenobarbitol: decreased levels of tinidazole

Phenytoin: decreased levels of tinidazole

Rifampin: decreased levels of tinidazole

Antibiotics Manual: A Guide to Commonly Used Antimicrobials, Second Edition. David Schlossberg and Rafik Samuel.
© 2017 John Wiley & Sons Ltd. Published 2017 by John Wiley & Sons Ltd.

Tacrolimus: increased effect of tacrolimus

Warfarin: increased effect of warfarin

Tinidazole may interfere with determinations of serum chemistry values, such as AST, ALT, LDH, triglycerides, and hexokinase glucose.

 DOSING

Tinidazole is administered as 250 mg and 500 mg tablets.

Trichomoniasis: a single 2 g oral dose taken with food.

Giardiasis: a single 2 g dose taken with food.

Amebiasis:

Mild to moderate intestinal disease: 2 g once PO daily × 3 d taken with food.

Severe intestinal and extraintestinal disease:

Amebic liver abscess: 2 g dose per day for 5 days taken with food.

Bacterial vaginosis: 2 g oral dose once daily for 2 days taken with food or a 1 g oral dose once daily for 5 days taken with food.

 SPECIAL POPULATIONS

RENAL IMPAIRMENT: If tinidazole is administered on the same day as and prior to hemodialysis, it is recommended that an additional dose of tinidazole equivalent to one-half of the recommended dose be administered after the end of the hemodialysis.

HEPATIC DYSFUNCTION: Usual recommended doses of tinidazole should be administered cautiously in patients with hepatic dysfunction.

PEDIATRICS:

Giardiasis: In pediatric patients older than three years of age, the recommended dose is a single dose of 50 mg/kg (up to 2 g) with food.

Amebiasis: *Mild to moderate intestinal disease:* In pediatric patients older than three years of age, the recommended dose is 50 mg/kg/day (up to 2 g per day) for 3 days with food.

Severe intestinal and extraintestinal disease: In pediatric patients older than three years of age, the recommended dose is 50 mg/kg/day (up to 2 g per day) for 5 days with food.

 THE ART OF ANTIMICROBIAL THERAPY

Clinical Pearls

1. Ethanol should be avoided when taking tinidazole.
2. For those unable to swallow tablets, tinidazole tablets may be crushed in artificial cherry syrup to be taken with food.
3. Tinidazole should not be used in the first trimester of pregnancy.

BASIC CHARACTERISTICS

Class: Integrase inhibitor.

Mechanism of Action: Dolutegravir is an HIV-1 integrase strand transfer inhibitor (INSTI). Inhibition of integrase prevents the integration of HIV-1 DNA into host genomic DNA, blocking propagation of the viral infection.

Mechanism of Resistance: Dolutegravir changes the structure of HIV integrase. Development of mutations on the enzyme integrase prevents dolutegravir from binding the active site of the enzyme and allowing integrase activity to continue. Resistance mutations that affect dolutegravir include E92Q, G118R, S153F or Y, G193E, R263K, Q148R or H, T97A, E138K, G140S, M154I, L74M, and N155H.

Metabolic Route: Dolutegravir is primarily metabolized via UGT1A1 with some contribution from CYP3A in the liver and excreted.

 ## FDA-APPROVED INDICATIONS

In combination with other antiretroviral drugs for the treatment of HIV-1 infection.

 ## SIDE EFFECTS/TOXICITY

Dolutegravir has been shown to increase serum creatinine due to inhibition of tubular secretion of creatinine without affecting renal glomerular function.

Immune reconstitution syndrome.

Redistribution/accumulation of body fat has been observed in patients receiving antiretroviral therapy.

Hypersensitivity reaction.

Hepatitis B immune reconstitution syndrome.

In less than 2 %: abdominal pain, flatulence, vomiting, hepatitis, myositis, suicidal ideation, attempt, behavior, or completion, renal impairment, and pruritus.

 ## DRUG INTERACTIONS/FOOD INTERACTIONS

Dolutegravir can be taken with or without food.

Dolutegravir is metabolized by UGT1A1 with some contribution from CYP3A. Drugs that induce or inhibit these enzymes can affect dolutegravir levels. Do not coadminister with nevirapine, oxcarbazepine, phenytoin, phenobarbital, or St John's wort. If dosed with etravirine, a protease inhibitor must be given with it.

Increase dose of dolutegravir to 50 mg twice daily if given with efavirenz, fosamprenavir, tipranavir, orcarbamazepine, or (if no INSTI mutation) rifampin.

Can be given with rifabutin with no dosage adjustment in either, even if INSTI mutation is present. If administered with magnesium, calcium, aluminum, or iron containing supplements, administer dolutegravir 2 hours before or 6 hours after these agents.

If administered with metformin, do not exceed a dose of 1000 mg daily.

Antibiotics Manual: A Guide to Commonly Used Antimicrobials, Second Edition. David Schlossberg and Rafik Samuel.
© 2017 John Wiley & Sons Ltd. Published 2017 by John Wiley & Sons Ltd.

DOSING

50 mg daily in patients without integrase-resistant virus.

50 mg twice daily in patients with integrase-resistant virus.

 SPECIAL POPULATIONS

RENAL IMPAIRMENT: No dose adjustment necessary.

HEPATIC DYSFUNCTION: Not indicated in Child Pugh class C.

PEDIATRICS: Not recommended for those under the age of 12 or those who weigh less than 40 kg.

 THE ART OF ANTIMICROBIAL THERAPY

Clinical Pearls

1. Dolutegravir should not be used with Triumeq.
2. Dolutegravir should not be used with other integrase inhibitors, including Isentress, Stribild, or Genvoya.
3. Dolutegravir still maintains activity against HIV integrase if integrase mutations are present.
4. Dolutegravir can increase serum creatinine by inhibiting its secretion in the distal tubules.

BASIC CHARACTERISTICS

Class: Aminoglycoside.

Mechanisms of Action:

1. Rearranges lipopolysaccharide in the outer membrane of the bacterial cell wall, resulting in disruption of the cell wall.
2. Binds the 30S subunit of the bacterial ribosome, which terminates protein synthesis.

Mechanism of Resistance:

1. Gram-negative bacteria inactivate aminoglycosides by acetylation.
2. Some bacteria alter the 30S ribosomal subunit, which prevents tobramycin's interference with protein synthesis.
3. Low-level resistance may result from inhibition of tobramycin uptake by the bacteria.

Metabolic Route: The drug is excreted unchanged in the urine.

 FDA-APPROVED INDICATIONS

Treatment of susceptible gram-negative bacteria causing bacteremia, pneumonia, osteomyelitis, arthritis, meningitis, skin and soft tissue infection, intra-abdominal infections, in burns and postoperative infections, and urinary tract infections.

Also Used for: Combination therapy with beta-lactams for the treatment of gram-positive endovascular infections and treatment of nontuberculous mycobacterial infections.

 SIDE EFFECTS/TOXICITY

> **WARNINGS:**
>
> **Ototoxicity**: vestibular toxicity and auditory ototoxicity, especially in patients with renal damage, those treated with higher doses, and those with prolonged treatment. Avoid use with potent diuretics such as ethacrynic acid because of additive ototoxicity.
>
> Other manifestations of neurotoxicity may include numbness, skin tingling, muscle twitching, and convulsions.
>
> **Nephrotoxicity**: especially in patients with impaired renal function and those treated with higher doses or prolonged treatment. Avoid concurrent use with other nephrotoxic agents and potent diuretics, which can cause dehydration.
>
> Prolonged serum concentrations above 12 mcg/mL should be avoided. Rising trough levels (above 2 mcg/mL) may indicate tissue accumulation.

Other adverse effects include anemia, granulocytopenia and thrombocytopenia, fever, rash, nausea, vomiting, diarrhea, confusion, abnormal liver function tests, neuromuscular blockade (especially in those receiving anesthetics, neuromuscular blocking agents or massive transfusions), decreased serum calcium, magnesium, sodium, and potassium, leukopenia, and leukocytosis.

 DRUG INTERACTIONS

Tobramycin should not be administered with other medications that are nephrotoxic or ototoxic.

Antibiotics Manual: A Guide to Commonly Used Antimicrobials, Second Edition. David Schlossberg and Rafik Samuel.
© 2017 John Wiley & Sons Ltd. Published 2017 by John Wiley & Sons Ltd.

DOSING

3–5 mg/kg/day IM or IV divided q 8 h; desired serum levels are peak 6–12 μg/mL and trough <2 μg/mL. Can also be given once daily as 5–7 mg/kg/24 h; desired serum levels are peak 16–24 μg/mL and trough < 1 μg/mL. Infuse over 60 minutes to avoid neuromuscular blockade.

Intrathecal dose: 4–8 mg/day.

SPECIAL POPULATIONS

RENAL IMPAIRMENT: Adjust dose either by increased interval (serum creatinine multiplied by 8), or by lowering the dose by dividing the dose by the serum creatinine. With either approach, adjustments should be made by following serum assays for q 8 h dosing, above.

Hemodialysis: 3 mg/kg loading dose followed by 1–1.7 mg/kg after hemodialysis.

Peritoneal dialysis: 1 mg/2 L dialysate removed.

CRRT: 3 mg/kg loading dose followed by 2 mg/kg q 24–48 h.

HEPATIC DYSFUNCTION: No dose adjustment necessary.

PEDIATRICS: 3–6 mg/kg/day; divide IV q 8 h (newborn: 0–7 d: <4 mg/kg/d q 12 h; 1–4 weeks: 3–5 mg/kg/d q 8 h).

THE ART OF ANTIMICROBIAL THERAPY

Clinical Pearls

1. Aminoglycosides require oxygen to be active and thus are less effective in anaerobic environment such as an abscess or infected bone.
2. Aminoglycosides have decreased activity in low pH environments such as respiratory secretions or abscesses.
3. When dosing aminoglycosides, use the ideal body weight not true body weight.
4. Tobramycin has a postantibiotic effect that allows it to be used once daily.
5. Renal and eighth-nerve function should be closely monitored.

BASIC CHARACTERISTICS

Class: Derivative of isonicotinic acid.

Mechanisms of Action: Blocks mycolic acid synthesis.

Mechanisms of Resistance: Incompletely understood.

Metabolic Route: Metabolism is presumed to occur in the liver and 6 metabolites have been isolated.

 FDA-APPROVED INDICATIONS

Treatment of active tuberculosis in patients with *M. tuberculosis* resistant to isoniazid or rifampin, or when there is intolerance on the part of the patient to other drugs.

 SIDE EFFECTS/TOXICITY

Contraindicated in patients with severe hepatic impairment and in patients who are hypersensitive to the drug.

Adverse events: hepatitis, hypoglycemia, hypothyroidism, nausea, vomiting, diarrhea, abdominal pain, excessive salivation, metallic taste, stomatitis, anorexia, weight loss, headache, psychotic disturbances, rash, photosensitivity, thrombocytopenia, gynecomastia, impotence, peripheral neuritis, optic neuritis, diplopia, blurred vision, and a pellagra-like syndrome.

 DRUG INTERACTIONS/FOOD INTERACTIONS

Ethionamide tablets may be administered without regard to the timing of meals.

Ethionamide has been found to raise serum concentrations of isoniazid.

Convulsions have been reported when ethionamide is administered with cycloserine. Excessive ethanol ingestion should be avoided because a psychotic reaction has been reported.

 DOSING

Ethionamide is supplied as 250 mg tablets. The usual adult dose is 15–20 mg/kg/day frequently divided (maximum dose 1 gm per day); usually 500–750 mg per day in 2 divided doses or a single daily dose.

A single daily dose can sometimes be given at bedtime or with the main meal.

 SPECIAL POPULATIONS

RENAL IMPAIRMENT: No dose adjustment is necessary.

HEPATIC DYSFUNCTION: Contraindicated in patients with severe hepatic dysfunction.

PEDIATRICS: Should not be used in pediatric patients under 12 years of age except when the organisms are definitely resistant to primary therapy and systemic dissemination of the disease, or other life-threatening complications of tuberculosis, is judged to be imminent. Dose is 15–20 mg/kg/day usually divided into 2–3 doses (maximum dose 1 gm per day).

Antibiotics Manual: A Guide to Commonly Used Antimicrobials, Second Edition. David Schlossberg and Rafik Samuel.
© 2017 John Wiley & Sons Ltd. Published 2017 by John Wiley & Sons Ltd.

THE ART OF ANTIMICROBIAL THERAPY

Clinical Pearls

1. Ethionamide should never be used alone in the treatment of active tuberculosis.
2. Ethionamide should only be used if resistance or intolerance of the first-line antituberculosis medications occur.
3. Ethionamide may cause increased side effects when used with cycloserine.
4. Pyridoxine should be given to all patients receiving ethionamide to prevent or relieve neurotoxic effects. Adults need 100 mg (more if also taking cycloserine) and children should receive a dose proportionate to their weight.
5. Alcohol should be avoided in patients receiving ethionamide.
6. Monitor TSH and liver function tests.
7. Cross-resistance may occur with INH and thiacetazone.
8. Should be taken with food to minimize gastrointestinal distress.
9. Some patients tolerate ethionamide best if it is begun with a small dose that is gradually increased over a few days to a week (ramping).

BASIC CHARACTERISTICS

Class: Nucleoside reverse transcriptase inhibitors + integrase inhibitor.

Mechanism of Action: Abacavir and lamivudine are converted by cellular enzymes to its active drugs lamivudine triphosphate (a cytosine analog) and carbavir triphosphate (a guanasine triphosphate). These triphosphate analogs compete with the naturally occurring nucleotides for incorporation in newly forming HIV DNA. Since the triphosphate analogs do not have terminal hydroxyl groups, they halt transcription and replication of the virus.

Dolutegravir is an HIV-1 integrase strand transfer inhibitor (INSTI). Inhibition of integrase prevents the integration of HIV-1 DNA into host genomic DNA, blocking propagation of the viral infection.

Mechanism of Resistance: Lamivudine and abacavir change the structure of HIV reverse transcriptase, leading to preferred incorporation of cytosine and guanasine triphosphate; this results in decreased incorporation of lamivudine and carbavir triphosphate, which allows transcription of DNA to continue. Resistance mutations that emerge in those on abacavir and lamivudine include M184V, K65R, and L74V.

Dolutegravir changes the structure of HIV integrase. Development of mutations on the enzyme integrase prevents dolutegravir from binding the active site of the enzyme and allowing integrase activity to continue. Resistance mutations that affect dolutegravir include E92Q, G118R, S153F or Y, G193E, R263K, Q148R or H, T97A, E138K, G140S, M154I, L74M, and N155H.

Metabolic Route: The majority of lamivudine is eliminated unchanged in urine by active organic cationic secretion. Abacavir is metabolized by alcohol dehydrogenase and glucuronyl transferase into inactive metabolites that are eliminated primarily in the feces. Dolutegravir is primarily metabolized via UGT1A1 with some contribution from CYP3A in the liver and excreted.

FDA-APPROVED INDICATIONS

Treatment of human immunodeficiency virus type 1 (HIV-1) infection.

SIDE EFFECTS/TOXICITY

WARNINGS: Hypersensitivity to Triumeq or any agents containing abacavir can be fatal. The hypersensitivity syndrome is a multiorgan clinical syndrome with 2 or more of the following: fever, rash, gastrointestinal symptoms, constitutional symptoms, and respiratory symptoms. Triumeq or any agents containing abacavir should be discontinued immediately and never restarted. Reintroduction can lead to serious or fatal reactions. Hypersensitivity occurs in up to 8% of patients, usually within the first month of therapy. Determining patient's HLA-B5701 status may screen for the risk of reaction: if the HLA-B5701 test is negative, the risk of hypersensitivity is near zero; if positive, the risk is 50%.

Lactic acidosis and severe hepatomegaly with steatosis, including fatal cases, have been reported with the use of nucleoside analogs alone or in combination, including abacavir and lamivudine.

Severe acute exacerbations of hepatitis B have been reported in patients who are coinfected with hepatitis B and HIV and have discontinued Triumeq or any medication containing lamivudine. Hepatic function should be monitored closely with both clinical and laboratory follow-up for at least several months in patients who discontinue Triumeq or any medication containing lamivudine and are coinfected with HIV and HBV. If appropriate, initiation of antihepatitis B therapy may be warranted.

Antibiotics Manual: A Guide to Commonly Used Antimicrobials, Second Edition. David Schlossberg and Rafik Samuel.
© 2017 John Wiley & Sons Ltd. Published 2017 by John Wiley & Sons Ltd.

Other side effects: Immune reconstitution inflammatory syndrome, fat redistribution including central obesity and dorsocervical fat enlargement, peripheral wasting, facial wasting, breast enlargement, GGT elevation, and pancreatitis.

Triumeq has been shown to increase serum creatinine due to inhibition of tubular secretion of creatinine without affecting renal glomerular function.

In less than 2 %: abdominal pain, flatulence, vomiting, hepatitis, myositis, suicidal ideation, attempt, behavior, or completion, renal impairment, and pruritus.

 ## DRUG INTERACTIONS/FOOD INTERACTIONS

Triumeq can be taken with or without food and is unaffected by pH.

Triumeq should not be used with emtricitabine because both lamivudine and emtricitabine are cytosine analogs and may be antagonistic.

Triumeq should not be given with other antiretrovirals containing lamivudine, abacavir, or dolutegravir. These include Epivir, Combivir, Ziagen, Epzicom, Trizivir, and Tivicay.

Do not coadminister with nevirapine, oxcarbazepine, phenytoin, phenobarbital, St John's wort, efavirenz, fosamprenavir, tipranavir, orcarbamazepine. If dosed with etravirine, a protease inhibitor must be given with it.

Can be given with rifabutin with no dosage adjustment in either, even if INSTI mutation is present. If given with rifampin, adjust dolutegravir dose to 50 mg twice daily. An additional 50 mg dose of dolutegravir should be taken, separated by 12 hours from Triumeq. If administered with magnesium, calcium, aluminum, or iron containing supplements, administer dolutegravir 2 hours before or 6 hours after these agents.

If administered with metformin, do not exceed a dose of 1000 mg daily.

 ## DOSING

A fixed dose combination of abacavir 600 mg, lamivudine 300 mg, and dolutegravir 50 mg given once daily.

 ## SPECIAL POPULATIONS

RENAL IMPAIRMENT: In patients with renal insufficiency, this formulation should not be used.

HEPATIC DYSFUNCTION: In patients with hepatic insufficiency, this formulation should not be used.

PEDIATRICS: Not recommended for those under the age of 18.

 ## THE ART OF ANTIMICROBIAL THERAPY

Clinical Pearls

1. Triumeq should not be used with other medications that contain abacavir, lamivudine, or dolutegravir. These include Epivir, Combivir, Ziagen, Epzicom, Trizivir, and Tivicay.
2. Triumeq should not be used with other integrase inhibitors, including Isentress, Stribild, or Genvoya.
3. Dolutegravir still maintains activity against HIV integrase if integrase mutations are present.
4. Dolutegravir can increase serum creatinine by inhibiting its secretion in the distal tubules.

5. An HLA-B5701 test should be done prior to starting and medication containing abacavir; if positive, abacavir should be avoided.

6. If a person has suspected hypersensitivity, abacavir and any medication containing abacavir should not be used.

7. Since lamivudine has activity against hepatitis B it is important to check for hepatitis B since using lamivudine or any medication containing lamivudine alone in hepatitis B-infected individuals leads to rapid resistance to lamivudine.

■ TRIZIVIR (Zidovudine, Lamivudine, and Abacavir)

 BASIC CHARACTERISTICS

Class: Nucleoside reverse transcriptase inhibitors (NRTI) with activity against HIV.

Mechanism of Action: Converted by cellular enzymes to its active drugs lamivudine triphosphate (a cytosine analog), zidovudine triphosphate (a thymadine analog), and carbavir triphosphate (a guanasine triphosphate). These triphosphate analogs compete with the naturally occurring nucleotides for incorporation in newly forming HIV DNA. Since the triphosphate analogs do not have terminal hydroxyl groups, they halt transcription and replication of the virus.

Mechanism of Resistance: Zidovudine mutations change the structure of HIV reverse transcriptase, which leads to pyrophosphorolysis of the nucleoside analogs, allowing transcription of DNA to continue. Lamivudine mutations change the structure of HIV reverse transcriptase, leading to preferred incorporation of cytosine triphosphate and decreased incorporation of lamivudine triphosphate, which allows transcription of DNA to continue.

Abacavir mutations change the structure of HIV reverse transcriptase, leading to preferred incorporation of guanasine triphosphate and decreased incorporation of carbavir triphosphate, which allows transcription of DNA to continue.

Resistance mutations that emerge in those on Trizivir include M184V and the "TAMS": 41 L, 67 N, 70R, 210 W, 215 F, and 219E.

Metabolic Route: Zidovudine is primarily eliminated by hepatic metabolism. The major metabolite of zidovudine is 3'-azido-3'-deoxy-5'-*O*-β-D-glucopyranuronosylthymidine (GZDV).

The majority of lamivudine is eliminated unchanged in urine by active organic cationic secretion.

Abacavir is metabolized by alcohol dehydrogenase and glucuronyl transferase into inactive metabolites that are eliminated primarily in the feces.

 FDA-APPROVED INDICATIONS

Trizivir is approved to be used in combination with other antiretrovirals or alone for the treatment of HIV infection. However, although it is approved for use alone, its preferred use is in combination with other antiretrovirals.

 SIDE EFFECTS/TOXICITY

> **WARNING:**
>
> **Hypersensitivity reactions**: Serious and sometimes fatal hypersensitivity reactions, with multiple organ involvement, have occurred with abacavir, a component of Trizivir. Patients who carry the HLA-B*5701 allele are at a higher risk of a hypersensitivity reaction to abacavir, although hypersensitivity reactions have occurred in patients who do not carry the HLA-B*5701 allele. Trizivir is **contraindicated** in patients with a prior hypersensitivity reaction to abacavir and in HLA-B*5701-positive patients. All patients should be screened for the HLA-B*5701 allele prior to initiating therapy with Trizivir or reinitiation of therapy with Trizivir, unless patients have a previously documented HLA-B*5701 allele assessment. Discontinue Trizivir immediately if a hypersensitivity reaction is suspected, regardless of HLA-B*5701 status and even when other diagnoses are possible.
>
> Following a hypersensitivity reaction to Trizivir, **never** restart Trizivir or any other abacavir-containing product because more severe symptoms, including death, can occur within hours. Similar severe reactions have also occurred rarely following the reintroduction of abacavir-containing products in patients who have no history of abacavir hypersensitivity.

Antibiotics Manual: A Guide to Commonly Used Antimicrobials, Second Edition. David Schlossberg and Rafik Samuel.
© 2017 John Wiley & Sons Ltd. Published 2017 by John Wiley & Sons Ltd.

Hematologic toxicity: Zidovudine, a component of Trizivir, has been associated with hematologic toxicity, including neutropenia and severe anemia, particularly in patients with advanced human immunodeficiency virus (HIV-1) disease.

Myopathy: Prolonged use of zidovudine has been associated with symptomatic myopathy.

Lactic acidosis and severe hepatomegaly with steatosis: Lactic acidosis and severe hepatomegaly with steatosis, including fatal cases, have been reported with the use of nucleoside analogs and other antiretrovirals. Discontinue Trizivir if clinical or laboratory findings suggestive of lactic acidosis or pronounced hepatotoxicity occur.

Exacerbations of hepatitis B: Severe acute exacerbations of hepatitis B have been reported in patients who are coinfected with hepatitis B virus (HBV) and HIV-1 and have discontinued lamivudine, a component of Trizivir. Hepatic function should be monitored closely with both clinical and laboratory follow-up for at least several months in patients who discontinue Trizivir and are coinfected with HIV-1 and HBV. If appropriate, initiation of antihepatitis B therapy may be warranted.

Other side effects: Immune reconstitution inflammatory syndrome, fat redistribution including central obesity and dorsocervical fat enlargement, peripheral wasting, facial wasting, breast enlargement, fever, rash, headache, malaise and fatigue, nausea, vomiting, diarrhea, and dreams/sleep.

 DRUG INTERACTIONS/FOOD INTERACTIONS

Trizivir can be taken with or without food and is unaffected by pH.

Trizivir should not be used with stavudine, since zidovudine and stavudine are both thymidine analogs and may be antagonistic.

Trizivir should not be administered with ribavirin because of additive effects on anemia.

Trizivir should not be administered with doxorubicin.

Trizivir should not be used with emtricitabine or any medication containing emtricitabine because both lamivudine and emtricitabine are cytosine analogs and may be antagonistic. These include Emtriva, Truvada, Descovy, Atripla, Complera, Odefsey, Stribild, and Genvoya.

Trizivir should not be given with other antiretrovirals containing lamivudine, abacavir, or zidovudine. These include Epivir, Combivir, Ziagen, Epzicom, Triumeq, and Retrovir.

 DOSING

Trizivir is administered in a fixed dose combination of zidovudine 300 mg, lamivudine 150 mg, and abacavir 300 mg. The recommended adult dose is one tablet twice daily.

 SPECIAL POPULATIONS

RENAL IMPAIRMENTS: Do not use in patients with creatinine clearance under 50 mL/min.

HEPATIC DYSFUNCTION: In patients with hepatic insufficiency, this formulation should not be used.

PEDIATRICS: Not recommended for children who weigh less than 40 kg.

THE ART OF ANTIMICROBIAL THERAPY

Clinical Pearls

1. Even though Trizivir contains 3 antiretrovirals, it should be used in combination with other antiretroviral agents because of less efficacy compared to other antiretroviral regimens.

2. Trizivir contains lamivudine, abacavir, and zidovudine and should not be used with medications containing these components, including Retrovir, Combivir, Epzicom, Ziagen, Triumeq, and Epivir.

3. Unlike other NRTIs, pharmacokinetic studies do not support a once daily dosing of Trizivir.

4. An HLA-B5701 test should be done prior to starting any medication containing abacavir; if positive, Trizivir or any medication containing abacavir should be avoided.

5. If a person has suspected hypersensitivity, Trizivir and any medication containing abacavir should not be used.

6. Since Trizivir has activity against hepatitis B, it is important to check for hepatitis B infection, since using Trizivir or any medication containing lamivudine alone in hepatitis B-infected individuals leads to rapid resistance to lamivudine.

BASIC CHARACTERISTICS

Class: Aminocyclitol antibiotic.

Mechanism of Action: An inhibitor of protein synthesis in the bacterial cell; the site of action is the 30S ribosomal subunit.

Metabolic Route: Excreted unchanged in the urine.

 FDA-APPROVED INDICATIONS

Treatment of acute gonorrheal urethritis and proctitis in the male and acute gonorrheal cervicitis and proctitis in the female when due to susceptible strains of *Neisseria gonorrhoeae*.

 SIDE EFFECTS/TOXICITY

Contains benzyl alcohol. Benzyl alcohol has been reported to be associated with a fatal "gasping syndrome" in premature infants and an increased incidence of neurologic and other complications.

Also seen: anaphylaxis, soreness at the injection site, urticaria, dizziness, nausea, chills, fever, insomnia, a decrease in hemoglobin, hematocrit and creatinine clearance, elevation of alkaline phosphatase, BUN, and SGPT.

 DRUG INTERACTIONS/FOOD INTERACTIONS

None reported.

 DOSING

2-gram dose administered intramuscularly.

In geographic areas where antibiotic resistance is known to be prevalent, initial treatment with 4 grams intramuscularly is preferred.

 SPECIAL POPULATIONS

RENAL IMPAIRMENT: No dose adjustment is necessary.

HEPATIC DYSFUNCTION: No dose adjustment is necessary.

PEDIATRICS: Safety and effectiveness in the pediatric population have not been established.

 THE ART OF ANTIMICROBIAL THERAPY

Clinical Pearls

1. Spectinomycin hydrochloride is not effective in the treatment of syphilis.
2. The 4-gram dose contains 10 mL and may be divided into two intramuscular (gluteal) sites.
3. Spectinomycin is not currently being produced in the United States.

Antibiotics Manual: A Guide to Commonly Used Antimicrobials, Second Edition. David Schlossberg and Rafik Samuel.
© 2017 John Wiley & Sons Ltd. Published 2017 by John Wiley & Sons Ltd.

TRUVADA (Tenofovir and Emtricitabine)

 ## BASIC CHARACTERISTICS

Class: Nucleotide reverse transcriptase inhibitor (NRTI) with activity against HIV and hepatitis B.

Mechanism of Action: Tenofovir and emtricitabine are converted by cellular enzymes to their active drugs tenofovir biphosphate (an analog of adenosine triphosphate) and emtricitabine triphosphate (an analog of cytosine triphosphate). These drugs compete with the naturally occurring nucleotides for incorporation in newly forming HIV DNA. Since they do not have a terminal hydroxyl group, they halt transcription and replication of the virus.

Mechanism of Resistance: Changes in the structure of HIV reverse transcriptase leads to preferred incorporation of adenosine triphosphate and decreased incorporation of tenofovir biphosphate, which allows transcription of DNA to continue. Resistance mutations include K65R, M184V, and "TAMS": 41 L, 67 N, 70R, 210 W, 215 F, and 219E.

Metabolic Route: Tenofovir and emtricitabine are excreted in the urine unchanged.

 ## FDA-APPROVED INDICATIONS

Treatment of HIV infection, in combination with other antiretrovirals.

Preexposure prophylaxis to reduce the risk of sexually acquired HIV in patients at high risk.

Also Used for: Truvada is active against hepatitis B.

 ## SIDE EFFECTS/TOXICITY

> **WARNING: Lactic acidosis and severe hepatomegaly with steatosis**, including fatal cases, have been reported with the use of nucleoside analogs, including tenofovir, a component of Truvada, in combination with other antiretrovirals.
>
> Truvada is not approved for the treatment of chronic hepatitis B virus (HBV) infection and the safety and efficacy of Truvada have not been established in patients coinfected with HBV and HIV-1. Severe acute exacerbations of hepatitis B have been reported in patients who are coinfected with HBV and HIV-1 and have discontinued Truvada. Therefore, hepatic function should be monitored closely with both clinical and laboratory follow-up for at least several months in patients who are infected with HBV and discontinue Truvada. If appropriate, initiation of antihepatitis B therapy may be warranted.
>
> Truvada used for a PrEP indication must only be prescribed to individuals confirmed to be HIV-negative immediately prior to initiating and periodically (at least every 3 months) during use. Drug-resistant HIV-1 variants have been identified with use of Truvada for a PrEP indication following undetected acute HIV-1 infection. Do not initiate Truvada for a PrEP indication if signs or symptoms of acute HIV-1 infection are present unless negative infection status is confirmed.

Other adverse events: Immune reconstitution inflammatory syndrome, fat redistribution including central obesity and dorso-cervical fat enlargement, peripheral wasting, facial wasting, breast enlargement, diarrhea, nausea, fatigue, headache, dizziness, depression, insomnia, abnormal dreams, rash, renal impairment, including acute renal failure and Fanconi syndrome, and decreased bone mineral density.

DRUG INTERACTIONS/FOOD INTERACTIONS

Truvada can be administered with or without food.

Truvada should not be administered with adefovir.

Antibiotics Manual: A Guide to Commonly Used Antimicrobials, Second Edition. David Schlossberg and Rafik Samuel.
© 2017 John Wiley & Sons Ltd. Published 2017 by John Wiley & Sons Ltd.

Truvada should not be given with didanosine because of decreased CD4 counts in patients maintained on this regimen. If didanosine is given with Truvada or any medication containing tenofovir, the didanosine should be decreased to 250 mg daily.

Truvada or any medication containing tenofovir decreases the levels of atazanavir. If given together, atazanavir must be given with ritonavir or cobicistat.

Truvada should not be administered with any medication containing lamivudine because lamivudine and emtricitabine are both cytosine analogs and may be antagonistic. These include Epivir, Combivir, Trizivir, Epzicom, and Triumeq.

Truvada should not be administered with Viread, Vemlidy, Emtriva, Descovy, Atripla, Complera, Odefsey, Genvoya, or Stribild.

 ## DOSING

Truvada is formulated as follows: Tablets: 200 mg/300 mg, 167 mg/250 mg, 133 mg/200 mg, and 100 mg/150 mg of emtricitabine and tenofovir disoproxil fumarate, respectively. The recommended adult dose is one 200 mg/300 mg tablet once daily.

 ## SPECIAL POPULATIONS

RENAL IMPAIRMENT: Do not use in patients with a creatinine clearance less than 60 mL/min.

HEPATIC DYSFUNCTION: No dose adjustment is necessary.

PEDIATRICS: Do not use in children less than 17 kg.

Truvada low-strength tablets

Body weight, kg	Dosing of FTC/TDF, mg/mg
17 to less than 22	One 100/150 tablet once daily
22 to less than 28	One 133/200 tablet once daily
28 to less than 35	One 167/250 tablet once daily

 ## THE ART OF ANTIMICROBIAL THERAPY

Clinical Pearls

1. Truvada should be used in combination with other antiretroviral agents.
2. Truvada contains both tenofovir and emtricitabine and should not be administered with Viread, Vemlidy, Emtriva, Descovy, Atripla, Complera, Odefsey, Genvoya, or Stribild.
3. Patients with HIV-1 should be tested for hepatitis B virus before initiating antiretroviral therapy with Truvada.
4. Truvada and didanosine combinations should be administered with caution.
5. Atazanavir should be boosted with ritonavir or cobicistat if given with Truvada.
6. Do not use Truvada for preexposure prophylaxis in individuals with unknown or positive HIV-1 status.
7. When using Truvada for preexposure prohylaxis, check HIV status every 3 months.

■ TYBOST (Cobicistat)

 BASIC CHARACTERISTICS

Class: CYP3A inhibitor.

Mechanism of Action: Mechanism-based CYP3A inhibitor.

Mechanism of Resistance: N/A.

Metabolic Route: Metabolized by CYP3A and to a minor extent by CYP2D6 enzymes in the liver and excreted in the feces and urine.

 FDA-APPROVED INDICATIONS

CYP3A inhibitor indicated to increase systemic exposure of atazanavir or darunavir (once daily dosing regimen) in combination with other antiretroviral agents in the treatment of HIV-1 infection.

 SIDE EFFECTS/TOXICITY

Decreases estimated creatinine clearance due to inhibition of tubular secretion of creatinine without affecting actual renal glomerular function.

Renal impairment, including cases of acute renal failure and Fanconi syndrome, has been reported when cobicistat was used in an antiretroviral regimen that contained tenofovir DF.

Other side effects reported include jaundice, rash, scleral icterus, nausea, diarrhea, and headache.

In less than 2 %: abdominal pain, vomiting, fatigue, rhabdomyolysis, depression, abnormal dreams, insomnia, nephropathy, and nephrolithiasis.

 DRUG INTERACTIONS/FOOD INTERACTIONS

Cobicistat should be given with food because Prezista or Reyataz must be given with food.

Cobicistat is metabolized by CYP3A and, to a minor extent, by CYP2D6. Drugs that induce or inhibit CYP3A activity may affect the levels of cobicistat.

Do not administer with nevirapine, Kaletra, saquinavir, fosamprenavir, tipranavir, etravirine, alfuzosin, dronedarone, carbamazapine, phenobarbatol, phenytoin, rifampin, rivaroxaban, irinotecan, dihydroergotamine, ergotamine, methylergonovine, cisapride, St John's wort, lovastatin, simvastatin, pimozide, nevirapine, avanafil, sildenafil, indinavir, triazolam, or midazolam.

Medication	Adjustment or action
Maraviroc	Maraviroc dose 150 bid
Efavirenz	**Contraindicated** if used with darunavir atazanavir 400 mg + efavirenz 600 mg + cobicistat 150 mg
Antacid	Administer 2 hours apart if used with atazanavir
Famotidine	If given with atazanavir, give at least 10 hours apart
Omeprazole	If given with atazanavir, must be separated by 12 hours

Antibiotics Manual: A Guide to Commonly Used Antimicrobials, Second Edition. David Schlossberg and Rafik Samuel.
© 2017 John Wiley & Sons Ltd. Published 2017 by John Wiley & Sons Ltd.

Medication	Adjustment or action
Colchicine	Not recommended in renal or hepatic impairment
Rifabutin	Rifabutin dose 150 mg qod
Bosentan	Bosentan dose 62.5 mg daily or qod
Cyclosporine, tacrolimus	Monitor levels of the immunosuppressants
Sildenafil	25 mg every 48 hours
Tadalafil	No more than 10 mg in 72 hours
Vardenafil	No more than 2.5 mg in 24 hours

 ## DOSING

150 mg daily coadministered with either Prezista 800 mg or Reyataz 300 mg daily.

 ## SPECIAL POPULATIONS

RENAL IMPAIRMENT: No dose adjustment necessary.

HEPATIC DYSFUNCTION: No dose adjustment necessary.

PEDIATRICS: Not recommended for those under the age of 18.

 ## THE ART OF ANTIMICROBIAL THERAPY

Clinical Pearls

1. Tybost is only indicated to be used with once daily Prezista or Reyataz.
2. Tybost should not be used with other agents that contain cobicistat: Prezcobix, Evotaz, Stribild, or Genvoya.
3. Tybost can increase serum creatinine due to inhibition of creatinine secretion in the distal tubules.
4. Tybost is not recommended with Prezista 600 mg twice daily.

TYZEKA (Telbivudine)

 ## BASIC CHARACTERISTICS

Class: Nucleoside reverse transcriptase inhibitor for hepatitis B.

Mechanism of Action: Telbivudine is a synthetic thymidine nucleoside analog with activity against hepatitis B virus (HBV). It is phosphorylated by cellular kinases to the active triphosphate form that inhibits HBV DNA polymerase (reverse transcriptase) by competing with the natural substrate, thymidine 5′-triphosphate. Incorporation of telbivudine 5′-triphosphate into viral DNA causes DNA chain termination.

Mechanism of Resistance: Mutations rtM204I/V with or without rtL180M on HBV DNA polymerase lead to decreased incorporation of telbivudine triphosphate.

Metabolic Route: Excreted unchanged in the urine.

 ## FDA-APPROVED INDICATIONS

Telbivudine is indicated for the treatment of chronic hepatitis B in adult patients (16 years or older) with evidence of viral replication and either persistent elevations in serum aminotransferases or histologically active disease.

 ## SIDE EFFECTS/TOXICITY

> **WARNING: Lactic acidosis and severe hepatomegaly with steatosis**, including fatal cases, have been reported with the use of nucleoside analogs alone or in combination with antiretrovirals.
>
> **Severe acute exacerbations of hepatitis B** have been reported in patients who have discontinued antihepatitis B therapy, including telbivudine. Hepatic function should be monitored closely with both clinical and laboratory follow-up for at least several months in patients who discontinue antihepatitis B therapy. If appropriate, resumption of hepatitis B therapy may be warranted.

Other adverse events include cases of myopathy/myositis several weeks to months after starting therapy, myalgia, peripheral neuropathy, risk for which is increase with concomitant interferon administration, fever, rash, fatigue, insomnia, headache, cough, nausea, diarrhea, fatigue, arthralgia, increased ALT, and increased CK.

 ## DRUG INTERACTIONS/FOOD INTERACTIONS

Telbivudine can be taken with or without food.

Telbivudine should not be given with pegylated interferon alfa-2a.

Because telbivudine is eliminated primarily by renal excretion, coadministration of telbivudine with drugs that alter renal function may alter plasma concentrations of telbivudine.

DOSING

Telbivudine is supplied as 600 mg tablets and a solution containing 100 mg/5 mL. The recommended dose of telbivudine for the treatment of chronic hepatitis B is 600 mg once daily.

Antibiotics Manual: A Guide to Commonly Used Antimicrobials, Second Edition. David Schlossberg and Rafik Samuel.
© 2017 John Wiley & Sons Ltd. Published 2017 by John Wiley & Sons Ltd.

SPECIAL POPULATIONS

RENAL IMPAIRMENT:

Creatinine

clearance, mL/min	Dose (oral solution)	Dose (tablet)
>50	30 mL daily	600 mg daily
30–49	20 mL daily	600 mg q 48 hours
<30	10 mL daily	600 mg q 72 hours
HD	6 mL daily	600 mg q 96 hours (if on HD day, administer after HD)

HEPATIC DYSFUNCTION: No adjustment to the recommended dose of telbivudine is necessary in patients with hepatic impairment.

PEDIATRICS: Telbivudine is not recommended to be used in children.

 THE ART OF ANTIMICROBIAL THERAPY

Clinical Pearls

1. Telbivudine should be used with caution in hepatitis B patients coinfected with HIV, HCV, or HDV, as it has not been investigated in patients with these coinfections.
2. May be taken with or without food.
3. Resistance mutations are similar between entecavir and telbivudine.

UNASYN (Ampicillin Sodium–Sulbactam Sodium)

BASIC CHARACTERISTICS

Class: Aminopenicillin/beta-lactamase inhibitor combination.

Mechanism of Action: Binds penicillin-binding protein, disrupting cell wall synthesis.

Mechanisms of Resistance:

1. The PBP can be altered, with reduced affinity.
2. Production of a beta-lactamase, resulting in hydrolysis of the beta-lactam ring.
3. Decreased ability of the antibiotic to reach the PBP when bacteria decrease porin production, resulting in a decrease of the drug concentration within the cell.

Metabolic Route: Ampicillin and sulbactam are excreted unchanged in the urine.

FDA-APPROVED INDICATIONS

Ampicillin sulbactam is indicated in the treatment of infections due to susceptible strains of microorganisms in the conditions listed below:

Skin and skin structure infections

Intra-abdominal infections

Gynecological infections

SIDE EFFECTS/TOXICITY

A history of allergic reaction to any of the penicillins is a **contraindication.**

Side effects include *Clostridium difficile*-associated diarrhea (CDAD), hypersensitivity reactions, including rashes, erythema multiforme, toxic epidermal necrolysis, and Stevens–Johnson syndrome, mucocutaneous candidiasis, black hairy tongue, nausea, vomiting, diarrhea, hepatic and renal dysfunction, seizures with high CNS levels, crystalluria, anemia, thrombocytopenia, eosinophilia, and leucopenia.

DRUG INTERACTIONS/FOOD INTERACTIONS

Concurrent use of ampicillin/sulbactam and probenecid may result in increased and prolonged blood levels of ampicillin/sulbactam.

Chloramphenicol, macrolides, sulfonamides, and tetracyclines may interfere with the bactericidal effects of penicillins. High urine concentrations of ampicillin may result in false-positive reactions when testing for the presence of glucose in urine using *Clinitest®*. It is recommended that glucose tests based on enzymatic glucose oxidase reactions (such as *Clinistix®*) be used.

DOSING

Ampicillin/sulbactam contains ampicillin to sulbactam in a 2:1 ratio.

Ampicillin/sulbactam may be administered by either the IV or the IM routes.

The recommended adult dosage is 1.5 g to 3 every six hours.

Antibiotics Manual: A Guide to Commonly Used Antimicrobials, Second Edition. David Schlossberg and Rafik Samuel.
© 2017 John Wiley & Sons Ltd. Published 2017 by John Wiley & Sons Ltd.

SPECIAL POPULATIONS

RENAL IMPAIRMENT:

Creatinine clearance, mL/min	Dose
10–50	1.5 g q 12 hours
<10	1.5 g q 24 hours
Hemodialysis	1.5 g q 24 hours and 1.5 grams after HD
CAPD	1.5 g q 24 hours (no supplemental dose)
CRRT	1.5 g q 12 hours

HEPATIC DYSFUNCTION: No dose adjustment is necessary.

PEDIATRICS: **Patients 1 year of age or older**: The recommended daily dose is 75 mg per kg every 6 hours.

Pediatric patients weighing 40 kg or more should be dosed according to adult recommendations.

 THE ART OF ANTIMICROBIAL THERAPY

Clinical Pearls

1. Ampicillin–sulbactam needs to be dose adjusted for renal dysfunction.
2. A high percentage of patients with mononucleosis who receive ampicillin develop a skin rash.

VALCYTE (Valganciclovir)

 ## BASIC CHARACTERISTICS

Class: Nucleoside analog.

Mechanism of Action: Valganciclovir is a valyl ester of ganciclovir. After oral administration, valganciclovir is converted to ganciclovir, which is a synthetic guanine nucleoside analog of 2′-deoxyguanosine that inhibits replication of herpes viruses. Ganciclovir is active against CMV and HSV. Ganciclovir is phosphorylated and inhibits viral DNA synthesis by (1) competitive inhibition of viral DNA polymerases and (2) incorporation into viral DNA, resulting in eventual termination of viral DNA elongation.

Mechanism of Resistance: Resistance to ganciclovir in CMV is the decreased ability to form the active triphosphate moiety; resistant viruses have been described that contain mutations in the UL97 gene of CMV that controls phosphorylation of ganciclovir. Mutations in the viral DNA polymerase have also been reported to confer viral resistance to ganciclovir.

Metabolic Route: Valganciclovir is a valyl ester of ganciclovir. After oral administration, valganciclovir is converted to ganciclovir by intestinal and hepatic esterases. Ganciclovir is excreted in the urine.

 ## FDA-APPROVED INDICATIONS

Treatment of cytomegalovirus retinitis in patients with acquired immunodeficiency syndrome.

Also indicated for the prevention of cytomegalovirus (CMV) disease in kidney, heart, and kidney–pancreas transplant patients at high risk (donor CMV seropositive/recipient CMV seronegative (D+/R−)).

Not indicated for use in liver transplant patients.

Prevention of CMV disease in kidney (4 months to 16 years of age) and heart transplant recipients (1 month to 16 years of age).

SIDE EFFECTS/TOXICITY

> **WARNING:**
>
> **Hematologic toxicity**: Severe leukopenia, neutropenia, anemia, thrombocytopenia, pancytopenia, bone marrow aplasia, and aplastic anemia have been reported in patients treated with valganciclovir.
>
> **Impairment of fertility**: Based on animal data, valganciclovir may cause temporary or permanent inhibition of spermatogenesis
>
> **Fetal toxicity**: Based on animal data, valganciclovir has the potential to cause birth defects in humans.
>
> **Mutagenesis and carcinogenesis**: Based on animal data, valganciclovir has the potential to cause cancers in humans.

Other adverse events include hepatic dysfunction, elevated creatinine, stomatitis, seizures, tinnitus, intestinal perforation, pancreatitis, pulmonary fibrosis, torsades de pointes, fever, diarrhea, vomiting, neuropathy, seizures, sweating, and pruritus.

 ## DRUG INTERACTIONS/FOOD INTERACTIONS

Valganciclovir should be administered with food.

Drug interactions: Both zidovudine and valganciclovir have the potential to cause neutropenia and anemia; some patients may not tolerate concomitant therapy with these drugs at full dosage. Generalized seizures have been reported in patients who

Antibiotics Manual: A Guide to Commonly Used Antimicrobials, Second Edition. David Schlossberg and Rafik Samuel.
© 2017 John Wiley & Sons Ltd. Published 2017 by John Wiley & Sons Ltd.

received ganciclovir and imipenem–cilastatin. These drugs should not be used concomitantly unless the potential benefits outweigh the risks.

Because of the possibility of additive toxicity, drugs such as dapsone, pentamidine, flucytosine, vincristine, vinblastine, adriamycin, amphotericin B, trimethoprim/sulfamethoxazole combinations or other nucleoside analogs, should be considered for concomitant use with valganciclovir only if the potential benefits are judged to outweigh the risks.

Increases in serum creatinine were observed in patients treated with valganciclovir plus either cyclosporine or amphotericin B, drugs with known potential for nephrotoxicity.

DOSING

Valganciclovir is administered in 450 mg tablets.

An oral solution of 50 mg/mL can be made by a pharmacist.

For treatment of CMV retinitis in patients with normal renal function

Induction: For patients with active CMV retinitis, the recommended dosage is 900 mg (two 450 mg tablets) twice a day for 21 days with food.

Maintenance: Following induction treatment, or in patients with inactive CMV retinitis, the recommended dosage is 900 mg (two 450 mg tablets) once daily with food.

For the prevention of CMV disease in heart, kidney, and kidney–pancreas transplantation

For patients who have received a kidney, heart, or kidney–pancreas transplant, the recommended dose is 900 mg (two 450 mg tablets) once daily with food starting within 10 days of transplantation until 100 days posttransplantation.

SPECIAL POPULATIONS

RENAL IMPAIRMENT:

Creatinine clearance, mL/min	Induction dose, mg/kg	Maintenance dose, mg/kg
≥60	900 mg q 12 hours	900 mg q day
40–59	450 mg q 12 hours	450 mg q day
25–39	450 mg daily	450 mg every 2 days
10–24	450 mg every 2 days	450 mg twice weekly
Hemodialysis	Do not administer	

HEPATIC DYSFUNCTION: No dose adjustment is needed.

PEDIATRICS: For the prevention of CMV disease in the pediatric kidney transplant recipient: $7 \times (BSA^*) \times (CrCl^{**})$ start within 10 days after transplant until 200 days after transplant.

For the prevention of CMV disease in the pediatric heart transplant recipient: $7 \times (BSA^*) \times (CrCl^{**})$ start within 10 days after transplant until 100 days after transplant.

*Mostellar BSA formula is located in Helpful Formulas, Equations, and Definitions.

$$**\text{Schwartz creatinine clearance} = \frac{k \times \text{Height}(\text{cm})}{\text{Serum Creatinine (mg/dL)}}.$$

THE ART OF ANTIMICROBIAL THERAPY

Clinical Pearls

1. Valganciclovir should not be administered if the absolute neutrophil count is less than 500 cells/µL or the platelet count is less than 25 000 cells/µL.

2. Valganciclovir is effective against HSV, VZV, and CMV. It may also have activity against EBV and HHV8, although its FDA-approved indications are for specific CMV infections, as detailed above.

3. Oral ganciclovir is not well absorbed; if using an oral therapy, valganciclovir is more reliable.

4. Adults should only use valganciclovir tablets, not the solution.

BASIC CHARACTERISTICS

Class: Nucleoside analog.

Mechanism of Action: Valacyclovir is the valine ester of the nucleoside analog acyclovir. After hydrolysis, it is phosphorylated by thymadine kinase to the active triphosphate form. Acyclovir triphosphate stops replication of herpes viral DNA in three ways: (1) competitive inhibition of viral DNA polymerase, (2) incorporation into and termination of the growing viral DNA chain, and (3) inactivation of the viral DNA polymerase. The greater antiviral activity of acyclovir against HSV compared to VZV is due to its more efficient phosphorylation by the viral thymidine kinase.

Mechanism of Resistance: Resistance of HSV and VZV to valacyclovir can result from qualitative or quantitative changes in the viral TK or DNA polymerase.

Metabolic Route: After oral administration, valacyclovir hydrochloride is rapidly absorbed from the gastrointestinal tract and nearly completely converted to acyclovir and *L*-valine by first-pass intestinal and/or hepatic metabolism. The acyclovir is metabolized to 9-[(carboxymethoxy)methyl]guanine and excreted in the urine.

 FDA-APPROVED INDICATIONS

Valacyclovir is indicated for the treatment of herpes zoster, the treatment or suppression of genital herpes in immunocompetent individuals, suppression of recurrent genital herpes in HIV-infected individuals and the treatment of cold sores (herpes labialis).

 SIDE EFFECTS/TOXICITY

Thrombotic thrombocytopenic purpura/hemolytic uremic syndrome (TTP/HUS) has occurred in patients with advanced HIV disease and also in allogeneic bone marrow transplant and renal transplant recipients at doses of 8 grams per day.

Nausea, vomiting and diarrhea were the most common side effects in those receiving oral valacyclovir. Central nervous system side effects including confusion, ataxia, altered behavior, seizure, and coma have been seen, particularly in older adults or in patients with renal impairment. Precipitation of acyclovir in renal tubules may occur when the solubility (2.5 mg/mL) is exceeded in the intratubular fluid. This has resulted in elevated BUN and serum creatinine and subsequent renal failure. Excessive doses of valacyclovir have been associated with acute renal failure in patients with underlying renal disease.

Other reported adverse events include anaphylaxis, angioedema, fever, headache, peripheral edema, diarrhea, anemia, leucopenia, thrombocytopenia, hepatitis, rash including toxic epidermal necrolysis and Stevens–Johnson syndrome, and visual disturbances.

 DRUG INTERACTIONS/FOOD INTERACTIONS

Valacyclovir can be administered orally with or without food.

There are no drug interactions.

 DOSING

Valacyclovir is dispensed in 500 mg and 1000 mg tablets. It is also available as an oral suspension in 25 mg/mL and 50 mg/mL.

Antibiotics Manual: A Guide to Commonly Used Antimicrobials, Second Edition. David Schlossberg and Rafik Samuel.
© 2017 John Wiley & Sons Ltd. Published 2017 by John Wiley & Sons Ltd.

Herpes zoster	1 gram 3 times daily for 7 days
Initial treatment of genital ulcers	1 gram twice daily for 10 days
Recurrent episodes of genital ulcers	500 mg twice daily for 3 days
Suppressive therapy	1 gram once daily
Suppressive therapy in HIV patients	500 mg twice daily
Reduction of transmission	500 mg once daily
Cold sores (herpes labialis)	2 grams twice daily for 1 day

 SPECIAL POPULATIONS

RENAL IMPAIRMENT:

	Creatinine Clearance, mL/min		
Indication	30–49	10–29	<10
Herpes zoster	1 g q 12 h	1 g q 24 h	500 mg q 24 h
Initial genital herpes	1 g q 12 h	1 g q 24 h	500 mg q 24 h
Recurrent genital herpes	500 mg q 12 h	500 mg q 24 h	500 mg q 24 h
Suppression genital herpes	1 g q 24 h	500 mg q 24 h	500 mg q 24 h
Suppression in HIV	500 mg q 12 h	500 mg q 24 h	500 mg q 24 h
Herpes labialis	Two 1 g doses 12 h apart	Two 500 mg doses 12 h apart	500 mg 1 time dose

Hemodialysis: Patients requiring hemodialysis should receive the dose for creatinine clearance <10 mL/min in the table above.

Peritoneal dialysis: Supplemental dose not required following peritoneal dialysis.

CRRT: Dose as for creatinine clearance 30–49 mL/min in the table above; supplemental dose following CRRT not required.

HEPATIC DYSFUNCTION: No dose adjustment is needed.

PEDIATRICS: For children with cold sores over the age of 12, the recommended dose is 2 g every 12 hours for 1 day.

For children 2 years of age and older, the recommended treatment for chickenpox is 20 mg/kg three times a day for 5 days, but not to exceed 1 g three times daily.

 THE ART OF ANTIMICROBIAL THERAPY

Clinical Pearls

1. Valacyclovir is effective against HSV and VZV. It has no activity against the other herpes viruses.
2. Valacyclovir can cause confusion or renal insufficiency, especially in the elderly.
3. Valacyclovir doses of 8 grams a day have been associated with TTP/HUS in AIDS patients and transplant recipients.

BASIC CHARACTERISTICS

Class: Glycopeptide.

Mechanism of Action: Vancomycin inhibits synthesis and assembly of the cell wall peptidoglycan polymers by complexing with their *d*-alanyl-*d*-alanine precursor, preventing its binding to the peptidoglycan terminus.

Vancomycin may impair RNA synthesis and injure protoplasts by altering the permeability of their cytoplasmic membrane.

Mechanisms of Resistance: The main mechanisms of resistance are carried by gene complexes (Van A, Van B, and Van C) mainly found in Enterococci (VRE) and have been found in Staphylococci, including *S. aureus* (VRSA):

1. Van A is plasmid mediated. It is the most common type and results in the synthesis of peptidoglycan cell wall precursors containing a pentapeptide ending with *d*-alanine-*d*-lactate.
2. Van B is encoded on a transposon and leads to resistance.
3. Van C is chromosomally encoded and leads to low-level resistance to vancomycin.

Intermediate resistance (VISA) in Staphylococci results when there is an abnormally thickened cell wall.

Metabolic Route: Oral vancomycin is poorly absorbed from the GI tract.

 FDA-APPROVED INDICATIONS

Treatment of enterocolitis caused by *Staphylococcus aureus* and *C. difficile*-associated diarrhea.

 SIDE EFFECTS/TOXICITY

Some patients with inflammation of the intestinal mucosa may have significant systemic absorption of oral vancomycin and, therefore, may be at risk for the development of adverse reactions usually associated with parenteral vancomycin, e.g., ototoxicity, nephrotoxicity, neutropenia, thrombocytopenia, anaphylaxis, vasculitis, rash, and Red Man syndrome (hypotension, urticaria, flushing, muscle spasm, dyspnea).

 DRUG INTERACTIONS/FOOD INTERACTIONS

None.

 DOSING

Vancomycin is administered as 125 mg and 250 mg tablets.

C. difficile-associated diarrhea: 125 mg orally 4 times daily for 10 days.

Staphylococcal enterocolitis: Total daily dosage is 500 mg to 2 g administered orally in 3 or 4 divided doses for 7 to 10 days.

 SPECIAL POPULATIONS

RENAL IMPAIRMENT: No dose adjustment is necessary.

Antibiotics Manual: A Guide to Commonly Used Antimicrobials, Second Edition. David Schlossberg and Rafik Samuel.
© 2017 John Wiley & Sons Ltd. Published 2017 by John Wiley & Sons Ltd.

HEPATIC DYSFUNCTION: No dose adjustment is necessary.

PEDIATRICS: 40 mg/kg in 3 or 4 divided doses for 7 to 10 days. The total daily dosage should not exceed 2 g.

 THE ART OF ANTIMICROBIAL THERAPY

Clinical Pearls

1. Oral vancomycin should not be used for any systemic infection since it is not well absorbed.

2. Intravenous vancomycin is not effective in treating *C. difficile* diarrhea.

3. Resin binders such as cholestyramine may bind oral vancomycin.

For oral vancomycin, see Vancocin (vancomycin-PO).

 BASIC CHARACTERISTICS

Class: Glycopeptide.

Mechanism of Action: Vancomycin inhibits synthesis and assembly of the cell wall peptidoglycan polymers by complexing with their *d*-alanyl-*d*-alanine precursor, preventing its binding to the peptidoglycan terminus.

Vancomycin may impair RNA synthesis and injure protoplasts by altering the permeability of their cytoplasmic membrane.

Mechanisms of Resistance: The main mechanisms of resistance are carried by gene complexes (Van A, Van B, and Van C) mainly found in Enterococci (VRE) and in Staphylococci, including *S. aureus* (VRSA):

1. Van A is plasmid mediated. It is the most common type and results in the synthesis of peptidoglycan cell wall precursors containing a pentapeptide ending with *d*-alanine-*d*-lactate.
2. Van B is encoded on a transposon and leads to resistance.
3. Van C is chromosomally encoded and leads to low-level resistance to vancomycin.

Intermediate resistance (VISA) in Staphylococci results when there is an abnormally thickened cell wall.

Metabolic Route: Vancomycin is excreted in the urine.

 FDA-APPROVED INDICATIONS

Treatment of serious or severe infections caused by susceptible strains of methicillin-resistant staphylococci in patients who are penicillin-allergic, who cannot receive or who have failed to respond to other drugs (including penicillins or cephalosporins), and for infections caused by vancomycin-susceptible organisms that are resistant to other antimicrobial drugs. It is indicated for initial therapy when methicillin-resistant staphylococci are suspected, but after susceptibility data are available, therapy should be adjusted accordingly.

Also Used for: the treatment of staphylococcal endocarditis and other staphylococcal infections, including septicemia, osteomyelitis, pneumonia, and skin and skin structure infections. In addition, it is used for the treatment of enterococcal (in combination with aminoglycosides), streptococcal, and diphtheroid endocarditis. In combination with rifampin, an aminoglycoside, or both, vancomycin has been used in early-onset prosthetic valve endocarditis caused by *S. epidermidis* or diphtheroids. Vancomycin has also been used for prophylaxis against bacterial endocarditis in penicillin-allergic patients.

 SIDE EFFECTS/TOXICITY

Pseudomembranous colitis, infusion-related toxicity (including anaphylactoid reactions, hypotension, wheezing, dyspnea, urticaria, or pruritus; rapid infusion may also cause flushing of the upper body ("Red Man syndrome") or pain and muscle spasm of the chest and back), anaphylaxis, drug fever, chills, rash (including exfoliative dermatitis, linear IgA bullous dermatosis, Stevens–Johnson syndrome, toxic epidermal necrolysis, and vasculitis), nephrotoxicity, ototoxicity including hearing loss, vertigo, dizziness, and tinnitus, neutropenia, and thrombocytopenia.

 DRUG INTERACTIONS/FOOD INTERACTIONS

Concomitant administration of vancomycin and anesthetic agents has been associated with erythema and histamine-like flushing and anaphylactoid reactions.

Antibiotics Manual: A Guide to Commonly Used Antimicrobials, Second Edition. David Schlossberg and Rafik Samuel.
© 2017 John Wiley & Sons Ltd. Published 2017 by John Wiley & Sons Ltd.

Concurrent and/or sequential systemic or topical use of other potentially neurotoxic and/or nephrotoxic drugs, such as amphotericin B, aminoglycosides, bacitracin, polymyxin B, colistin, viomycin, or cisplatin, when indicated, requires careful monitoring.

 ## DOSING

The usual daily intravenous dose is 2 g divided either as 500 mg every six hours or 1 g every 12 hours. Each dose should be administered at no more than 10 mg/min or over a period of at least 60 minutes, whichever is longer.

 ## SPECIAL POPULATIONS

RENAL IMPAIRMENT: Dosage adjustment must be made in patients with impaired renal function.

Creatinine Clearance, mL/min	Dose
50–80	500 mg every 12 hours
10–50	500 mg every 24 hours
0–10	1 gram weekly
Hemodialysis	1 gram weekly
CAPD	1 gram weekly
CRRT	1 gram every 24 hours
Intrathecal dose	5–10 mg q 48–72 hours

HEPATIC DYSFUNCTION: No dose adjustment is necessary.

PEDIATRICS: The usual intravenous dosage of vancomycin is 10 mg/kg per dose given every six hours.

Infants and neonates: an initial dose of 15 mg/kg, followed by 10 mg/kg every 12 hours for the first week of life and every eight hours thereafter up to the age of one month.

 ## THE ART OF ANTIMICROBIAL THERAPY

Clinical Pearls

1. Red Man's syndrome is not a true allergy: if a patient develops Red Man's syndrome, slowing the infusion, diluting the vancomycin, and administration of diphenhydramine may be of benefit.

2. Conventional dosage of vancomycin is 1 gram every 12 hours; more recently the dose of 15 mg/kg every 12 hours has been suggested.

3. Although the cut-off for vancomycin susceptibility is 4 mcg/mL, many experts believe that an MIC of 2 or greater is associated with failures of vancomycin.

4. Tolerance to vancomycin has been reported during the use of vancomycin (continued growth of *S. aureus* despite MIC suggesting it is still susceptible).

5. The vancomycin trough should be measured after 4 doses and 1 hour prior to the fifth dose. The recommended trough is 5–12 mcg/mL.

6. In patients with renal insufficiency, troughs should be monitored.

7. In patients on hemodialysis or peritoneal dialysis, levels should guide dosing, since patients metabolize vancomycin at different rates.

BASIC CHARACTERISTICS

Class: Hydroquinoline,

Mechanism of Action: Unknown,

Metabolic Route: Oxidized in the liver and is excreted in the urine.

 FDA-APPROVED INDICATIONS

Used for: *Schistosoma mansoni* infections.

Not active against: *Schistosoma hematobium* or *Schistosoma japonicum*.

 SIDE EFFECTS/TOXICITY

Abdominal pain, nausea, vomiting and diarrhea, fever, elevations of ALT and AST, seizures, dizziness, drowsiness, severe head-aches, hallucinations, syncope, amnesia, disorientation and confusion, and orange to red discoloration of the urine.

 DRUG INTERACTIONS/FOOD INTERACTIONS

Oxamniquine should not be taken with food because food delays its absorption.

 DOSING

15 mg/kg PO once. In East Africa, the dose should be increased to 30 mg/kg PO and in Egypt and South Africa to 30 mg/kg/d PO × 2 d. Some experts recommend 40–60 mg/kg PO over 2–3 d in all of Africa.

 SPECIAL POPULATIONS

RENAL IMPAIRMENT: There is no dose adjustment.

HEPATIC DYSFUNCTION: There is no dose adjustment.

PEDIATRICS: 20 mg/kg/d PO in 2 doses × 1 d. In East Africa, the dose should be increased to 30 mg/kg PO and in Egypt and South Africa to 30 mg/kg/d PO × 2 d. Some experts recommend 40–60 mg/kg PO over 2–3 d in all of Africa.

 THE ART OF ANTIMICROBIAL THERAPY

Clinical Pearls

1. Oxamniquine is not available in the US. It may be available through a compounding pharmacy: Call the National Association of Compounding Pharmacies (800-687-7850) or Professional Compounding Centers of America (800-331-2498, www.pccarx.com).

2. Oxamniquine is active only against *Schistosoma mansoni* but not against *Schistosoma hematobium* or *Schistosoma japonicum*.

Antibiotics Manual: A Guide to Commonly Used Antimicrobials, Second Edition. David Schlossberg and Rafik Samuel.
© 2017 John Wiley & Sons Ltd. Published 2017 by John Wiley & Sons Ltd.

■ VANTIN (Cefpodoxime)

 BASIC CHARACTERISTICS

Class: Third generation cephalosporin.

Mechanism of Action: Binds penicillin-binding protein, disrupting cell wall synthesis.

Mechanisms of Resistance:

1. The PBP can be altered, with reduced affinity.

2. Production of a beta-lactamase, resulting in hydrolysis of the beta-lactam ring.

3. Decreased ability of the antibiotic to reach the PBP when bacteria decrease porin production, resulting in a decrease of the drug concentration within the cell.

Metabolic Route: Cefpodoxime is excreted unchanged in the urine.

 FDA-APPROVED INDICATIONS

Mild to moderate infections caused by susceptible strains of microorganisms in the conditions listed below:

Acute otitis media

Pharyngitis and/or tonsillitis

Community-acquired pneumonia

Acute bacterial exacerbation of chronic bronchitis

Acute, uncomplicated urethral and cervical gonorrhea

Acute, uncomplicated anorectal infections in women due to *Neisseria gonorrhoeae*

Uncomplicated skin and skin structure infections

Acute maxillary sinusitis

Uncomplicated urinary tract infections (cystitis)

 SIDE EFFECTS/TOXICITY

Cefpodoxime proxetil is **contraindicated** in patients with a known allergy to cefpodoxime or to the cephalosporin group of antibiotics.

Cefpodoxime should be used with caution if hypersensitivity exists to penicillin.

Toxicity includes fever, anaphylaxis, rash including Stevens–Johnson syndrome, erythema multiforme and toxic epidermal necrolysis, angioedema, flushing, serum-sickness-like reactions, encephalopathy, seizures, hallucination, hyperkinesias, diarrhea, *Clostridium difficile*-associated diarrhea and pseudomembranous colitis, oral candidiasis, anorexia, taste perversion, nausea, vomiting, stomach cramps, flatulence, hepatitis, renal impairment, genital moniliasis, vaginitis, hemorrhage, epistaxis prolonged prothrombin time, pancytopenia, hemolytic anemia, positive Coombs' test, hyperglycemia, hypoglycemia, hypoalbuminemia, hypoproteinemia, hyperkalemia, and hyponatremia.

 DRUG INTERACTIONS/FOOD INTERACTIONS

Cefpodoxime proxetil for oral suspension may be given without regard to food.

Concomitant administration of high doses of antacids or H2 blockers reduces peak plasma levels by 24 % to 42 %.

Antibiotics Manual: A Guide to Commonly Used Antimicrobials, Second Edition. David Schlossberg and Rafik Samuel.
© 2017 John Wiley & Sons Ltd. Published 2017 by John Wiley & Sons Ltd.

Cephalosporins may cause false-positive urine glucose determinations when using cupric sulfate solution (Benedict's solution, *Clinitest®*). Tests utilizing glucose oxidase (*Tes-Tape®*, *Clinistix®*) are not affected by cephalosporins.

Probenecid increases levels of cefpodoxime.

Close monitoring of renal function is advised when cefpodoxime proxetil is administered concomitantly with compounds of known nephrotoxic potential.

 ## DOSING (PO)

Infection	Dose	Duration
Pharyngitis/tonsillitis	100 mg q 12 hours	5–10 days
Community acquired pneumonia	200 mg q 12 hours	14 days
Gonorrhea	200 mg	Single dose
Skin and skin structure	400 mg q 12 hours	7–14 days
Acute maxillary sinusitis	200 mg q 12 hours	10 days
Urinary tract infections	100 mg q 12 hours	7 days

 ## SPECIAL POPULATIONS

RENAL IMPAIRMENT:

Creatinine clearance, mL/min	Dose
<30	Usual dose once daily
Hemodialysis	200 mg after dialysis only
CAPD	Usual dose once daily
CRRT	N/A

HEPATIC DYSFUNCTION: Dose adjustment is not necessary.

PEDIATRICS: Safety and efficacy in infants less than 2 months of age have not been established.

Infection	Dose	Duration
Acute otitis media	5 mg/kg (max. 200 mg) q 12 h	5 days
Pharyngitis/tonsillitis	5 mg/kg (max. 100 mg) q 12 h	5–10 days
Acute maxillary sinusitis	5 mg/kg (max. 200 mg) q 12 h	10 days

 ## THE ART OF ANTIMICROBIAL THERAPY

Clinical Pearls

1. Cefpodoxime is dose adjusted for renal dysfunction.
2. Cross allergy with penicillins is <10%.
3. Antacids or H2 blockers may decrease serum concentrations.

■ VEMLIDY (Tenofovir Alafenamide Fumarate (TAF))

 BASIC CHARACTERISTICS

Class: Nucleotide reverse transcriptase inhibitor for hepatitis B.

Mechanism of Action: Tenofovir alafenamide is a phosphonamidate prodrug of tenofovir. Tenofovir is an acyclic nucleotide analog of adenosine monophosphate, which is phosphorylated to the active metabolite tenofovir diphosphate by cellular kinases. Tenofovir diphosphate inhibits HBV replication through incorporation into viral DNA by the HBV reverse transcriptase, which results in DNA chain-termination.

Mechanism of Resistance: No specific substitutions occurred at a sufficient frequency to be associated with resistance to TAF.

Metabolic Route: TAF is rapidly converted to tenofovir alafenamide, which is then metabolized by the liver CES 1 and excreted.

 FDA-APPROVED INDICATIONS

TAF is indicated for the treatment of chronic hepatitis B with compensated liver disease.

 SIDE EFFECTS/TOXICITY

> **WARNING:** Lactic acidosis and severe hepatomegaly with steatosis, including fatal cases, have been reported with the use of nucleoside analogs. Discontinuation of antihepatitis B therapy, including TAF, may result in severe acute exacerbations of hepatitis B. Hepatic function should be monitored closely with both clinical and laboratory follow-up for at least several months in patients who discontinue antihepatitis B therapy, including TAF. If appropriate, resumption of antihepatitis B therapy may be warranted.

Other side effects include: headache, abdominal pain, fatigue, cough, nausea, back pain, and elevations in ALT. Renal impairment has been seen with other formulations of tenofovir, but that has not been reported with TAF.

 DRUG INTERACTIONS/FOOD INTERACTIONS

TAF should be taken with food.

TAF is a substrate of P-gp and BCRP. Drugs that strongly affect P-gp and BCRP activity may lead to changes in tenofovir alafenamide absorption.

TAF should not be coadministered with St John's wort, rifampin, rifabutin, or rifapentine.

If coadministering TAF with carbamazepine, oxcarbazepine, phenobarbital, or phenytoin, the TAF dose should be 50 mg once daily.

TAF should not be used with any other compound that includes tenofovir. These include Viread, Truvada, Complera, Odefsey, Descovy, Stribild, Atripla, or Genvoya.

 DOSING

TAF is dispensed as a 25 mg tablet. The recommended dose is 25 mg once daily with food.

Antibiotics Manual: A Guide to Commonly Used Antimicrobials, Second Edition. David Schlossberg and Rafik Samuel.
© 2017 John Wiley & Sons Ltd. Published 2017 by John Wiley & Sons Ltd.

SPECIAL POPULATIONS

RENAL IMAIRMENT: Not recommended in patients with a creatinine clearance less than 15 mg/mL.

HEPATIC DYSFUNCTION: Not recommended in patients with moderate or severe hepatic impairment.

PEDIATRICS: No recommendations for those under 18 years of age.

 THE ART OF ANTIMICROBIAL THERAPY

Clinical Pearls

1. All patients should be tested for HIV before initiating TAF for hepatitis B treatment.
2. Although tenofovir disoproxil fumarate has been associated with fanconi syndrome and bone mineral loss, tenofovir alafenamide fumarate has not been shown to cause these side effects in studies.
3. TAF is available in combination with other antiretrovirals; however, this formulation is not indicated for the treatment of HIV.
4. TAF should not be used in combination with any medication that contains tenofovir. These include Viread, Truvada, Complera, Odefsey, Descovy, Stribild, Atripla, and Genvoya.

■ VFEND (Voriconazole)

 BASIC CHARACTERISTICS

Class: Triazole.

Mechanism of Action: Inhibition of lanosterol 14-α-demethylase, which is involved in the synthesis of ergosterol, an essential component of fungal cell membranes.

Mechanisms of Resistance:

1. Point mutations in the gene (*ERG11*) encoding for the target enzyme lead to an altered target with decreased affinity for azoles.

2. Overexpression of *ERG11* results in the production of high concentrations of the target enzyme, creating the need for higher intracellular drug concentrations to inhibit all of the enzyme molecules in the cell.

3. Active efflux of itraconazole out of the cell through the activation of two types of multidrug efflux transporters.

Metabolic Route: Voriconazole is metabolized by cytochrome P450 CYP2C19, CYP2C9, and CYP3A4 and is excreted primarily in the urine.

 FDA-APPROVED INDICATIONS

Invasive aspergillosis.

Candidemia in nonneutropenic patients.

Disseminated candida infections in skin and infections in abdomen, kidney, bladder wall, and wounds.

Esophageal candidiasis.

Serious fungal infections caused by *Scedosporium apiospermum* (*Pseudoallescheria boydii*) and *Fusarium* spp.

 SIDE EFFECTS/TOXICITY

Voriconazole is **contraindicated** in patients with known hypersensitivity to voriconazole or its excipients. Caution should be used when prescribing voriconazole to patients with hypersensitivity to other azoles.

Adverse events include rare but severe hepatotoxicity, optic neuritis, papilledema, hepatotoxicity, fever, rash, photosensitivity, anaphylaxis, vomiting, nausea, diarrhea, headache, sepsis, peripheral edema, abdominal pain, respiratory disorder, adrenal insufficiency, diabetes insipidus, dysthyroidism, cardiac toxicity including QT prolongation and torsade de pointes, seizures, aplastic anemia, and electrolyte disturbances.

 DRUG INTERACTIONS/ADMINISTRATION

Oral voriconazole should be taken at least one hour before, or one hour following, a meal. Gastric pH does not affect drug levels.

Voriconazole is metabolized by the human hepatic cytochrome P450 enzymes CYP2C19, CYP2C9, and CYP3A4. Inhibitors or inducers of these enzymes may increase or decrease voriconazole plasma concentrations, respectively. In addition, voriconazole inhibits the metabolic activity of the cytochrome P450 enzymes CYP2C19, CYP2C9, and CYP3A, so that voriconazole may increase plasma concentrations of other drugs metabolized by these CYP450 enzymes, resulting in toxicity.

Antibiotics Manual: A Guide to Commonly Used Antimicrobials, Second Edition. David Schlossberg and Rafik Samuel.
© 2017 John Wiley & Sons Ltd. Published 2017 by John Wiley & Sons Ltd.

The following medications are **contraindicated** with voriconazole: terfenadine, astemizole, cisapride, pimozide, quinidine, sirolimus, rifabutin, rifampin, carbamazapine, long-acting barbiturates, efavirenz, high-dose ritonavir, ergot alkaloids (ergotamine and dihydroergotamine), St. John's Wort

The following list comprises significant drug interactions with voriconazole:

Alfentanil: Reduction in the dose of alfentanil and other opiates metabolized by CYP3A4 (e.g., sufentanil) should be considered.

Benzodiazepines: Monitor for increased benzodiazepine effects.

Calcium channel blockers: Monitor for increased calcium channel effects.

Cyclosporine: Reduce the cyclosporine dose to one-half of the starting dose and monitor cyclosporine blood levels.

HMG–CoA reductase inhibitors (statins): Monitor for increased statin effects.

Methadone: Monitor. Dose reduction of methodone may be necessary.

Omeprazole: When initiating therapy with VFEND in patients already receiving omeprazole doses of 40 mg or greater, reduce the omeprazole dose by one-half.

Oral contraceptives: Increased levels of both oral contraceptives and voriconazole.

Phenytoin: Monitor for phenytoin toxicity; increase voriconazole maintenance dose from 4 mg/kg to 5 mg/kg IV every 12 hours or from 200 mg to 400 mg orally every 12 hours (100 mg to 200 mg orally every 12 hours in patients weighing less than 40 kg).

Protease inhibitors: Low dose (100 mg q 12 h) may be given and where benefit outweighs risk. With other protease inhibitors, levels of both the PI and voriconazole may be elevated.

Sulfonylurea oral hypoglycemics: Monitor for hypoglycemia.

Tacrolimus: Reduce the tacrolimus dose to one-third of the starting dose and monitor tacrolimus blood levels.

Warfarin: Monitor for increased warfarin effects.

Vinca alkaloids: Monitor for increased vinca alkaloid effects.

 ## DOSING

Voriconazole is dispensed in 50 mg and 200 mg tablets; a powder for oral ingestion containing 45 mg/vial; and a powder for intravenous administration.

For treatment of aspergillosis, scedosporiosis, fusariosis, and invasive candidiasis: Loading dose of 6 mg/kg IV every 12 hours first day followed by 4 mg/kg every 12 hours or 200 mg orally q 12 hours.

Adult patients who weigh less than 40 kg should receive an oral maintenance dose of 100 mg every 12 hours.

For esophageal candidiasis: 200 mg orally every 12 hours.

 ## SPECIAL POPULATIONS

RENAL IMPAIRMENT: In patients with creatinine clearance <50 mL/min, accumulation of the intravenous vehicle, SBECD, occurs. Oral voriconazole should be administered to these patients, unless an assessment of the benefit/risk to the patient justifies the use of intravenous voriconazole. There is no dose adjustment for oral voriconazole.

HEPATIC DYSFUNCTION: The maintenance dose should be 100 mg every 12 hours in those with Child Pugh* Class A and B. Voriconazole has not been studied in patients with severe cirrhosis (Child Pugh* Class C). Patients with hepatic insufficiency must be carefully monitored for drug toxicity.

PEDIATRICS: Safety and effectiveness in pediatric patients below the age of 12 years have not been established.

In children 12 years and older, the maintenance dose of 4 mg/kg q 12 h can be given.

*Child Pugh categories, see Helpful Formulas, Equations, and Definitions.

 ## THE ART OF ANTIMICROBIAL THERAPY

Clinical Pearls

1. Voriconazole is active against most molds except *Zygomycete* spp.
2. Voriconazole should not be administered by the IV route in patients with renal insufficiency; oral voriconazole is recommended instead.
3. Voriconazole is an inhibitor of cytochrome P450 and can enhance the activity of many commonly used drugs, e.g., oral hypoglycemics and anticoagulants.
4. Voriconazole should be administered with caution to patients with potentially proarrhythmic conditions.
5. Voriconazole levels should be monitored in patients with severe life-threatening infections or those who do not respond to therapy.
6. Recent reports have shown an association between voriconazole and melanoma/squamous cell carcinoma of the skin in transplant recipients.
7. Recent reports have shown an association between voriconazole and pancreatitis in children.

BASIC CHARACTERISTICS

Class: Lipoglycopeptide.

Mechanism of Action: Telavancin inhibits bacterial cell wall synthesis by interfering with the polymerization and crosslinking of peptidoglycan. Telavancin binds to the bacterial membrane and disrupts membrane barrier function.

Mechanisms of Resistance: Unknown.

Metabolic Route: Excreted unchanged in the urine.

 FDA-APPROVED INDICATIONS

Complicated skin and skin structure infections (cSSSIs) caused by susceptible gram-positive organisms, including methicillin-susceptible and -resistant *Staphylococcus aureus*.

Hospital-acquired and ventilator-associated bacterial pneumonia (HABP/VABP), caused by susceptible isolates of *Staphylococcus aureus* (both methicillin-susceptible and -resistant isolates).

 SIDE EFFECTS/TOXICITY

> **WARNING:** Patients with preexisting moderate/severe renal impairment (creatinine clearance ≤50 mL/min) who were treated with telavancin for hospital-acquired bacterial pneumonia/ventilator-associated bacterial pneumonia (HABP/VABP) had increased mortality observed versus vancomycin. Use of VIBATIV in patients with preexisting moderate/severe renal impairment (creatinine clearance ≤50 mL/min) should be considered only when the anticipated benefit to the patient outweighs the potential risk of nephrotoxicity and new-onset or worsening renal impairment has occurred. Monitor renal function in all patients.
>
> Women of childbearing potential should have a serum pregnancy test prior to administration of telavancin. Avoid use of telavancin during pregnancy unless the potential benefit to the patient outweighs the potential risk to the fetus. Adverse developmental outcomes observed in 3 animal species at clinically relevant doses raise concerns about potential adverse developmental outcomes in humans.

Toxicity includes increases in serum creatinine, "Red Man's syndrome", *Clostridium difficile*-associated diarrhea, prolongation of the QTc interval, nausea, vomiting, taste disturbance, and foamy urine.

 DRUG INTERACTIONS/FOOD INTERACTIONS

Elevations in the test results for prothrombin time, international normalized ratio, activated partial thromboplastin time, activated clotting time, and coagulation-based factor Xa tests. D-dimer, bleeding time, and whole blood clotting time are not affected.

 DOSING

Telavancin dosing is 10 mg/kg daily.

Antibiotics Manual: A Guide to Commonly Used Antimicrobials, Second Edition. David Schlossberg and Rafik Samuel.
© 2017 John Wiley & Sons Ltd. Published 2017 by John Wiley & Sons Ltd.

SPECIAL POPULATIONS

RENAL IMPAIRMENT:

Creatinine clearance, mL/min	Telavancin dosage regimen
>50	10 mg/kg every 24 hours
30–50	7.5 mg/kg every 24 hours
10–<30	10 mg/kg every 48 hours
<10	Not recommended

HEPATIC DYSFUNCTION: No dose adjustment is necessary.

PEDIATRICS: Safety and efficacy in patients under the age of 18 have not been established.

 ## THE ART OF ANTIMICROBIAL THERAPY

Clinical Pearls

1. Telavancin should be renally adjusted.
2. Women of childbearing potential should have a serum pregnancy test prior to administration.
3. Telavancin may cause false elevation of PT/INR results.
4. Telavancin is not active against vancomycin-resistant enterococci.

BASIC CHARACTERISTICS

Class:

Dasabuvir is a hepatitis C virus nonnucleoside NS5B polymerase inhibitor.

Ombitasvir is a hepatitis C virus NS5A inhibitor.

Paritaprevir is a hepatitis C virus NS3/4A protease inhibitor.

Ritonavir is a CYP3A inhibitor.

Mechanism of Action:

Dasabuvir is a non-nucleoside inhibitor of the HCV RNA-dependent RNA polymerase, which is essential for replication of the viral genome.

Ombitasvir is an inhibitor of HCV NS5A, which is essential for viral RNA replication and virion assembly.

Paritaprevir is an inhibitor of the HCV NS3/4A protease, which is necessary for the proteolytic cleavage of the HCV encoded polyprotein and is essential for viral replication.

Ritonavir is a CYP3A inhibitor that inhibits CYP3A mediated metabolism of paritaprevir.

Mechanism of Resistance:

Dasabuvir activity is decreased by mutations on the polymerase protein: C316Y, M414I/T, E446K/Q, Y448C/H, A553T, G554S, S556G/R, and Y561H.

Ombitasvir activity is decreased by mutations on the NS5A protein: M28T/V, Q30E/R, L31V, H58D, and Y93C/H/L/N.

Paritaprevir activity is decreased by mutations on the protease enzyme: F43L, R155G/K/S, A156T, D168A/E/F/H/N/V/Y, and Q80K.

Metabolic Route:

Dasabuvir is metabolized by CYP 2C8.

Ombitasvir is metabolized by amide hydrolysis.

Pariteprevir is metabolized by CYP 3A4.

Ritonavir is metabolized by the CYP 3A4.

 FDA-APPROVED INDICATIONS

Viekira Pak is indicated for:

1. The treatment of adult patients with chronic hepatitis C virus (HCV) genotype 1b without cirrhosis or with compensated cirrhosis.

2. The treatment of adult patients with HCV genotype 1a without cirrhosis or with compensated cirrhosis for use in combination with ribavirin.

 SIDE EFFECTS/TOXICITY

Hepatic decompensation and hepatic failure, including liver transplantation or fatal outcomes, increased the risk of ALT elevations.

Other side effects include fatigue, nausea, pruritis, rash, insomnia, and asthenia.

Antibiotics Manual: A Guide to Commonly Used Antimicrobials, Second Edition. David Schlossberg and Rafik Samuel.
© 2017 John Wiley & Sons Ltd. Published 2017 by John Wiley & Sons Ltd.

DRUG INTERACTIONS/FOOD INTERACTIONS

Ombitasvir, paritaprevir, and dasabuvir are inhibitors of UGT1A1, and ritonavir is an inhibitor of CYP3A4. Paritaprevir is an inhibitor of OATP1B1 and OATP1B3 and paritaprevir, ritonavir, and dasabuvir are inhibitors of BCRP. Coadministration of Viekira Pak with drugs that are substrates of CYP3A, UGT1A1, BCRP, OATP1B1, or OATP1B3 may result in increased plasma concentrations of such drugs.

If Viekira Pak is administered with ribavirin, the **contraindications** to ribavirin also apply to this combination regimen. Refer to the ribavirin prescribing information for a list of **contraindications**.

Viekira Pak should not be administered with alfuzosin, ranolazine, dronedarone, carbamazepine, phenobarbital, phenytoin, colchicine, gemfibrozil, rifampin, rifapentine, lurasidone, pimozide, ergotamine, dihydroergotamine, methylergonovine, ethinyl estradiol, St John's wort, cisapride, lovastatin, pravastatin, efavirenz, sildenafil, triazolam, midazolam, voriconazole, fluticasone, darunavir, Kaletra, rilpivirine, or salmeterol.

Medication	Adjustment or action
Valsartan, losartan, candesartan	Lower the dose of the ARB
Antiarrhythmics	Monitor levels
Ketoconazole	Maximum dose of ketoconazole should be 200 mg
Quetiapine	Decrease the dose of quetiapine to one-sixth.
Calcium channel blockers	Decrease the calcium channel blocker by 50 %
Atazanavir/ritonavir	Atazanavir 300 mg should be given in the morning only
Rosuvastatin	Maximum dose of rosuvastatin is 10 mg
Pravastatin	Maximum dose of pravastatin is 40 mg
Cyclosporine	Decrease cyclosporine to one-fifth of the dose and monitor levels
Tacrolimus	Reduce dose to 0.5 mg every 7 days and monitor levels
Buprenorphine/naloxone	Monitor closely
Alprazolam	Monitor closely
Rifabutin	150 mg/d or 300 mg 3 ×/week and monitor

 DOSING

Viekira Pak is ombitasvir 12.5 mg, paritaprevir 75 mg, and ritonavir 50 mg fixed dose combination tablets copackaged with dasabuvir 250 mg tablets. The recommended oral dosage of is two ombitasvir, paritaprevir, ritonavir tablets once daily (in the morning) and one dasabuvir tablet twice daily (morning and evening). Take Viekira Pak with a meal without regard to fat or calorie content.

Patient population	Medication	Duration
Genotype 1 without cirrhosis	Viekira Pak + ribavirin	12 weeks
Genotype 1 with compensated cirrhosis	Viekira Pak + ribavirin	24 weeks
Genotype 1b with or without compensated cirrhosis	Viekira Pak	12 weeks
Transplant patients with Genotype 1 (a or b)	Viekira Pak + ribavirin	24 weeks

SPECIAL POPULATIONS

RENAL IMPAIRMENT: No dosage adjustment.

HEPATIC DYSFUNCTION: Not recommended for patients with moderate or severe hepatic dysfunction.

PEDIATRICS: Do not use in those under 18 years of age.

 THE ART OF ANTIMICROBIAL THERAPY

Clinical Pearls

1. Viekira Pak is active against HCV genotype 1 only.
2. All patients should have HCV resistance testing prior to initiation of Viekira Pak. An alternative therapy should be considered for patients with those that have the Q80K mutation.
3. Monitor liver chemistry tests before and during Viekira Pak therapy.
4. Viekira Pak contains ritonavir, so all patients with HIV must be on treatment to prevent HIV resistance.
5. Review the most current hepatitis C treatment guidelines because they are changing rapidly: http://www.cdc.gov/hepatitis/HCV/index.htm.

■ VIRAMUNE (Nevirapine)

 ## BASIC CHARACTERISTICS

Class: Nonnucleoside reverse transcriptase inhibitor.

Mechanism of Action: Nevirapine inhibits reverse transcriptase activity by binding the enzyme.

Mechanism of Resistance: Changes in the structure of reverse transcriptase leads to the inability of nevirapine to bind the enzyme and allow transcription to continue. The most frequent resistance mutations include K103N and Y181C.

Metabolic Route: Metabolized by the cytochrome P450 system to hydroxylated metabolites.

 ## FDA-APPROVED INDICATIONS

Treatment of HIV-1 in combinations with other antiretroviral agents.

 ## SIDE EFFECTS/TOXICITY

> **WARNING:**
>
> **Hepatotoxicity:** Severe, life-threatening, and in some cases fatal hepatotoxicity, particularly in the first 18 weeks, has been reported in patients treated with nevirapine. In some cases, patients presented with nonspecific prodromal signs or symptoms of hepatitis and progressed to hepatic failure. These events are often associated with rash. Female gender and higher CD4+ cell counts at initiation of therapy place patients at increased risk; women with CD4+ cell counts greater than 250 cells/mm^3, including pregnant women receiving nevirapine in combination with other antiretrovirals for the treatment of HIV-1 infection, are at the greatest risk. However, hepatotoxicity associated with nevirapine use can occur in both genders, all CD4+ cell counts, and at any time during treatment. Hepatic failure has also been reported in patients without HIV taking nevirapine for postexposure prophylaxis (PEP). Use of nevirapine for occupational and nonoccupational PEP is **contraindicated**. Patients with signs or symptoms of hepatitis, or with increased transaminases combined with rash or other systemic symptoms, must discontinue nevirapine and seek medical evaluation immediately.
>
> **Skin reactions:** Severe, life-threatening skin reactions, including fatal cases, have occurred in patients treated with nevirapine. These have included cases of Stevens–Johnson syndrome, toxic epidermal necrolysis, and hypersensitivity reactions characterized by rash, constitutional findings, and organ dysfunction. Patients developing signs or symptoms of severe skin reactions or hypersensitivity reactions must discontinue nevirapine and seek medical evaluation immediately. Transaminase levels should be checked immediately for all patients who develop a rash in the first 18 weeks of treatment. The 14-day lead-in period with nevirapine 200 mg daily dosing has been observed to decrease the incidence of rash and must be followed.
>
> **Monitoring:** Patients must be monitored intensively during the first 18 weeks of therapy with nevirapine to detect potentially life-threatening hepatotoxicity or skin reactions. Extra vigilance is warranted during the first 6 weeks of therapy, which is the period of greatest risk of these events. Do not restart nevirapine following clinical hepatitis, or transaminase elevations combined with rash or other systemic symptoms, or following severe skin rash or hypersensitivity reactions. In some cases, hepatic injury has progressed despite discontinuation of treatment.

Other adverse events **include elevated cholesterol, fat redistribution, immune reconstitution syndrome, fever, anemia, neutropenia, rhabdomyolysis, and paresthesias.**

Antibiotics Manual: A Guide to Commonly Used Antimicrobials, Second Edition. David Schlossberg and Rafik Samuel.
© 2017 John Wiley & Sons Ltd. Published 2017 by John Wiley & Sons Ltd.

DRUG INTERACTIONS/FOOD INTERACTIONS

Food: no significant effect.

Nevirapine should not be administered concurrently with astemizole, bepridil, cisapride, midazolam, pimozide, triazolam, ketoconazole, ergot derivatives, St John's wort, atazanavir, or etravirine.

Nevirapine is principally metabolized by the liver via the cytochrome P450 isoenzymes, 3A and 2B6. Nevirapine causes hepatic enzyme induction of CYP3A4; coadministration of nevirapine with drugs primarily metabolized by 3A4 and 2B6 isozymes may result in altered plasma concentrations of the coadministered drug. Drugs that induce CYP3A4 activity would be expected to increase the clearance of nevirapine, resulting in lowered plasma concentrations. Because of these metabolic activities, the following drug interactions warrant consideration of dosage adjustment and monitoring of clinical effects and serum levels of affected drugs:

Medication	*Adjustment or action*
Fluconazole	Risk of hepatotoxicity, monitor for toxicity
Voriconazole	Monitor for toxicity
Clarithromycin	Consider alternative agent
Rifampin	Use rifabutin and monitor for rifabutin toxicity
Contraceptives	Use alternative or additional method
Methadone	Opiate withdrawal common, titrate methadone
Indinavir	IDV 1000 mg q 8 h + RTV 100 bid
Lopinavir/ritonavir	Use 600/150 mg lopinavir/ritonavir bid
Warfarin	Monitor warfarin effect

In addition, **potential** drug interactions warrant monitoring for decreased effects of the following when given with nevirapine: antiarrhythmics, anticonvulsants, calcium channel blockers, immunosuppressants, and cancer chemotherapeutic agents.

 DOSING

Nevirapine is administered in 200 mg tablets and a white oral suspension containing 50 mg nevirapine in each 5 mL. The recommended dose for nevirapine is one 200 mg tablet daily for the first 14 days, followed by one 200 mg tablet twice daily, in combination with other antiretroviral agents.

Nevirapine XR is formulated as 100 mg and 400 mg tablets.

 SPECIAL POPULATIONS

RENAL IMPAIRMENT: There is no adjustment needed.

HEPATIC DYSFUNCTION: Nevirapine is contraindicated in patients with moderate or severe (Child Pugh* Class B or C, respectively) hepatic impairment.

PEDIATRICS: **for treatment:** The recommended oral dose for pediatric patients 15 days and older is 150 mg/m^2 once daily for 14 days followed by 150 mg/m^2 twice daily thereafter. The total daily dose should not exceed 400 mg for any patient. Body surface area may be calculated using the Mosteller formula.*

*Child Pugh determination and Mosteller formula: see Helpful Formulas, Equations and Definitions.

THE ART OF ANTIMICROBIAL THERAPY

Clinical Pearls

1. Nevirapine should always be used in combination with other antiretrovirals.

2. Nevirapine should not be initiated in women with CD4 counts greater than 250 or men with CD4 counts greater than 400.

3. Patients must be monitored intensively during the first 18 weeks of therapy with nevirapine to detect potentially life-threatening hepatotoxicity or skin reactions.

4. Nevirapine should be administered as 200 mg daily for 2 weeks prior to the full dose of nevirapine 200 mg twice daily or nevirapine XR 400 mg once daily.

5. Nevirapine has a very long half-life. If stopping antiretroviral regimen, to decrease resistance, the other medications should be continued for at least another 48 hours.

6. Whenever initiating nevirapine, make sure to review all medications the patient is receiving, to limit drug interactions.

BASIC CHARACTERISTICS

Class: Nucleoside analog.

Mechanism of Action: Not known.

Mechanism of Resistance: Not known.

Metabolic Route: Ribavirin is metabolized by phosphorylation or deribosylation/hydrolysis to yield a triazole carboxylic acid metabolite and is excreted renally.

 FDA-APPROVED INDICATIONS

Inhaled ribavirin is indicated for the treatment of hospitalized infants and young children with severe lower respiratory tract infections due to respiratory syncytial virus. Treatment early in the course of severe lower respiratory tract infection may be necessary to achieve efficacy.

Also Used for: Some authorities recommend consideration of ribavirin therapy for any patient with viral hemorrhagic fever caused by arenavirus (Lassa fever, New World hemorrhagic fevers) or bunyavirus (Hantavirus, Rift Valley fever, Crimean–Congo hemorrhagic fever), or for suspected VHF if the etiology is unknown.

 SIDE EFFECTS/TOXICITY

> **WARNING:** Aerosolized ribavirin in patients requiring mechanical ventilator assistance should be undertaken only by physicians and support staff familiar with the specific ventilator being used and this mode of administration of the drug. Strict attention must be paid to procedures that have been shown to minimize the accumulation of drug precipitate, which can result in mechanical ventilator dysfunction and associated increased pulmonary pressures.
>
> Sudden deterioration of respiratory function has been associated with initiation of aerosolized ribavirin use in infants. Respiratory function should be carefully monitored during treatment. If initiation of aerosolized ribavirin treatment appears to produce sudden deterioration of respiratory function, treatment should be stopped and reinstituted only with extreme caution, continuous monitoring, and consideration of concomitant administration of bronchodilators.
>
> Inhaled ribavirin is not indicated for use in adults. Physicians and patients should be aware that ribavirin has been shown to produce testicular lesions in rodents and to be teratogenic in all animal species in which adequate studies have been conducted.
>
> Ribavirin is **contraindicated** in patients with a history of hypersensitivity, autoimmune hepatitis, hemoglobinopathies (e.g., thalassemia major, sickle-cell anemia).

Other toxicities of aerosolized ribavirin: Sudden deterioration of respiratory function has been associated with initiation of aerosolized ribavirin use in infants. Respiratory function should be carefully monitored during treatment. If sudden deterioration of respiratory function is noted, treatment should be stopped and reinstituted only with extreme caution, continuous monitoring, and consideration of concomitant administration of bronchodilators. Use of aerosolized ribavirin in patients requiring mechanical ventilator assistance should be undertaken only by physicians and support staff familiar with this mode of administration and the specific ventilator being used. Strict attention must be paid to procedures that have been shown to minimize the accumulation of drug precipitate, which can result in mechanical ventilator dysfunction and associated increased pulmonary pressures.

Antibiotics Manual: A Guide to Commonly Used Antimicrobials, Second Edition. David Schlossberg and Rafik Samuel.
© 2017 John Wiley & Sons Ltd. Published 2017 by John Wiley & Sons Ltd.

DRUG INTERACTIONS/FOOD INTERACTIONS

None.

 DOSING

Ribavirin for inhalation is supplied in 100 mL glass vials with 6 grams of sterile, lyophilized drug, which is to be reconstituted with 300 mL of sterile water and administered only by a small particle aerosol generator (SPAG-2). The recommended treatment regimen is 20 mg/mL with continuous aerosol administration for 12–18 hours per day for 3 to 7 days.

 SPECIAL POPULATIONS

RENAL IMPAIRMENT: No adjustment is necessary.

HEPATIC DYSFUNCTION: No adjustment is necessary.

PEDIATRICS: Inhaled ribavirin dosage is as above.

 THE ART OF ANTIMICROBIAL THERAPY

Clinical Pearls
1. Treatment early with inhaled ribavirin for severe lower respiratory tract infection may be necessary to achieve efficacy.
2. Ribavirin is pregnancy category X; women should use 2 barriers of protection for birth control. This caution extends to **men as well**.

Also available in Truvada, Atripla, Complera, and Stribild.

 BASIC CHARACTERISTICS

Class: Nucleotide reverse transcriptase inhibitor (NRTI) with activity against HIV and Hepatitis B.

Mechanism of Action: Converted by cellular enzymes to its active drug tenofovir biphosphate, an analog of adenosine triphosphate. The tenofovir biphosphate competes with the naturally occurring nucleotides for incorporation in newly forming HIV DNA. Since tenofovir biphosphate does not have a terminal hydroxyl group, it halts transcription and replication of the virus.

Mechanism of Resistance: Changes in the structure of HIV reverse transcriptase leads to preferred incorporation of adenosine triphosphate and decreased incorporation of tenofovir biphosphate, which allows transcription of DNA to continue. Resistance mutations include K65R and TAMS.

Metabolic Route: Tenofovir is excreted in the urine unchanged.

 FDA-APPROVED INDICATIONS

Treatment of HIV infection, in combination with other antiretrovirals.

Treatment of chronic Hepatitis B in adults.

 SIDE EFFECTS/TOXICITY

> **WARNING: Severe acute exacerbations of hepatitis** have been reported in hepatitis B-infected patients who have discontinued antihepatitis B therapy, including tenofovir. Hepatic function should be monitored closely with both clinical and laboratory follow-up for at least several months in patients who discontinue antihepatitis B therapy, including tenofovir. If appropriate, resumption of anti-hepatitis B therapy may be warranted.
>
> **Lactic acidosis and severe hepatomegaly with steatosis**, including fatal cases, have been reported with the use of nucleoside analogs, including tenofovir, in combination with other antiretrovirals.

Other side effects: Immune reconstitution inflammatory syndrome, fat redistribution including central obesity and dorsocervical fat enlargement, peripheral wasting, facial wasting, breast enlargement, renal impairment, including cases of acute renal failure and Fanconi syndrome, decreased bone mineral density, rash, nausea, diarrhea, headache, pain, depression, and asthenia.

 DRUG INTERACTIONS/FOOD INTERACTIONS

Tenofovir should be administered with food.

Tenofovir should not be administered with adefovir.

Tenofovir should not be given with didanosine because of decreased CD4 counts in patients maintained on this regimen. If didanosine is given with tenofovir, the didanosine should be decreased to 250 mg daily.

Tenofovir decreases the levels of atazanavir. If given together, atazanavir must be given with ritonavir or cobicistat.

Coadministration of tenofovir and ledipasvir/sofosbuvir has been shown to increase tenofovir exposure.

Antibiotics Manual: A Guide to Commonly Used Antimicrobials, Second Edition. David Schlossberg and Rafik Samuel.
© 2017 John Wiley & Sons Ltd. Published 2017 by John Wiley & Sons Ltd.

Tenofovir should not be administered with other medications containing tenofovir (Truvada, Atripla, Complera, Stribild, Descovy, Odefsey, or Genvoya).

 DOSING

Tenofovir is administered in a 150 mg, 200 mg, 250 mg, and 300 mg tablet. It is also available in an oral powder consisting of white, taste-masked, coated granules containing 40 mg of tenofovir disoproxil fumarate, which is equivalent to 33 mg of tenofovir disoproxil, per level scoop. Each level scoop contains 1 gram of oral powder. The recommended adult dose is 300 mg once daily.

 SPECIAL POPULATIONS

RENAL IMPAIRMENT: Tenofovir should be adjusted based on renal function. For creatinine clearance of 30–49 cc/min, tenofovir should be administered every 48 hours. For clearance less than 30 cc/min, it should be administered every 72–96 hours. For those on hemodialysis, it is administered once weekly.

HEPATIC DYSFUNCTION: No dose adjustment is necessary.

PEDIATRICS: For pediatric patients 2 years of age and older, the recommended oral dose of tenofovir is 8 mg of tenofovir disoproxil fumarate per kilogram of body weight (up to a maximum of 300 mg) once daily administered as oral powder or tablets.

 THE ART OF ANTIMICROBIAL THERAPY

Clinical Pearls

1. Tenofovir should be used in combination with other antiretroviral agents.
2. Tenofovir (disoproxil or alafenamide) is present in nine different medications: Viread, Vemlidy, Truvada, Descovy, Atripla, Complera, Odefsey, Stribild, and Genvoya.
3. Patients with HIV-1 should be tested for hepatitis B virus before initiating antiretroviral therapy with tenofovir.
4. Tenofovir and didanosine combinations should be administered with caution (see above).
5. Atazanavir should be boosted with ritonavir or cobicistat if given with tenofovir.
6. A newer formulation of tenofovir is tenofovir alafenamide. This newer formulation may have less renal and bone side effects.
7. The daily dose of tenofovir disoproxil is different from the tenofovir alafenamide; use caution when prescribing.

BASIC CHARACTERISTICS

Class: Antiviral.

Mechanism of Action: Incorporation of cidofovir diphosphate into the growing CMV viral DNA chain results in reductions in the rate of viral DNA synthesis.

Mechanism of Resistance: Insufficient data.

Metabolic Route: Cidofovir must be administered with probenecid. Cidofovir is cleared unchanged in the urine.

 FDA-APPROVED INDICATIONS

Treatment of CMV retinitis in patients with acquired immunodeficiency syndrome (AIDS).

Also Used for: Some authorities recommend cidofovir for smallpox and complications of smallpox vaccination, i.e., eczema vaccinatum, progressive vaccinia and inadvertent inoculation, and for monkeypox. It may also have activity against polyoma-viruses and adenovirus.

 SIDE EFFECTS/TOXICITY

> **WARNING:** Renal impairment is the major toxicity of cidofovir. Cases of acute renal failure resulting in dialysis and/or contributing to death have occurred with as few as one or two doses of cidofovir. To reduce possible nephrotoxicity, intravenous prehydration with normal saline and administration of probenecid must be used with each cidofovir infusion. Renal function (serum creatinine and urine protein) must be monitored within 48 hours prior to each dose of cidofovir and the dose of cidofovir modified for changes in renal function as appropriate. Cidofovir is **contraindicated** in patients who are receiving other nephrotoxic agents.
>
> Neutropenia has been observed in association with cidofovir treatment. Therefore, neutrophil counts should be monitored during cidofovir therapy.
>
> Cidofovir is indicated only for the treatment of CMV retinitis in patients with acquired immunodeficiency syndrome.
>
> In animal studies cidofovir was carcinogenic, teratogenic, and caused hypospermia.

Other toxic effects include proximal tubular cell injury with metabolic acidosis with Fanconi's syndrome, glycosuria, decreased in serum phosphate, uric acid, and bicarbonate, and decreased intraocular pressure with impaired visual acuity, uveitis, or iritis, liver dysfunction, and pancreatitis.

 DRUG INTERACTIONS/FOOD INTERACTIONS

Probenecid: Probenecid is known to interact with the metabolism or renal tubular excretion of many drugs (e.g., acetaminophen, acyclovir, angiotensin-converting enzyme inhibitors, aminosalicylic acid, barbiturates, benzodiazepines, bumetanide, clofibrate, methotrexate, famotidine, furosemide, nonsteroidal anti-inflammatory agents, theophylline, and zidovudine). Concomitant medications should be carefully assessed.

Zidovudine should either be temporarily discontinued or decreased by 50 % when coadministered with probenecid on the day of cidofovir infusion.

Nephrotoxic agents: Concomitant administration of cidofovir and agents with nephrotoxic potential is contraindicated.

Antibiotics Manual: A Guide to Commonly Used Antimicrobials, Second Edition. David Schlossberg and Rafik Samuel.
© 2017 John Wiley & Sons Ltd. Published 2017 by John Wiley & Sons Ltd.

DOSING

The recommended induction dose of cidofovir is 5 mg/kg body weight once weekly for two consecutive weeks. The recommended maintenance dose of cidofovir is 5 mg/kg administered once every 2 weeks.

 SPECIAL POPULATIONS

RENAL IMPAIRMENT: The maintenance dose of cidofovir must be reduced from 5 mg/kg to 3 mg/kg for an increase in serum creatinine of 0.3–0.4 mg/dL above baseline. Cidofovir therapy must be discontinued for an increase in serum creatinine of $\geq$ 0.5 mg/dL above baseline or development of $\geq$3+ proteinuria.

Cidofovir is **contraindicated** in patients with a serum creatinine concentration >1.5 mg/dL, a calculated creatinine clearance* $\leq$55 mL/min, or a urine protein $\geq$100 mg/dL (equivalent to $\geq$ 2+ proteinuria).

HEPATIC DYSFUNCTION: No adjustment is needed.

PEDIATRICS: Cidofovir has not been studied in children.

 THE ART OF ANTIMICROBIAL THERAPY

Clinical Pearls

1. To minimize potential nephrotoxicity, probenecid and intravenous saline prehydration must be administered with each cidofovir infusion. Probenecid is administered orally with each cidofovir dose: two grams 3 hours prior to the cidofovir dose and one gram 2 and again at 8 hours after completion of the 1 hour cidofovir infusion (for a total of 4 grams). Patients should be warned of potential adverse events caused by probenecid (e.g., headache, nausea, vomiting, and hypersensitivity reactions, including rash, fever, chills, and anaphylaxis).
2. Cidofovir is **contraindicated** in patients with creatinine >1.5, those with CrCl <55 or a urine protein of >100.
3. Cidofovir should not be administered with other nephrotoxic agents.
4. Cidofovir should not be administered intraocularly.
5. Patients should be monitored for neutropenia.

BASIC CHARACTERISTICS

Class: Integrase inhibitor.

Mechanism of Action: Elvitegravir is an HIV-1 integrase strand transfer inhibitor (INSTI). Inhibition of integrase prevents the integration of HIV-1 DNA into host genomic DNA, blocking propagation of the viral infection.

Mechanism of Resistance: Elvitegravir changes the structure of HIV integrase. Development of mutations on the enzyme integrase prevents elvitegravir from binding to the active site of the enzyme and allowing integrase activity to continue. Resistance mutations that emerge in patients taking elvitegravir include T66A/I, E92G/Q, S147G, and Q148R.

Metabolic Route: Elvitegravir undergoes primarily oxidative metabolism via CYP3A and is secondarily glucuronidated via UGT1A1/3 enzymes in the liver and excreted.

 FDA-APPROVED INDICATIONS

In combination with an HIV protease inhibitor coadministered with ritonavir and with other antiretroviral drug(s) for the treatment of HIV-1 infection in antiretroviral treatment-experienced adults.

 SIDE EFFECTS/TOXICITY

Immune reconstitution syndrome.

Other side effects reported include diarrhea, nausea, and headache.

In less than 2%: abdominal pain, dyspepsia, vomiting, fatigue, depression, insomnia, suicidal ideation and suicide attempt, and rash.

 DRUG INTERACTIONS/FOOD INTERACTIONS

Elvitegravir must be taken with food.

Elvitegravir is metabolized by CYP3A. Drugs that induce or inhibit CYP3A activity are expected to affect the clearance of elvitegravir.

Do not coadminister elvitegravir with efavirenz, nevirapine, indinavir, saquinavir, nelfinavir, phenobarbital, phenytoin, carbamazepine, oxcarbazepine, rifampin, rifapentine, dexamethasone, St John's wort, or norgestimate/ethinyl estradiol.

If administered with antacids, separate by at least 2 hours.

Rifabutin: for elvitegravir given with PI, rifabutin should be dosed at 300 mg 3 times a week or 150 mg daily.

If administered with bosentan, bosentan should be dosed at 62.5 mg daily or every other day.

 DOSING

85 mg daily when administered with Kaletra or Reyataz/Norvir.

150 mg daily when administered with Prezista/Norvir, Lexiva/Norvir, or Aptivus/Norvir.

Antibiotics Manual: A Guide to Commonly Used Antimicrobials, Second Edition. David Schlossberg and Rafik Samuel.
© 2017 John Wiley & Sons Ltd. Published 2017 by John Wiley & Sons Ltd.

SPECIAL POPULATIONS

RENAL IMPAIRMENT: No dose adjustment necessary.

HEPATIC DYSFUNCTION: Not indicated in Child Pugh class C.

PEDIATRICS: Not recommended for those under the age of 12.

 THE ART OF ANTIMICROBIAL THERAPY

Clinical Pearls

1. Vitekta is only approved in combination with protease inhibitors that include Norvir.
2. Vitekta should not be used with other medications containing elvitegravir such as Stribild, or Genvoya.
3. Elvitegravir should not be used with other integrase inhibitors, including Isentress, Tivicay, or Triumeq.
4. Caution should be used when prescribing Vitekta because different doses are used with different protease inhibitors.

BASIC CHARACTERISTICS

Class: Analog of rifampin.

Mechanism of Action: Rifaximin acts by binding to the beta-subunit of bacterial DNA-dependent RNA polymerase, resulting in inhibition of bacterial RNA synthesis.

Metabolic Route: Rifaximin is excreted in the feces.

FDA-APPROVED INDICATIONS

Treatment of patients (≥12 years of age) with travelers' diarrhea caused by noninvasive strains of *Escherichia coli*.

Also Used for: Prophylaxis of traveler's diarrhea, treatment of *Clostridium difficile*, and treatment of hepatic encephalopathy.

SIDE EFFECTS/TOXICITY

Contraindicated in patients with hypersensitivity to any of the rifamycins.

Side effects include hypersensitivity reactions, including exfoliative dermatitis, rash, angioneurotic edema, urticaria, flushing, sunburn, neck pain, ear pain, gingival disorder, dry throat, anorexia, loss of taste, abdominal distension, diarrhea, blood in stool, nasopharyngitis, respiratory tract infection, chest pain, dyspnea, fatigue, malaise, dehydration, arthralgia, myalgia, abnormal dreams, dizziness, motion sickness, tinnitus, migraine, syncope, insomnia, dysuria, hematuria, polyuria, proteinuria, urinary frequency, hot flashes, lymphocytosis, monocytosis, neutropenia, and aspartate aminotransferase increase.

DRUG INTERACTIONS/FOOD INTERACTIONS

Rifaximin can be administered with or without food. No significant drug interactions have been reported.

DOSING

Rifaximin tablets are supplied as 200 mg tablets. The usual dose is 1 tablet taken three times a day for 3 days.

SPECIAL POPULATIONS

RENAL IMPAIRMENT: No dose adjustment is necessary.

HEPATIC DYSFUNCTION: No dose adjustment is necessary.

PEDIATRICS: The safety and effectiveness of rifaximin in pediatric patients less than 12 years of age have not been established.

Antibiotics Manual: A Guide to Commonly Used Antimicrobials, Second Edition. David Schlossberg and Rafik Samuel.
© 2017 John Wiley & Sons Ltd. Published 2017 by John Wiley & Sons Ltd.

THE ART OF ANTIMICROBIAL THERAPY

Clinical Pearls

1. Rifaximin has no significant interactions with other medications.

2. Rifaximin should not be used in patients with diarrhea complicated by fever or blood in the stool or diarrhea due to pathogens other than *Escherichia coli*.

3. Rifaximin is not suitable for treating systemic bacterial infections because less than 0.4 % of the drug is absorbed after oral administration.

4. Pseudomembranous colitis has been reported with nearly all antibacterial agents; it is important to consider this diagnosis in patients who present with diarrhea subsequent to the administration of antibacterial agents, including rifaximin.

BASIC CHARACTERISTICS

Class: Halogenated hydroxyquinoline.

Mechanism of Action: Unknown.

Metabolic Route: Iodoquinol is poorly absorbed from the GI tract and most of it is excreted in the feces.

Used for: Treatment of intestinal amebiasis.

For asymptomatic disease, it is given as monotherapy.

If the patient has invasive (intestinal or extraintestinal) disease, it is given a following treatment with metronidazole or tinidazole.

Treatment of balantidiasis.

Treatment of *Blastocystis hominis*.

Treatment of *Dientamoeba fragilis*.

 SIDE EFFECTS/TOXICITY

Iodoquinol is **contraindicated** in patients with known hypersensitivity to iodine and halogenated hydroxyquinolines.

Toxic effects include rash, hypersensitivity, nausea, vomiting, diarrhea, rare optic atrophy, neuritis, and blindness.

 DRUG INTERACTIONS/FOOD INTERACTIONS

None reported.

Iodoquinol may interfere with thyroid function tests because of its high iodine content.

 DOSING

650 mg three times a day for 20 days.

 SPECIAL POPULATIONS

RENAL IMPAIRMENT: **Contraindicated.**

HEPATIC DYSFUNCTION (NOT DUE TO AMEBIASIS): **Contraindicated.**

PEDIATRICS: 10 mg/kg q 8 hours doses for 20 days with a maximum of 2 grams per day.

 THE ART OF ANTIMICROBIAL THERAPY

Clinical Pearls

1. Iodoquinol should be avoided in children if possible.
2. For extraluminal or severe cases of amebiasis, iodoquinol should be used with another agent such as metronidazole.
3. Iodoquinone is not available commercially in the US. It may be available through a compounding pharmacy: Call the National Association of Compounding Pharmacies (800-687-7850) or Professional Compounding Centers of America (800-331-2498, www.pccarx.com).

Antibiotics Manual: A Guide to Commonly Used Antimicrobials, Second Edition. David Schlossberg and Rafik Samuel.
© 2017 John Wiley & Sons Ltd. Published 2017 by John Wiley & Sons Ltd.

YOMESAN (Niclosamide)

 ## BASIC CHARACTERISTICS

Class: Salicylanilide.

Mechanism of Action: Blocks the uptake of glucose by the intestinal tapeworms, resulting in death.

Metabolic Route: Minimal absorption occurs.

Used for: Niclosamide is effective against intestinal tapeworms including *Taenia saginata*, *T. solium*, *Diphyllobothrium latum*, and *Hymenolepis nana* and *Dipylidium caninum*.

 ## SIDE EFFECTS/TOXICITY

Nausea, vomiting, diarrhea, light-headedness, malaise, and pruritus.

 ## DRUG INTERACTIONS/FOOD INTERACTIONS

Alcohol should be avoided when taking this drug as it increases absorption, increasing the risk of side effects.

 ## DOSING

Taenia and *Diphyllobothrium* **infections**: A single 2 gram dose should be used. The tablets should be thoroughly chewed and washed down with a small amount of water.

H. nana: 2 g PO daily × 7 d.

 ## SPECIAL POPULATIONS

RENAL IMPAIRMENT: No data available.

HEPATIC DYSFUNCTION: No data available.

PEDIATRICS:

Taenia and *Diphyllobothrium* **infections**: 50 mg/kg PO once.

H. nana: 11–34 kg: 1 g PO on day 1 then 500 mg/d PO × 6 days.

>34 kg: 1.5 g PO on day 1 then 1 g/d PO 6 days.

The tablet should be crushed and then mixed with water.

THE ART OF ANTIMICROBIAL THERAPY

Clinical Pearls

1. Niclosamide is not available commercially in the US. It may be obtained from a compounding pharmacy: Call the National Association of Compounding Pharmacies (800-687-7850) or Professional Compounding Centers of America (800-331-2498, www.pccarx.com).

2. Niclosamide is not active against the larval form of *T. solium* (cysticercosis) because it is poorly absorbed.

3. Niclosamide should be chewed thoroughly before swallowing.

4. For children, the pill should be crushed and mixed with water.

Antibiotics Manual: A Guide to Commonly Used Antimicrobials, Second Edition. David Schlossberg and Rafik Samuel.
© 2017 John Wiley & Sons Ltd. Published 2017 by John Wiley & Sons Ltd.

BASIC CHARACTERISTICS

Class:

Elbasvir is an inhibitor of HCV NS5A.

Grazoprevir is an inhibitor of the HCV NS3/4A protease.

Mechanism of Action:

Elbasvir is an inhibitor of HCV NS5A, which is essential for viral RNA replication and virion assembly.

Grazoprevir is an inhibitor of the HCV NS3/4A protease, which is necessary for the proteolytic cleavage of the HCV encoded polyprotein.

Mechanism of Resistance:

For elbasvir, single NS5A substitutions at positions 28, 30, 31, 58, 93 reduce its activity.

For grazoprevir, single NS3 substitutions at positions 36, 43, 56, 80, 107, 155, 156, 168 reduce its activity.

Metabolic Route: Elbasvir and grazoprevir are partially eliminated by oxidative metabolism, primarily by CYP3A and excreted in the feces.

 FDA-APPROVED INDICATIONS

Zepatier is indicated with or without ribavirin for the treatment of chronic hepatitis C virus (HCV) genotypes 1 or 4 infection in adults.

 SIDE EFFECTS/TOXICITY

Fatigue, headache, nausea, and diarrhea.

Lab abnormalities including elevated ALT and bilirubin; decreased hemoglobin.

 DRUG INTERACTIONS/FOOD INTERACTIONS

Zepatier may be taken without regard to food.

When Zepatier is used in combination with ribavirin, the **contraindications** applicable to ribavirin are applicable to combination therapies.

Do not coadminister Zepatier with carbamazepine, phenytoin, rifampin, rifabutin, rifapentine, St John's wort, cyclosporine, efavirenz, atazanavir, darunavir, lopinavir, saquinavir, tipranavir, etravirine, Stribild, Genvoya, nafcillin, ketoconazole, bosentan, or modafenil.

Dose adjustments that are needed are as follows:

Medication	Adjustment or action
Tacrolimus	Monitor levels closely
Rosuvastatin	Maximum dose of rosuvastatin is 10 mg
Atorvastatin	Maximum dose of atorvastatin is 20 mg
Fluvastatin, lovastatin, simvastatin	Use lowest dose necessary

Antibiotics Manual: A Guide to Commonly Used Antimicrobials, Second Edition. David Schlossberg and Rafik Samuel.
© 2017 John Wiley & Sons Ltd. Published 2017 by John Wiley & Sons Ltd.

DOSING

Zepatier is a two-drug, fixed-dose combination product containing 50 mg of elbasvir and 100 mg of grazoprevir in a single tablet. The recommended dosage is one tablet taken orally once daily with or without food.

Patient population	Medication	Duration
Genotype 1a PI treatment naive Without NS5A polymorphisms	Zepatier	12 weeks
Genotype 1a PI treatment naive With NS5A polymorphisms	Zepatier + ribavirin	16 weeks
Genotype 1b PI treatment naive	Zepatier	12 weeks
Genotype 1a or 1b PI treatment Experienced	Zepatier + ribavirin	12 weeks
Genotype 4 treatment naïve	Zepatier	12 weeks
Genotype 4 treatment experienced	Zepatier + ribavirin	16 weeks

 SPECIAL POPULATIONS

RENAL IMPAIRMENT: No dose adjustment.

HEPATIC DYSFUNCTION: Do not use in moderate to severe hepatic dysfunction.

PEDIATRICS: Do not use in patients under 18 years of age.

 THE ART OF ANTIMICROBIAL THERAPY

Clinical Pearls

1. Zepatier is active against HCV genotypes 1 and 4 only.
2. NS5A resistance testing must be done prior to using Zepatier in genotype 1a infected patients.
3. NS5A resistance-associated polymorphisms at amino acid positions 28, 30, 31, or 93 require coadministration of ribavirin to improve efficacy.
4. Zepatier can be used in HIV coinfected patients.
5. Review the most current hepatitis C treatment guidelines because they are changing rapidly: http://www.cdc.gov/hepatitis/HCV/index.htm.

BASIC CHARACTERISTICS

Class: Cephalosporin and beta-lactamase inhibitor.

Mechanism of Action: Binds penicillin-binding protein, disrupting cell wall synthesis.

Mechanisms of Resistance:

1. The PBP can be altered, with reduced affinity.
2. Production of a beta-lactamase, resulting in hydrolysis of the beta-lactam ring. (Not all beta-lactamases are inhibited.)
3. Decreased ability of the antibiotic to reach the PBP when bacteria decrease porin production, resulting in a decrease of the drug concentration within the cell.

Metabolic Route: Primarily excreted by the kidneys.

 FDA-APPROVED INDICATIONS

Complicated intra-abdominal infections caused by susceptible microorganism, used in combination with metronidazole.
Complicated urinary tract infections, including pyelonephritis, caused by a susceptible microorganism.

 SIDE EFFECTS/TOXICITY

Contraindicated in patients who have shown serious hypersensitivity to ceftolozane/tazobactam or to other beta-lactams. If other forms of hypersensitivity to beta-lactams exist, use with caution.

Toxicity includes **nausea**, **diarrhea**, **headache**, and **pyrexia**, *Clostridium difficile*-associated diarrhea (CDAD) tachycardia, angina pectoris ileus, gastritis, abdominal distension, dyspepsia, flatulence, infusion site reactions, candidiasis, oropharyngeal, fungal urinary tract infection, increased serum (GGT), alkaline phosphatase, positive Coombs' test, hyperglycemia, hypomagnesemia, hypophosphatemia, ischemic stroke, renal impairment, dyspnea, urticaria, and venous thrombosis.

 DRUG INTERACTIONS/FOOD INTERACTIONS

No significant drug–drug interactions are anticipated between ceftolozane/tazobactam and substrates, inhibitors, and inducers of cytochrome P450 enzymes (CYPs).

 DOSING

Type of infection	Dose	Duration
Intra-abdominal infections	1.5 g q 8 hours	4–14 days (plus metronidazole 500 mg q 8 hours)
Urinary tract infection	1.5 g q 8 hours	7 days

Antibiotics Manual: A Guide to Commonly Used Antimicrobials, Second Edition. David Schlossberg and Rafik Samuel.
© 2017 John Wiley & Sons Ltd. Published 2017 by John Wiley & Sons Ltd.

SPECIAL POPULATIONS

RENAL INPAIRMENT:

Creatinine clearance	Dose
30–50 mL/min	750 mg (500 and 250) q 8 hours
15–29 mL/min	375 mg (250 and 125) q 8 hours
ESRD on HD	Single loading dose of 750 (500 and 250) followed by 150 mg (100 and 50) q 8 hours; give after dialysis

HEPATIC DYSFUNCTION: No dose adjustment necessary.

PEDIATRICS: Safety and effectiveness in patients younger than 18 has not been established.

GERIATRICS: Higher incidence of adverse reactions was observed in patients aged 65 years and older. In complicated intra-abdominal infections, cure rates were lower in patients aged 65 years and older.

 THE ART OF ANTIMICROBIAL THERAPY

Clinical Pearls

1. Efficacy may be reduced in patients with creatinine clearance of 30–50 mL/min compared to those with clearance of 50 mL/min or greater.

2. Monitor creatinine clearance at least daily in patients with changing renal function and adjust the dose of ceftolozane/tazobactam accordingly.

3. Ceftolozane/tazobactam is an extremely active antipseudomonal agent, even when the organism is resistant to ceftazidime.

4. Ceftolozane/tazobactam is not active against carbapenem-resistant enterobacteriaceae.

Also available in Epzicom, Trizivir, and Triumeq.

 BASIC CHARACTERISTICS

Class: Nucleoside reverse transcriptase inhibitor (NRTI) with activity against HIV.

Mechanism of Action: Converted by cellular enzymes to its active drug carbavir triphosphate, an analog of guanasine triphosphate. The carbavir triphosphate competes with the naturally occurring nucleotide for incorporation in newly forming HIV DNA. Since carbavir triphosphate does not have a terminal hydroxyl group, it halts transcription and replication of the virus.

Mechanism of Resistance: Changes in the structure of HIV reverse transcriptase leads to preferred incorporation of guanasine triphosphate and decreased incorporation of carbavir triphosphate, which allows transcription of DNA to continue. Resistance mutations include L74V, K65R, and 3 "TAMS" (41 L, 67 N, 70R, 210 W, 215 F, and 219E) + M184V.

Metabolic Route: Metabolized by alcohol dehydrogenase and glucuronyl transferase into inactive metabolites that are eliminated primarily in the feces.

 FDA-APPROVED INDICATIONS

Abacavir is approved to be used in combination with other antiretrovirals for the treatment of HIV infection.

 SIDE EFFECTS/TOXICITY

> **WARNING:**
>
> **Hypersensitivity reactions**: Serious and sometimes fatal hypersensitivity reactions, with multiple organ involvement, have occurred with abacavir tablets (abacavir).
>
> Patients who carry the HLA-B*5701 allele are at a higher risk of a hypersensitivity reaction to abacavir, although hypersensitivity reactions have occurred in patients who do not carry the HLA-B*5701 allele. Abacavir tablets are **contraindicated** in patients with a prior hypersensitivity reaction to abacavir and in HLA-B*5701-positive patients. All patients should be screened for the HLA-B*5701 allele prior to initiating therapy with abacavir tablets or reinitiation of therapy with abacavir tablets, unless patients have a previously documented HLA-B*5701 allele assessment. Discontinue abacavir tablets immediately if a hypersensitivity reaction is suspected, regardless of HLA-B*5701 status and even when other diagnoses are possible. Following a hypersensitivity reaction to abacavir tablets, **never** restart abacavir tablets or any other abacavir-containing product because more severe symptoms, including death, can occur within hours. Similar severe reactions have also occurred rarely following the reintroduction of abacavir-containing products in patients who have no history of abacavir hypersensitivity.
>
> **Lactic acidosis and severe hepatomegaly with steatosis**: Lactic acidosis and severe hepatomegaly with steatosis, including fatal cases, have been reported with the use of nucleoside analogs and other antiretrovirals. Discontinue abacavir tablets if clinical or laboratory findings suggestive of lactic acidosis or pronounced hepatotoxicity occur.

Other side effects: Immune reconstitution inflammatory syndrome, fat redistribution (including central obesity and dorsocervical fat enlargement, peripheral wasting, facial wasting, and breast enlargement), GGT elevation, and pancreatitis.

Antibiotics Manual: A Guide to Commonly Used Antimicrobials, Second Edition. David Schlossberg and Rafik Samuel.
© 2017 John Wiley & Sons Ltd. Published 2017 by John Wiley & Sons Ltd.

DRUG INTERACTIONS/FOOD INTERACTIONS

Abacavir can be taken with or without food and is unaffected by pH.

Do not use abacavir with other medications containing abacavir, including Epzicom, Trizivir, and Triumeq.

 DOSING

Abacavir is administered in a 300 mg tablet or in a strawberry–banana flavored liquid, which contains 20 mg/cc. The recommended adult dose is 300 mg twice daily or 600 mg once daily.

 SPECIAL POPULATIONS

RENAL IMPAIRMENT: No dose adjustment is necessary.

HEPATIC DYSFUNCTION: Mild hepatic disease: 200 mg twice daily; avoid in patients with severe liver disease.

PEDIATRICS: The approved dose is 8 mg/kg twice daily up to 300 mg twice daily.

 THE ART OF ANTIMICROBIAL THERAPY

Clinical Pearls

1. Abacavir should be used in combination with other antiretroviral agents.
2. Abacavir is present in four different medications: Ziagen, Trizivir, Epzicom, and Triumeq.
3. An HLA-B5701 test should be done prior to starting abacavir; if positive, abacavir should be avoided.
4. If a person has suspected hypersensitivity, abacavir should not be used.

BASIC CHARACTERISTICS

Class: Azolide/macrolide.

Mechanism of Action: Azithromycin acts by binding to the 50S ribosomal subunit of susceptible microorganisms and, thus, interfering with microbial protein synthesis.

Mechanisms of Resistance:

1. Decreased permeability.
2. Active efflux.
3. Alteration of the 50S ribosomal unit.
4. Alteration of the 23S subunit of the 50S ribosomal unit.
5. Enzymatic inactivation of the macrolide.

Metabolic Route: Azithromycin is excreted in the bile.

 FDA-APPROVED INDICATIONS

1. **Azithromycin for injection:**

   Community-acquired pneumonia

   Pelvic inflammatory disease

2. **Azithromycin 250 mg or 500 mg tablets and solution:**

   Treatment of patients with mild to moderate infections caused by susceptible strains of the designated microorganisms in the specific conditions listed below:

   Acute bacterial exacerbations of chronic obstructive pulmonary disease

   Acute bacterial sinusitis

   Community-acquired pneumonia

   Pharyngitis/tonsillitis

   Uncomplicated skin and skin structure infections

   Urethritis and cervicitis

   Genital ulcer disease in men due to *Haemophilus ducreyi* (chancroid)

3. **Azithromycin 600 mg tablets** is indicated for the treatment of serious infections caused by susceptible strains of microorganisms in the conditions listed below:

   Prophylaxis of disseminated *Mycobacterium avium* complex (MAC)

   Treatment of disseminated *Mycobacterium avium* complex (MAC)

4. **Azithromycin 1 gram packets:**

   Sexually transmitted diseases due to *Chlamydia trachomatis* or *Neisseria ghonorrhea*

5. **Zmax** is indicated for the treatment with mild to moderate infections caused by susceptible isolates of the designated microorganisms in the specific conditions listed below:

   Acute bacterial sinusitis in adults

   Community-acquired pneumonia in adults and children 6 months and older

Antibiotics Manual: A Guide to Commonly Used Antimicrobials, Second Edition. David Schlossberg and Rafik Samuel.
© 2017 John Wiley & Sons Ltd. Published 2017 by John Wiley & Sons Ltd.

SIDE EFFECTS/TOXICITY

Contraindicated in patients with known hypersensitivity to azithromycin, erythromycin, and any macrolide or ketolide antibiotic.

Side effects include serious allergic reactions including anaphylaxis, rash, photosensitivity, angioedema, Stevens–Johnson syndrome and toxic epidermal necrolysis, *Clostridium difficile*-associated diarrhea, prolonged cardiac repolarization and QT interval, exacerbation of symptoms of myasthenia gravis and new onset of myasthenic syndrome, nausea, vomiting, diarrhea, abdominal pain, hepatitis, dyspepsia, flatulence, melena, cholestatic jaundice, palpitations, chest pain, monilia, vaginitis, nephritis, seizures, hearing loss, dizziness, headache, vertigo, somnolence, thrombocytopenia, and leucopenia.

 DRUG INTERACTIONS/FOOD INTERACTIONS

Azithromycin tablets and suspension can be administered with or without food.

The Zmax formulation should be taken on an empty stomach at least 1 hour before or 2 hours following a meal.

Concurrent use of macrolides and **theophylline** has been associated with increases in the serum concentrations of theophylline.

Concomitant administration of azithromycin may potentiate the effects of oral **anticoagulants**. Prothrombin times should be carefully monitored while patients are receiving azithromycin and oral anticoagulants concomitantly.

When azithromycin and these drugs are used concomitantly, careful monitoring of patients is advised:

Digoxin: elevated digoxin levels.

Ergotamine or dihydroergotamine: acute ergot toxicity characterized by severe peripheral vasospasm and dysesthesia.

Triazolam: decreases the clearance of triazolam and thus may increase the pharmacologic effect of triazolam.

Drugs metabolized by the cytochrome P450 system: elevations of serum carbamazepine, cyclosporine, hexobarbital, and phenytoin levels.

 DOSING

Azithromycin IV formulation: 500 mg as a single daily dose. For the treatment of severe community acquired pneumonia, conversion to oral therapy can occur after the second dose and continued at 500 mg daily. The timing of the switch to oral therapy should be done at the discretion of the physician.

Azithromycin tablets and suspension in the following strengths: 250 mg and 500 mg tablets in addition to a suspension in the following concentrations: 100 mg/5 mL or 200 mg/5 mL.

The recommended doses are as follows:

Infection	Recommended dose/duration of therapy
Community-acquired pneumonia (mild severity) Pharyngitis/tonsillitis Skin/skin structure (uncomplicated)	500 mg on day 1, then 250 mg for 4 more days
Acute bacterial exacerbations of chronic obstructive pulmonary disease	500 mg q d × 3 days OR 500 mg on day 1, then 250 mg for 4 more days
Acute bacterial sinusitis	500 mg q d × 3 days
Genital ulcer disease (chancroid)	One 1-gram dose
Nongonoccocal urethritis and cervicitis	One 1-gram dose
Gonococcal urethritis and cervicitis	One 2-gram dose

Zithromax 600 mg tablets:

Prevention of disseminated MAC infections: 1200 mg taken once weekly.

Treatment of disseminated MAC infections: daily dose of 600 mg, in combination with ethambutol at the recommended daily dose of 15 mg/kg.

Azithromycin for oral suspension (1 gram formulation): The recommended dose for the treatment of non-gonococcal urethritis and cervicitis due to *C. trachomatis* is a single 1 gram (1000 mg) packet. The entire contents of the packet should be mixed thoroughly with two ounces (approximately 60 mL) of water. Drink the entire contents immediately; add an additional two ounces of water, mix, and drink to ensure complete consumption of dosage. The single-dose packet should not be used to administer doses other than 1000 mg of azithromycin.

Zmax: Zmax should be taken as a single 2 g dose. Zmax provides a full course of antibacterial therapy in a single oral dose. It is recommended that Zmax be taken on an empty stomach (at least 1 hour before or 2 hours following a meal).

 ## SPECIAL POPULATIONS

RENAL IMPAIRMENT: Caution should be used when given to patients with a creatinine clearance of <10 mL/min.

HEPATIC DYSFUNCTION: Caution should be used.

PEDIATRICS:

Acute otitis media: Azithromycin for oral suspension of 30 mg/kg given as a single dose or 10 mg/kg once daily for 3 days or 10 mg/kg as a single dose on the first day followed by 5 mg/kg/day on days 2 through 5.

Community-acquired pneumonia: Azithromycin for oral suspension for the 10 mg/kg as a single dose on the first day followed by 5 mg/kg on days 2 through 5.

Pharyngitis/tonsillitis: Azithromycin for oral suspension of 12 mg/kg once daily for 5 days.

For pediatric patients 6 months and older, **Zmax** for community acquired pneumonia should be taken as a single dose of 60 mg/kg body weight. Pediatric patients weighing 34 kg or more should receive the adult dose of 2 g.

The azithromycin 1 gram packet is not for pediatric use.

 ## THE ART OF ANTIMICROBIAL THERAPY

Clinical Pearls

1. Multiple formulations of azithromycin are available; caution should be used to administer the appropriate formulation in the correct dosage.
2. When treating MAC, azithromycin must be combined with other agents to minimize resistance.
3. Macrolides prolong QT intervals and must be used with caution.
4. Despite successful symptomatic treatment of allergic symptoms, allergic symptoms have recurred in some patients upon discontinuation of symptomatic therapy, possibly due to the long tissue half-life of azithromycin.

    This possibility warrants prolonged observation.

■ ZOSYN (Piperacillin–Tazobactam)

 BASIC CHARACTERISTICS

Class: Ureodopenicillin and beta-lactamase inhibitor combination.

Mechanism of Action: Binds penicillin-binding protein, disrupting cell wall synthesis.

Mechanisms of Resistance:

1. The PBP can be altered, with reduced affinity.

2. Production of a beta-lactamase, resulting in hydrolysis of the beta-lactam ring.

3. Decreased ability of the antibiotic to reach the PBP when bacteria decrease porin production, resulting in reduced drug concentration within the cell.

Metabolic Route: Piperacillin is excreted unchanged in the urine. Tazobactam and its metabolite are excreted in the urine.

 FDA-APPROVED INDICATIONS

Piperacillin/tazobactam is indicated in the treatment of moderate to severe infections caused by piperacillin-resistant, piperacillin/tazobactam-susceptible, β-lactamase producing microorganisms in the conditions listed below:

Appendicitis

Uncomplicated and complicated skin and skin structure infections

Postpartum endometritis or pelvic inflammatory disease

Community-acquired pneumonia (moderate severity only)

Nosocomial pneumonia (moderate to severe)

 SIDE EFFECTS/TOXICITY

Contraindicated in patients with a history of allergic reactions to any of the penicillins, cephalosporins, or β-lactamase inhibitors.

Side effects include *Clostridium difficile*-associated diarrhea (CDAD), hypersensitivity reactions including anaphylaxis, rash including erythema multiforme and Stevens–Johnson syndrome, mucocutaneous candidiasis, nausea, vomiting, diarrhea, constipation, black hairy tongue, headache, arrhythmias, hyperactivity and seizures, confusion, hepatitis, renal dysfunction, crystalluria, anemia, thrombocytopenia, eosinophilia, leukopenia, abnormalities of coagulation, false-positive reaction for urinary glucose, and hypokalemia.

 DRUG INTERACTIONS/FOOD INTERACTIONS

Concurrent use of piperacillin/tazobactam and probenecid may result in increased and prolonged blood levels of piperacillin/tazobactam. Neuromuscular blockade produced by any of the nondepolarizing muscle relaxants could be prolonged in the presence of piperacillin. The clearance of methotrexate may be reduced.

Chloramphenicol, macrolides, sulfonamides, and tetracyclines may interfere with the bactericidal effects of penicillin.

High urine concentrations of piperacillin may result in false-positive reactions when testing for the presence of glucose in urine using *Clinitest®*. It is recommended that glucose tests based on enzymatic glucose oxidase reactions (such as *Clinistix®*) be used.

Antibiotics Manual: A Guide to Commonly Used Antimicrobials, Second Edition. David Schlossberg and Rafik Samuel.
© 2017 John Wiley & Sons Ltd. Published 2017 by John Wiley & Sons Ltd.

DOSING

The usual dose is 3.375 g IV every 6 hours.

For nosocomial pneumonia, the dose should be 4.5 g every six hours IV along with an aminoglycoside.

 SPECIAL POPULATIONS

RENAL IMPAIRMENT:

Creatinine clearance, mL/min	Usual dose	Nosocomial pneumonia
20–40	2.25 g q 6 hours	3.375 g q 6 hours
<20	2.25 g q 8 hours	2.25 g q 6 hours
Hemodialysis	2.25 g q 12 hours	2.25 g q 8 hours An additional 0.75 g should be administered following each dialysis
CAPD	2.25 g q 8 hours	2.25 g q 6 hours
CRRT	2.25 g q 12 hours	2.25 g q 8 hours

HEPATIC DYSFUNCTION: No dose adjustment is necessary.

PEDIATRICS: For patients 9 months and older, the recommended dose is 100 mg piperacillin/12.5 mg tazobactam/kg every 8 hours.

For patients between 2 months and 9 months of age, the recommended dose is 80 mg piperacillin/10 mg tazobactam/kg every 8 hours.

 THE ART OF ANTIMICROBIAL THERAPY

Clinical Pearls

1. Piperacillin/tazobactam needs to be dose adjusted for renal dysfunction.
2. Piperacillin/tazobactam is a monosodium salt of piperacillin and a monosodium salt of tazobactam and contains a total of 2.79 meq (64 mg) of Na^+ per gram of piperacillin in the combination product. This should be considered when treating patients requiring restricted salt intake.
3. As with other semisynthetic penicillins, piperacillin therapy has been associated with an increased incidence of fever and rash in cystic fibrosis patients.
4. Nosocomial pneumonia caused by *P. aeruginosa* should be treated in combination with an aminoglycoside.
5. Neuromuscular blockade produced by any of the nondepolarizing muscle relaxants could be prolonged in the presence of piperacillin.

ZOVIRAX (Acyclovir)

 ## BASIC CHARACTERISTICS

Class: Nucleoside analog.

Mechanism of Action: Acyclovir is a nucleoside analog that is phosphorylated by thymadine kinase to the active triphosphate form. Acyclovir triphosphate stops replication of herpes viral DNA in three ways: (1) competitive inhibition of viral DNA polymerase, (2) incorporation into and termination of the growing viral DNA chain, and (3) inactivation of the viral DNA polymerase. The greater antiviral activity of acyclovir against HSV compared to VZV is due to its more efficient phosphorylation by the viral thymadine kinase.

Mechanism of Resistance: Resistance of HSV and VZV to acyclovir can result from qualitative or quantitative changes in the viral TK or DNA polymerase.

Metabolic Route: Acyclovir is metabolized to 9-[(carboxymethoxy)methyl]guanine and excreted in the urine.

 ## FDA-APPROVED INDICATIONS

Oral acyclovir is indicated for the acute treatment of herpes zoster, initial and recurrent episodes of genital herpes, and the treatment of chickenpox.

Intravenous acyclovir is indicated for the treatment of initial and recurrent mucosal and cutaneous herpes simplex (HSV-1 and HSV-2) in immunocompromised patients, severe initial clinical episodes of herpes genitalis in immunocompetent patients, herpes simplex encephalitis, neonatal herpes infections, and varicella zoster infections in immunocompromised patients.

 ## SIDE EFFECTS/TOXICITY

Nausea, vomiting, and diarrhea were the most common side effects in those receiving oral acyclovir. Central nervous system side effects including confusion, ataxia, altered behavior, seizure, and coma have been seen, particularly in older adults or in patients with renal impairment. Precipitation of acyclovir in renal tubules may occur when the solubility (2.5 mg/mL) is exceeded in the intratubular fluid. This has resulted in elevated BUN and serum creatinine and subsequent renal failure.

Other reported adverse events include anaphylaxis, angioedema, rash including toxic epidermal necrolysis and Stevens-Johnson syndrome, fever, headache, hepatitis, diarrhea, peripheral edema, anemia, leucopenia, and thrombocytopenia.

 ## DRUG INTERACTIONS/FOOD INTERACTIONS

Oral acyclovir can be administered with or without food.

Coadministration of probenecid has been shown to reduce the urinary excretion and renal clearance of acyclovir.

DOSING

Acyclovir is supplied in a 200 mg capsule, 400 mg and 800 mg tablets, and a crystalline powder for solution for oral dosing and a white crystalline powder for injection.

Antibiotics Manual: A Guide to Commonly Used Antimicrobials, Second Edition. David Schlossberg and Rafik Samuel.
© 2017 John Wiley & Sons Ltd. Published 2017 by John Wiley & Sons Ltd.

Disease state	Dose
Herpes zoster	800 mg every 4 hours orally, five times daily for 7 to 10 days
Genital herpes	200 mg every 4 hours, five times daily for 10 days
Chronic suppressive therapy for **herpes**	400 mg bid or 200 mg tid for 5 days
Intermittent therapy of **HSV**	200 mg 5 × d for 5 days
Treatment of **chickenpox**	800 mg four times daily for 5 days
Mucosal and cutaneous **herpes simplex**	5 mg/kg IV every 8 hours for 7 daysin immunocompromised patients
Severe initial **herpes** genitalis	5 mg/kg IV every 8 hours for 5 days
Herpes simplex **encephalitis**	10 mg/kg IV every 8 hours for 10 days
Varicella zoster in immunocompromised patients	10 mg/kg IV every 8 hours for 7 days

 ## SPECIAL POPULATIONS

RENAL IMPAIRMENT:

For oral dose:

Normal dose	Creatinine clearance, mL/min	Adjusted dose	Interval
200 mg q 4 hours	0–10	200 mg	Every 12 hours
400 mg q 12 hours	0–10	200 mg	Every 12 hours
800 mg 5 days	10–25	800 mg	Every 8 hours
	<10	800 mg	Every 12 hours

For intravenous dose adjustment:

Creatine clearance, mL/min	% of dose	Dosing interval
>50	100 %	8 hours
25–50	100 %	12 hours
10–25	100 %	24 hours
0–10	50 %	24 hours

For patients who require hemodialysis, an additional dose is administered after each dialysis.

For patients receiving peritoneal dialysis, no supplemental dose appears to be necessary after adjustment of the dosing interval.

For patients receiving CRRT, the dose is 5–7.5 mg/kg daily.

HEPATIC DYSFUNCTION: No dose adjustment.

PEDIATRICS:

Disease state	Dosing
Chickenpox (children 2 years of age and older)	20 mg/kg per dose orally four times daily (80 mg/kg/day) for 5 days
Children over 40 kg should receive the adult dose	
Mucosal and cutaneous **herpes simplex** in immuno-compromised patients (under 12 years of age)	10 mg/kg IV every 8 hours for 7 days
Herpes simplex encephalitis	
Pediatrics (3 months to 12 years of age)	20 mg/kg IV every 8 hours for 10 days
Neonatal herpes (birth to 3 months)	10 mg/kg IV up to 20 mg/kg every 8 hours for 10 days
Varicella zoster in immunocompromised patients (under 12 years of age)	20 mg/kg IV every 8 hours for 7 days

 THE ART OF ANTIMICROBIAL THERAPY

Clinical Pearls

1. Acyclovir dose should be based on ideal body weight.
2. Acyclovir is effective against HSV and VZV. It has no activity against the other herpes viruses.
3. Oral acyclovir is not recommended for children under 2 years of age; intravenous acyclovir is recommended in this age group.
4. Acyclovir can cause confusion or renal insufficiency.

BASIC CHARACTERISTICS

Class: Oxazolidinone.

Mechanism of Action: Linezolid binds the bacterial 23S ribosomal RNA of the 50S subunit and prevents the formation of a functional 70S initiation complex, which is an essential component of the bacterial translation process.

Mechanisms of Resistance:

1. Mutations in the 23S ribosomal RNA is the major cause of linezolid resistance in VRE and MRSA.
2. Resistance can also be conveyed by the *cfr* rRNA methyltransferase conferring resistance to lincosamides, oxazolidinones, and streptogramins.

Metabolic Route: Linezolid is metabolized by oxidation and excreted in the urine as both linezolid and linezolid metabolites.

 FDA-APPROVED INDICATIONS

Vancomycin-resistant *Enterococcus faecium* infections

Nosocomial pneumonia caused by *Staphylococcus aureus* (including MRSA) or *Streptococcus pneumoniae*

Complicated skin and skin structure infections, including diabetic foot infections, without concomitant osteomyelitis, caused by *Staphylococcus aureus* (including MRSA), *Streptococcus pyogenes*, or *Streptococcus agalactiae*

Uncomplicated skin and skin structure infections caused by methicillin-susceptible *Staphylococcus aureus* or *Streptococcus pyogenes*

Community-acquired pneumonia caused by *Streptococcus pneumoniae* or methicillin-susceptible *Staphylococcus aureus*

Also used for: susceptible strains of *M. Tuberculosis*.

 SIDE EFFECTS/TOXICITY

Anaphylaxis, rash including Stevens–Johnson syndrome, **myelosuppression** (including anemia, leukopenia, pancytopenia, and thrombocytopenia), ***Clostridium difficile*-associated diarrhea (CDAD)**, **lactic acidosis**, **peripheral** and **optic neuropathy** (primarily in patients treated for longer than the maximum recommended duration of 28 days), nausea, vomiting, diarrhea, headache, tongue and tooth discoloration, taste alteration, oral and vaginal moniliasis, and seizures.

 DRUG INTERACTIONS/FOOD INTERACTIONS

Linezolid can be taken without regard to food.

Serotonin syndrome (cognitive dysfunction, fever, hyperreflexia, and incoordination): Unless patients are carefully observed for signs and/or symptoms of serotonin syndrome, linezolid should not be administered to patients with carcinoid syndrome and/or patients taking any of the following medications: serotonin reuptake inhibitors, tricyclic antidepressants, serotonin 5-HT1 receptor agonists (triptans), meperidine, or buspirone.

Monoamine oxidase inhibition: Linezolid is an inhibitor of monoamine oxidase and has the potential for interaction with adrenergic and serotonergic agents; it should not be used in patients taking MAO inhibitors (within 2 weeks) and should not be administered to patients with uncontrolled hypertension, pheochromocytoma, thyrotoxicosis, and/or patients taking any of the following types of medications: directly and indirectly acting sympathomimetic agents (e.g., pseudoephedrine or

Antibiotics Manual: A Guide to Commonly Used Antimicrobials, Second Edition. David Schlossberg and Rafik Samuel.
© 2017 John Wiley & Sons Ltd. Published 2017 by John Wiley & Sons Ltd.

phenylpropanolamine), vasopressive agents (e.g., epinephrine, norepinephrine), and dopaminergic agents (e.g., dopamine, dobutamine). Patients receiving linezolid need to avoid consuming large amounts of foods or beverages with high tyramine content.

DOSING

Linezolid is available in 400 mg and 600 mg tablets, as an oral suspension containing 100 mg/5 mL, and for intravenous administration.

Infection	Dose (12 years and older)	Duration
Complicated skin infections	600 mg oral or IV q 12 hours	10–14 days
Pneumonia	600 mg oral or IV q 12 hours	10–14 days
VRE infection	600 mg oral or IV q 12 hours	14–28 days
Uncomplicated skin infection	400–600 mg oral q 12 hours	10–14 days

SPECIAL POPULATIONS

RENAL IMPAIRMENT: No dose adjustment is necessary.

HEPATIC DYSFUNCTION: No dose adjustment is necessary.

PEDIATRICS:

Infection	Dose (up to 11 years of age; older pediatric patients should receive the adult dosage)	Duration
Complicated skin infections	10 mg/kg oral or IV q 8 hours	10–14 days
Pneumonia	10 mg/kg oral or IV q 8 hours	10–14 days
VRE infection	10 mg/kg oral or IV q 8 hours	14–28 days
Uncomplicated skin infection	10 mg oral q 8–12 hours	10–14 days

THE ART OF ANTIMICROBIAL THERAPY

Clinical Pearls

1. Linezolid is not approved and should not be used for the treatment of patients with catheter-related bloodstream infections or catheter-site infections.
2. Linezolid has no clinical activity against gram-negative pathogens and is not indicated for the treatment of gram-negative infections.
3. Use caution when linezolid is administered with SSRI, MAO inhibitors, or adrenergic agents.
4. Monitor CBC weekly when using linezolid for more than 2 weeks.
5. Peripheral and optic neuropathy can be seen with prolonged linezolid use; visual function should be monitored.
6. In the chronic treatment of resistant tuberculosis, linezolid (in combination with other drugs) is used at a dose of 600 mg daily.

1. Child Pugh classification of severity of liver disease

Parameter	Points assigned		
	1	2	3
Ascites	Absent	Slight	Moderate
Bilirubin	<2 mg/dL (<34.2 micromol/liter)	2–3 mg/dL (34.2 to 51.3 micromol/liter)	>3 mg/dL (>51.3 micromol/liter)
Albumin	>3.5 g/dL (35 g/liter)	2.8–3.5 g/dL (28 to 35 g/liter)	<2.8 g/dL (<28 g/liter)
Prothrombin time, seconds over control	<4	4–6	>6
INR	<1.7	1.7–2.3	>2.3
Encephalopathy	None	Grade 1–2	Grade 3–4

2. Estimating creatinine clearance (mL/min)

Cockcroft and Gault equation:

$$\text{Creatinine clearance} = (140 - \text{age}) \times \text{IBW}/(\text{Scr} \times 72) \qquad (\times 0.85 \text{ for females})$$

3. Estimate ideal body weight (in kg)

Males: IBW = 50 kg + 2.3 kg for each inch over 5 feet

Females: IBW = 45.5 kg + 2.3 kg for each inch over 5 feet

4. The pregnancy and lactation labeling final rule (PLLR)

The FDA is in the process of changing pregnancy risk categories. The older system of A, B, C, D, and X categories is being phased out and replaced with narrative sections in the package insert (or drug label), entitled **Pregnancy**, **Lactation** and **Females and Males of Reproductive Potential**. All previous letter categories will be removed by June 29, 2018, although medications approved prior to June 29, 2001 will not require the PLLR format. For the most current recommendations, please consult the drug's latest package insert.

5. CRRT, or continuous renal replacement therapy

CRRT is being used increasingly in patients with acute renal failure and comprises a variety of techniques, including continuous arteriovenous hemofiltration (CAVH), continuous venovenous hemofiltration (CVVH), continuous arteriovenous hemodialysis (CAVHD), continuous venovenous hemodialysis (CVVHD), and continuous venovenous hemodialfiltration (CVVHDF). For practical purposes of antibiotic administration, the arterial and venous samples can be assumed to be equal. In general, CRRT produces a CrCl of approximately 30 mL/min, though this is a rough estimate only, and, when possible, serum antibiotic assays should be monitored. SLEDD, or slow extended daily dialysis, is a related modality that is used for 6–12 hours/day; antibiotic replacement in patients treated with SLEDD are in general similar to those used for patients receiving CRRT; for antimicrobial agents that experience significant removal during dialysis, those normally administered every 24 hours can be given after SLEDD each day, and those normally given every 12 hours should be given after SLEDD and 12 hours later.

6. Body surface area (Mostellar formula)

$$\text{BSA}(m^2) = \sqrt{\frac{\text{Height (cm)} \times \text{Weight (kg)}}{3600}}$$

Antibiotics Manual: A Guide to Commonly Used Antimicrobials, Second Edition. David Schlossberg and Rafik Samuel.
© 2017 John Wiley & Sons Ltd. Published 2017 by John Wiley & Sons Ltd.

This list comprises antimicrobial agents that frequently cause the indicated toxicities. The list is not intended to be all-inclusive, and current literature and product inserts should always be referred to for complete information about adverse events.

Antibiotics that cause neuromuscular depression

Clindamycin

Aminoglycosides

Fluoroquinolones

Vancomycin

Polymyxins

Antimicrobials that affect glucose homeostasis

Classes:

Fluoroquinolones

HIV protease inhibitors

In addition, the following medications:

Pentamidine

Quinine

Antibiotics that are associated with significant bone marrow suppression

Classes:

Interferons

In addition, the following medications:

Chloramphenicol

Dapsone

Flucytosine

Ganciclovir

Linezolid

Ribavirin

Sulfadiazine

Tedizolid

Trimethoprim sulfamethoxazole

Trimetrexate

Valganciclovir

Zidovudine

Antibiotics Manual: A Guide to Commonly Used Antimicrobials, Second Edition. David Schlossberg and Rafik Samuel.
© 2017 John Wiley & Sons Ltd. Published 2017 by John Wiley & Sons Ltd.

Antimicrobials that are associated with significant hepatotoxicity

Classes:

Azoles

Echinocandins

Fluoroquinolones

Rifamycins

In addition, the following medications:

Ethionamide

Isoniazid

Nevirapine

Terbinafine

Pyrazinamide

Amoxicillin-clavulanate

TMP-SMX

Oxacillin

Antimicrobials that are associated with significant renal toxicity

Classes:

Aminoglycosides

Amphotericins

In addition, the following medications:

Acyclovir

Cidofovir

Colistin

Foscarnet

Tenofovir disoproxil-containing antiretrovirals

Trimetrexate

Valacyclovir

Antimicrobials that can cause seizures

Classes:

Beta-lactams

Fluoroquinolones

In addition, the following medications:

Acyclovir

Colistin

Cycloserine

Ethionamide

Isoniazid

Valacyclovir

Antibiotics that prolong the QT interval

Classes:

Azoles

Fluoroquinolones

Macrolides

HIV protease inhibitors

This list comprises antimicrobial agents with in vitro activity against specific pathogens and pathogen classes.

Antimicrobials with coverage against mucormycosis

Agent:

Amphotericin B deoxycholate

Amphotericin B lipid complex

Amphotericin B colloidal dispersion

Amphotericin B liposomal

Posaconazole

Isavuconazole

Antimicrobials with anaerobic coverage*

Agent:

Ampicillin sulbactam*

Amoxicillin clavulanate*

Piperacillin tazobactam*

Ticarcillin clavulanate*

Imipenem*

Meropenem*

Doripenem*

Ertapenem*

Cefotetan

Cefoxitin

Colistin

Polymyxin

Metronidazole* (misses some clinically significant gram-positive anaerobes)

Clindamycin

Moxifloxacin

Doxycycline

Minocycline

Tetracycline

Tigecycline

Chloramphenicol*

*Most complete anaerobic coverage for *B. fragilis*.

Antibiotics Manual: A Guide to Commonly Used Antimicrobials, Second Edition. David Schlossberg and Rafik Samuel.
© 2017 John Wiley & Sons Ltd. Published 2017 by John Wiley & Sons Ltd.

Antimicrobials with enterococcal coverage*

Agent:

Ampicillin

Ampicillin sulbactam

Amoxicillin

Amoxicillin clavulanate

Piperacillin

Piperacillin tazobactam

Ticarcillin clavulanate

Imipenem

Meropenem

Doripenem

Vancomycin

Dalbavancin

Telavancin

Oritavancin

Daptomycin

Linezolid

Tedizolid

Tigecycline

*No single antimicrobial is reliably bactericidal for enterococcus. For bactericidal coverage, e.g., for endocarditis, combination therapy is essential, typically with a cell-wall active agent such as ampicillin or vancomycin plus an aminoglycoside. Recent data support the combination of ampicillin plus ceftriaxone.

Antimicrobials with MRSA coverage

Agent:	Activity:
Vancomycin	Bactericidal
Dalbavancin	Bactericidal
Televancin	Bactericidal
Oritavancin	Bactericidal
Daptomycin	Bactericidal
Ceftaroline	Bactericidal
Moxifloxacin	Bactericidal
Levofloxacin	Bactericidal
Linezolid	Bacteriostatic
Tedizolid	Bacteriostatic
Trimethoprim-sulfamethoxazole	Bacteriostatic

Antimicrobials with MRSA coverage

Agent:	Activity:
Doxycycline	Bacteriostatic
Tetracycline	Bacteriostatic
Minocycline	Bacteriostatic
Tigecycline	Bacteriostatic
Clindamycin*	Bacteriostatic
Rifampin**	Bacteriostatic

*Only use if D test is negative.

**Only use in combination with other medications.

Antimicrobials with actitivity against *Pseudomonas*

Agent:

Piperacillin, piperacillin tazobactam, ticarcillin clavulanate

Aztreonam

Imipenem, meropenem, doripenem

Ceftazidime, ceftazidime avibactam

Cefepime, cefoperazone, cefpirome, ceftizoxime, ceftolozane tazobactam

Ciprofloxacin, levofloxacin

Amikacin, tobramycin, gentamicin

Colistin, polymyxin

BIBLIOGRAPHY AND REFERENCES

The Medical Letter, *Drugs for Parasitic Infections*, Vol. 11 (Suppl.), 2013.

Cunha, B.A. (ed.), *Antibiotic Essentials*, Jaypee Brothers Medical Publishers, New Dehli, 2015.

Gilbert, D.N., Chanbers, H.F., Eliopoulos, G.M., and Saag, M.S. *The Sanford Guide to Antimicrobial Therapy*, Antimicrobial Therapy, Inc., Sperryville, VA, 2014.

Francis, J. *Drug-Resistant Tuberculosis: A Survival Guide for Clinicians*, Third Edition, Curry National Tuberculosis Center and California Department of Public Health, 2015.

Bennett, J.E., Dolin, R., and Blaser, M.J. *Principles and Practice of Infectious Diseases*, Eighth Edition, Elsevier, Philadelphia, PA, 2015.

Schlossberg, D. (ed.) *Clinical Infectious Disease*, Second Edition, Cambridge University Press, London, 2015.

http://www.dailymed.nlm.nih.gov
http://www.accessdata.fda.gov/Scripts/cder/DrugsatFDA/
http://www.drugs.com/
http://www.rxlist.com/
http://www.PDR.net
http://labeldataplus.org
Drugs@FDA.com

Antibiotics Manual: A Guide to Commonly Used Antimicrobials, Second Edition. David Schlossberg and Rafik Samuel.
© 2017 John Wiley & Sons Ltd. Published 2017 by John Wiley & Sons Ltd.

The manufacturer's authorised representative in the EU for product safety is Oxford
University Press España S.A. of El Parque Empresarial San Fernando de Henares,
Avenida de Castilla, 2 – 28830 Madrid (www.oup.es/en or product.safety@oup.com).
OUP España S.A. also acts as importer into Spain of products made by the manufacturer.

Printed in the USA/Agawam, MA
January 13, 2025

880951.015